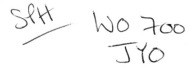

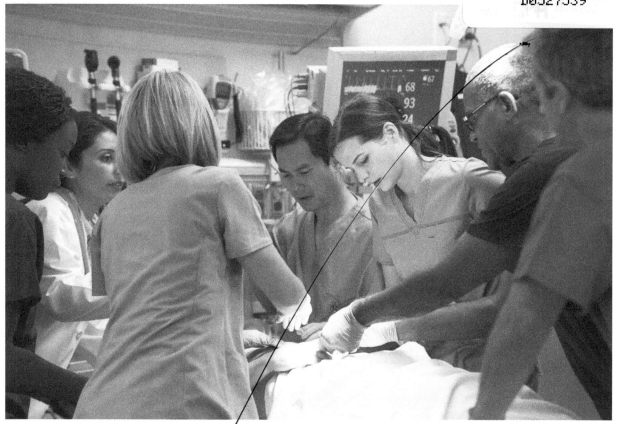

BMJ Clinical Review:

Emergency Medicine, Perioperative and Critical Care

Edited by
Babita Jyoti and Michail A. Karvelis

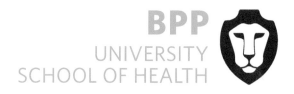

BPP
UNIVERSITY
SCHOOL OF HEALTH

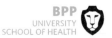

First edition August 2015

ISBN 9781 4727 3929 2
eISBN 9781 4727 4407 4
eISBN 9781 4727 4415 9

British Library Cataloguing-in-Publication Data
A catalogue record for this book is available
from the British Library

Published by
BPP Learning Media Ltd
BPP House, Aldine Place
London W12 8AA

www.bpp.com/health

Printed in the United Kingdom by
Ashford Colour Press Ltd

Unit 600, Fareham Reach,
Fareham Road,
Gosport, Hampshire,
PO13 0FW

Your learning materials, published by BPP Learning
Media Ltd, are printed on paper sourced from
sustainable, managed forests.

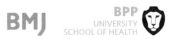

About the publisher

BPP Learning Media is dedicated to supporting aspiring professionals with top quality learning material. BPP Learning Media's commitment to success is shown by our record of quality, innovation and market leadership in paper-based and e-learning materials. BPP Learning Media's study materials are written by professionally-qualified specialists who know from personal experience the importance of top quality materials for success.

About The BMJ

The BMJ (formerly the British Medical Journal) in print has a long history and has been published without interruption since 1840. The BMJ's vision is to be the world's most influential and widely read medical journal. Our mission is to lead the debate on health and to engage, inform, and stimulate doctors, researchers, and other health professionals in ways that will improve outcomes for patients. We aim to help doctors to make better decisions. BMJ, the company, advances healthcare worldwide by sharing knowledge and expertise to improve experiences, outcomes and value.

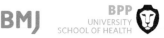

Contents

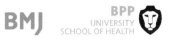

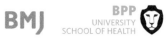

About the editors

Dr Babita Jyoti is a Radiation Oncologist with a special interest in Paediatric Proton Therapy. She graduated in Medicine in India followed by training in UK and obtained MRCP (UK) & FRCR (UK). She trained as a Clinical Oncologist at Clatterbridge Cancer Centre. She is currently working at the University of Florida Health Proton Therapy Institute in Paediatric Proton Therapy. She has been a PBL tutor and an OSCE examiner at Manchester Medical School.

Dr Michail A. Karvelis is a Pain Fellow at the Royal Liverpool and Broadgreen University Hospitals. He qualified from the Medical School of the Aristotle University of Thessaloniki, Greece in 2003. He trained as an anaesthetist both in Greece and the UK and he obtained his CCT in 2011. He was awarded a Masters degree in Pain management from Leicester University in 2011. He has worked as a consultant anaesthetist in the Naval Hospital of Athens and since 2014 he has been developing his special interest in regional anaesthesia and pain medicine in the NHS.

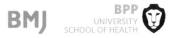

Introduction to Emergency Medicine, Perioperative and Critical Care

Physicians involved in emergency medicine, perioperative and critical care are confronted with challenging medical decision making every day; and each decision taken can be crucial for the patient. Keeping abreast of the evolutions in the field therefore is vital.

New developments are made constantly; with regular publication of results from clinical studies on topics such as cardiopulmonary resuscitation, diagnosis and treatment of life-threatening arrhythmias, initial resuscitation of trauma patients, mechanical ventilation, as well as perioperative fluid administration and pain management.

BMJ Clinical reviews represents an effort to contribute to delivering high-quality care to patients in the National Health Service and worldwide. In this book, we have carefully selected clinical reviews on emergency medicine, perioperative and critical care from The BMJ's rich database, in an effort to help refresh and update knowledge on topics relevant to direct patient care.

We encourage healthcare professionals to use this book, taking advantage of the simple format to consolidate understanding, use the references to further knowledge, and continue to practice evidence based medicine.

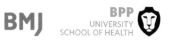

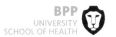
Anaphylaxis: the acute episode and beyond

F Estelle R Simons, professor, department of paediatrics and child health, professor, department of immunology[1],

Aziz Sheikh, professor of primary care research and development[2]

[1]Faculty of Medicine, University of Manitoba, Winnipeg, Canada R3A 1R9

[2]Allergy and Respiratory Research Group, Centre for Population Health Sciences, University of Edinburgh, Edinburgh, UK

Correspondence: F E R Simons lmcniven@hsc.mb.ca

Cite this as: *BMJ* 2013;346:f602

DOI: 10.1136/bmj.f602

http://www.bmj.com/content/346/bmj.f602

Anaphylaxis is an alarming medical emergency,[1][2][3] not only for the patient or caregiver, but also sometimes for the healthcare professionals involved. Although it is thought of as uncommon, the lifetime prevalence is estimated at 0.05-2%,[4][5] and the rate of occurrence is increasing. Hospital admissions, although uncommon, are also increasing, as are admissions to critical care units.[6][7] Many anaphylaxis episodes now occur in community settings.[8] Accurate community based population estimates are difficult to obtain because of underdiagnosis, under-reporting, and miscoding, as well as use of different anaphylaxis definitions and different methods of case ascertainment in the populations studied.[5] Although death from anaphylaxis seems to be uncommon, it is under-reported.[9]

In this article, we draw on evidence from randomised controlled trials, quasi-experimental and other observational studies, and systematic reviews. We also reference key evidence based international and national anaphylaxis guidelines and their updates.[1][2][10][11]

How is anaphylaxis defined?

The widely used definition of anaphylaxis—"a serious allergic reaction that is rapid in onset and may cause death"—is accompanied by clinical criteria for diagnosis,[3] which have been validated for use in clinical and research contexts (fig 1).[1][3][11][12][13] In emergency departments, this definition has high sensitivity (97%) and high negative predictive value (98%), with lower specificity (82%) and positive predictive value (67%), as anticipated in a multisystem disease.[3][12] Hypotension and shock are not prerequisites for making the diagnosis of anaphylaxis. Death occurs as often after respiratory arrest as it does after shock or cardiac arrest.[14]

SOURCES AND SELECTION CRITERIA

We based this review on Medline and other searches for publications relevant to human anaphylaxis, including Cochrane reviews and other systematic reviews, randomised controlled trials, and quasi-experimental and other observational studies. We also used World Allergy Organization guidelines for the assessment and management of anaphylaxis and UK Resuscitation Council guidelines for emergency treatment of anaphylactic reactions (both of which were not commercially sponsored).

SUMMARY POINTS

- Diagnosis is based on clinical presentation—sudden onset of characteristic symptoms in more than one body system, minutes to hours after exposure to a likely or known allergen
- Factors associated with increased risk of severe or fatal anaphylaxis include asthma, cardiovascular disease, mastocytosis, and drugs such as β blockers
- When anaphylaxis occurs, promptly call for help, inject adrenaline intramuscularly, and place the patient on the back or in a semi-reclining position with lower extremities raised
- During the episode, if needed, give high flow supplemental oxygen, establish intravenous access to provide high volume fluids, and perform cardiopulmonary resuscitation
- Provide at risk patients with adrenaline autoinjectors, personalised anaphylaxis emergency action plans, and medical identification
- Confirm the specific trigger so that it can be avoided or allergen specific immune modulation—such as venom immunotherapy to prevent anaphylaxis from insect stings—can be carried out

What are the mechanisms, triggers, and patient risk factors for anaphylaxis?

The clinical features of anaphylaxis result from sudden release of histamine, tryptase, leucotrienes, prostaglandins, platelet activating factor, and many other inflammatory mediators into the systemic circulation. Typically, this occurs through an immune mechanism involving interaction between an allergen and allergen specific IgE bound to high affinity IgE receptors on mast cells and basophils. However, IgE independent immune mechanisms and direct degranulation of mast cells are sometimes responsible, and other episodes, especially in adults, are idiopathic (box 1).[1]

Patient risk factors for anaphylaxis include vulnerability owing to age or physiological state (box 2).[1][11][15][16][17][18] Some diseases such as asthma and cardiovascular disease, and some drugs such as β adrenergic blockers and angiotensin converting enzyme inhibitors also increase the risk of severe or fatal anaphylaxis episodes (box 2).[1][11][14][18][19][20] Cofactors that can amplify or augment acute anaphylaxis episodes have been identified (box 2)[1][8][11][21][22] Doctors and patients should be aware of the relevant risk factors and cofactors in the context of long term management.

How do patients present with anaphylaxis?

Patients with anaphylaxis present with different scenarios. Some develop iatrogenic anaphylaxis after administration of a diagnostic or therapeutic agent. Others present to the emergency department after experiencing anaphylaxis in the community; in such patients, the duration of symptoms and signs varies from minutes to hours, and treatment with adrenaline (epinephrine), oxygen, intravenous fluids, an H1 antihistamine, a glucocorticoid, or other drug might have already been started. In addition, many patients present to their doctor with a history of anaphylaxis that occurred weeks, months, or even years earlier, which may or may not have been appropriately investigated or followed up. Regardless of the scenario, the clinical diagnosis of anaphylaxis is based on the history of the acute episode.[1][2]

How is an acute episode of anaphylaxis diagnosed?

Clinical presentation

Anaphylaxis is characterised by symptom onset within minutes to a few hours after exposure to a food, drug, insect sting, or other trigger (box 1). Target organ involvement varies. Two or more body organ systems (cutaneous, respiratory, gastrointestinal, cardiovascular, or central nervous system) are usually affected (box 3; fig 1).[1][3]

To some extent, symptoms and signs depend on age and physiological state.[1][3][15][17][18] As examples, infants and young children who cannot describe their symptoms typically develop sudden behavioural changes and become anxious, frightened, or clingy.[15] Children sometimes use terms such as "burning" or "tingly" to mean itching, and those with upper airway involvement sometimes scratch at their throat or gag. Pregnant women can experience intense itching of the genitalia, abdominal cramps, back pain, signs of fetal distress, and preterm labour.[17]

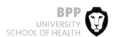

Skin symptoms and signs are reported in 80-90% of patients. In their absence, anaphylaxis can be difficult to recognise. Upper and lower respiratory tract symptoms and signs occur in up to 70% of those experiencing anaphylaxis and cardiovascular symptoms and signs in about 45%. Gastrointestinal symptoms occur in about 45% and central nervous system symptoms and signs in about 15%.

The patterns of target organ involvement vary between patients, and in the same patient from one episode to another (fig 1).[1][3] Symptoms and signs therefore differ from one patient to another and from one episode to another in the same patient in terms of type, number of organ systems affected, time of onset in relation to exposure to the inciting agent, and duration.

Anaphylaxis can range in severity from transient and unrecognised or undiagnosed episodes, to respiratory arrest, shock, cardiac arrest, and death within minutes.[1][2][3][14][23] At the onset of an episode, it can be difficult or

Anaphylaxis is highly likely when any one of the following three criteria is fulfilled:

1. Sudden onset of an illness (minutes to several hours), with involvement of skin, mucosal tissue, or both (for example, generalised hives, itch, or flush or swollen lips, tongue, or uvula)

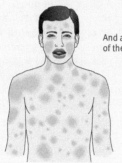

And at least one of the following:

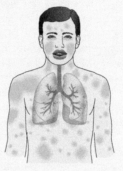

Sudden respiratory symptoms and signs
(for example, shortness of breath, wheeze, cough, stridor, hypoxaemia)

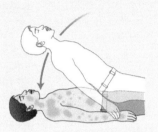

Sudden reduced blood pressure or symptoms of end organ dysfunction
(for example, hypotonia (collapse), incontinence)

Or

2. Two or more of the following that occur suddenly after exposure to a likely allergen or other trigger* for that patient (minutes to several hours):

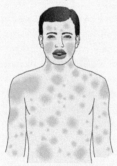

Sudden skin or mucosal symptoms and signs
(for example, generalised hives, itch, or flush or swollen lips, tongue, or uvula)

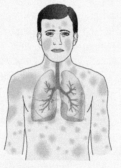

Sudden respiratory symptoms and signs
(for example, shortness of breath, wheeze, cough, stridor, hypoxaemia)

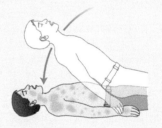

Sudden reduced blood pressure or symptoms of end organ dysfunction
(for example, hypotonia (collapse), incontinence)

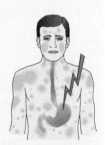

Sudden gastrointestinal symptoms
(for example, crampy abdominal pain, vomiting)

Or

3. Reduced blood pressure after exposure to a known allergen† for that patient (minutes to several hours):

Infants and children: low systolic blood pressure (age specific) or greater than 30% decrease in systolic blood pressure‡

Adults: systolic blood pressure of less than 90 mm Hg or greater than 30% decrease from that person's baseline

* For example, immunological but IgE independent, or non-immunological (direct mast cell activation)
† For example, after an insect sting, reduced blood pressure might be the only manifestation of anaphylaxis; or, after allergen immunotherapy, generalised hives might be the only initial manifestation of anaphylaxis
‡ Low systolic blood pressure for children is defined as less than 70 mm Hg from 1 month to 1 year, less than (70 mm Hg + (2 x age)) from 1 to 10 years, and less than 90 mm Hg from 11 to 17 years. Normal heart rate ranges from 80 to 140 beats/min at age 1-2 years; from 80 to 120 beats/min at age 3 years; and from 70 to 115 beats/min after age 3 years. In infants and children, respiratory compromise is more likely than hypotension or shock, and shock is more likely to be manifest initially by tachycardia than by hypotension

Fig 1 Clinical criteria for the diagnosis of anaphylaxis as illustrated in the 2011 World Allergy Organization anaphylaxis guidelines. These diagnostic criteria were developed by a National Institutes of Health sponsored international consensus group in 2004-06 to facilitate prompt recognition of anaphylaxis[1][3]

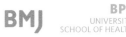

impossible to predict the rate of progression, the ultimate severity, or the likelihood of death.[1] [3] [14] In a UK registry study of anaphylaxis related deaths, median times to cardiac or respiratory arrest were five minutes in iatrogenic anaphylaxis, 15 minutes in insect sting anaphylaxis, and 30 minutes in food anaphylaxis.[23]

Some patients develop biphasic or multiphasic anaphylaxis, in which symptoms resolve, then reappear hours later despite no further exposure to the trigger.[24] Protracted anaphylaxis, in which uninterrupted symptoms recur for days despite treatment, is uncommon.[1] [2]

More than 40 differential diagnoses exist, including episodes of acute asthma, acute generalised urticaria, or acute angio-oedema, acute anxiety or panic attacks, and syncope (box 4).[1] [2] [8] [14] [15] [18]

What investigations should be considered?

Measurement of mast cell tryptase concentration—the most widely used laboratory test—is not universally available, takes hours to perform, is not available on an emergency basis, and is not helpful for confirming the clinical diagnosis of anaphylaxis in the initial minutes or hours after symptom onset. Treatment must therefore not be delayed to obtain a blood sample for tryptase measurement.

Total tryptase concentrations measured in serum during an anaphylaxis episode can, however, sometimes be helpful later to confirm the diagnosis, especially in patients with drug or insect sting induced anaphylaxis and those with hypotension.[1] [2] [10] [11] [25] [26] Tryptase concentrations are seldom raised in patients with anaphylaxis triggered by food, or in those whose blood pressure remains normal during the anaphylactic episode. Several factors may explain this: localised mast cell degranulation—for example, in the upper airway—with less tryptase entering the circulation than after generalised degranulation; involvement of respiratory epithelial mast cells rather than perivascular and cardiac mast cells that contain more tryptase; greater distance of respiratory epithelial mast cells than perivascular mast cells from the circulation; and involvement of basophils,

which release minimal tryptase.[26] [27] A serum tryptase concentration within the reference range of 1-11.4 ng/mL does not refute the clinical diagnosis of anaphylaxis, and an increased concentration is not specific for anaphylaxis.[1] [2]

Tryptase has a short elimination half life. Serial measurements are reported to improve test specificity and are ideally obtained 15-180 minutes after symptom onset, one to two hours later, and after resolution of the episode. A raised baseline value suggests the diagnosis of mastocytosis rather than anaphylaxis.[1] [2] [10] [11] [25] [26]

How should an acute episode of anaphylaxis initially be treated?

Figure 2 outlines a systematic approach to the basic initial management of anaphylaxis that emphasises the primary role of adrenaline.[1] [11] In healthcare settings, it is important to prepare for this medical emergency by using an anaphylaxis assessment and management protocol based on current national or international guidelines.[1] [2] [28] This protocol should be displayed in locations where all healthcare professionals and staff can access it and rehearse it.

BOX 1 MECHANISMS AND TRIGGERS OF ANAPHYLAXIS

Immune mechanism: IgE dependent*

- Foods: peanut, tree nuts (such as cashews), milk, eggs, shellfish, finned fish, wheat, soy, sesame, kiwi
- Drugs†: penicillins and other β lactam antibiotics
- Biologicals: monoclonal antibodies, vaccines (rare)
- Insect stings: bees, hornets, wasps, yellow jackets, some ants
- Natural rubber latex
- Seminal fluid (rare)

Other immune mechanisms: IgE independent*

- IgG mediated: infliximab, high molecular weight dextran (rare)
- Immune aggregates: intravenous immunoglobulin (rare)
- Drugs†: aspirin, ibuprofen, and other non-steroidal anti-inflammatory drugs
- Complement and coagulation pathways

Direct mast cell and basophil activation*

- Exercise, usually with a cofactor such as a food or drug
- Other physical factors: for example, cold air or cold water
- Drugs†: opioids such as codeine or morphine

Idiopathic anaphylaxis*‡

- No trigger can be identified

Examples of mechanisms and triggers are given; the number of triggers is infinite.
†Different classes of drugs induce anaphylaxis through different mechanisms.
‡Consider the possibility of an uncommon or novel trigger (such as galactose α-1,3-galactose, the carbohydrate moiety in red meat; saliva injected by biting insects; or topically applied allergens such as chlorhexidine) or a concurrent diagnosis of mastocytosis.

BOX 2 PATIENT RISK FACTORS FOR ANAPHYLAXIS

Age related factors

- Infants: anaphylaxis can be hard to recognise, especially if the first episode; patients cannot describe symptoms
- Adolescents and young adults: increased risk taking behaviours such as failure to avoid known triggers and to carry an adrenaline autoinjector consistently
- Pregnancy: risk of iatrogenic anaphylaxis—for example, from β lactam antibiotics to prevent neonatal group B streptococcal infection, agents used perioperatively during caesarean sections, and natural rubber latex
- Older people: increased risk of death because of concomitant disease and drugs

Concomitant diseases

- Asthma and other chronic respiratory diseases
- Cardiovascular diseases
- Mastocytosis
- Allergic rhinitis and eczema*
- Depression, cognitive dysfunction, substance misuse

Drugs

- β adrenergic blockers†
- Angiotensin converting enzyme (ACE) inhibitors†
- Sedatives, antidepressants, narcotics, recreational drugs, and alcohol may decrease the patient's ability to recognise triggers and symptoms

Cofactors that amplify anaphylaxis

- Exercise: anaphylaxis associated with exercise may be food dependent or food independent; non-steroidal anti-inflammatory drugs and other listed cofactors may also be relevant
- Acute infection such as an upper respiratory tract infection
- Fever
- Emotional stress
- Disruption of routine—for example, travel and jet lag
- Premenstrual status in women and girls

*Atopic diseases are a risk factor for anaphylaxis triggered by food, latex, and exercise, but not for anaphylaxis triggered by most drugs or by insect stings
†Patients taking β adrenergic blockers or ACE inhibitors seem to be at increased risk for severe anaphylaxis. In addition, those taking β adrenergic blockers may not respond optimally to adrenaline treatment and may need glucagon, a polypeptide with non-catecholamine dependent inotropic and chronotropic cardiac effects, atropine for persistent bradycardia, or ipratropium for persistent bronchospasm.

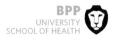

At the time of diagnosis, exposure to the trigger should be halted if possible—for example, by discontinuing an intravenously administered diagnostic or therapeutic agent. The patient's circulation, airway, breathing, mental status, skin, and body weight (mass) should be assessed.[1 2 3 10 11]

Simultaneously and promptly, call for help—from emergency medical services in a community setting or a resuscitation team in a hospital or other healthcare setting.[1 2 3 10 11] In an adult, inject adrenaline 0.3 mg (0.3 mL) by the intramuscular route in the mid-outer thigh, to a maximum of 0.5 mg (0.5 mL) of a 1 mg/mL (1:1000) solution; in a prepubertal child, inject adrenaline 0.15 mg (0.15 mL) to a maximum of 0.3 mg (0.3 mL).[1 2 3 10 11] Adrenaline is classified as an essential drug by the World Health Organization and

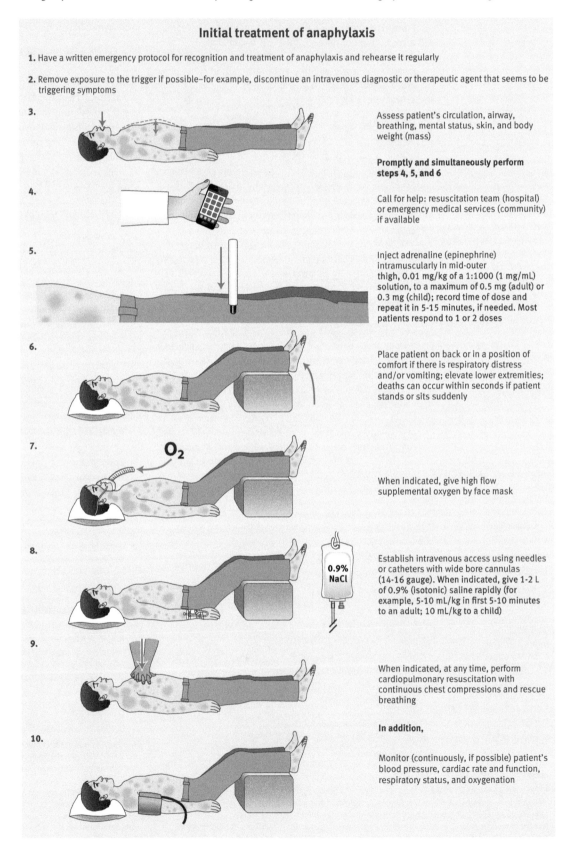

Initial treatment of anaphylaxis

1. Have a written emergency protocol for recognition and treatment of anaphylaxis and rehearse it regularly

2. Remove exposure to the trigger if possible—for example, discontinue an intravenous diagnostic or therapeutic agent that seems to be triggering symptoms

3. Assess patient's circulation, airway, breathing, mental status, skin, and body weight (mass)

Promptly and simultaneously perform steps 4, 5, and 6

4. Call for help: resuscitation team (hospital) or emergency medical services (community) if available

5. Inject adrenaline (epinephrine) intramuscularly in mid-outer thigh, 0.01 mg/kg of a 1:1000 (1 mg/mL) solution, to a maximum of 0.5 mg (adult) or 0.3 mg (child); record time of dose and repeat it in 5-15 minutes, if needed. Most patients respond to 1 or 2 doses

6. Place patient on back or in a position of comfort if there is respiratory distress and/or vomiting; elevate lower extremities; deaths can occur within seconds if patient stands or sits suddenly

7. When indicated, give high flow supplemental oxygen by face mask

8. Establish intravenous access using needles or catheters with wide bore cannulas (14-16 gauge). When indicated, give 1-2 L of 0.9% (isotonic) saline rapidly (for example, 5-10 mL/kg in first 5-10 minutes to an adult; 10 mL/kg to a child)

9. When indicated, at any time, perform cardiopulmonary resuscitation with continuous chest compressions and rescue breathing

In addition,

10. Monitor (continuously, if possible) patient's blood pressure, cardiac rate and function, respiratory status, and oxygenation

Fig 2 Initial treatment of anaphylaxis as illustrated in the 2011 World Allergy Organization anaphylaxis guidelines[1]

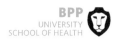

is available worldwide in a 1 mL ampoule (1 mg/mL), even in most low resource areas.[29]

As soon as the symptoms of anaphylaxis are recognised, the injection should be given by anyone trained or authorised to administer it. In healthcare settings, it is typically ordered or given by a doctor. However, in many immunisation clinics, infusion clinics, and allergen immunotherapy clinics, nurses are preauthorised to do this.[30] In community settings, adrenaline is often self injected through an autoinjector by the patient or injected by the parent, teacher, or other person responsible for the child. Delay in administration is associated with greater likelihood of biphasic and protracted

anaphylaxis, and of death[23][24]; in a UK series, only 14% of the patients who died from anaphylaxis received adrenaline before respiratory or cardiac arrest.[23]

The adrenaline injection can be repeated after five to 15 minutes, if needed. When the initial injection is given promptly after symptoms are recognised, patients seldom require more than two or three injections. Compared with the intravenous route, the intramuscular route has the advantages of rapid initial access and a considerably wider margin of safety.[1][2][10]

For ethical and practical reasons, no randomised controlled trials of adrenaline have been conducted during anaphylaxis. The recommendation for intramuscular injection of adrenaline is based on consistent clinical evidence supporting its use, observational studies, and objective measurements of adrenaline absorption in randomised controlled clinical pharmacology studies in people not experiencing anaphylaxis at the time of study.[31][32][33] The beneficial effects of adrenaline are time dependent.

BOX 3 SYMPTOMS AND SIGNS OF ANAPHYLAXIS

During an anaphylaxis episode, symptoms and signs can range from few to many. A comprehensive list is provided to aid in prompt recognition and to indicate the possibility of rapid progression to multiorgan system involvement.

Skin, subcutaneous tissue, and mucosa

Generalised flushing, itching, urticaria (hives), angio-oedema, morbilliform rash, pilor erection
Periorbital itching, erythema, oedema, conjunctival erythema, tearing
Itching or swelling (or both) of lips, tongue, palate, uvula, external auditory canals
Itching of the genitalia, palms, soles

Respiratory

- Nasal itching, congestion, rhinorrhoea, sneezing
- Throat itching, tightness, dysphonia, hoarseness, dry staccato cough, stridor
- Lower airways: cough, increased respiratory rate, shortness of breath, chest tightness, wheezing
- Cyanosis
- Respiratory arrest

Gastrointestinal

- Abdominal pain, dysphagia, nausea, vomiting (stringy mucus), diarrhoea

Cardiovascular system

- Chest pain (myocardial ischaemia)*
- Tachycardia, bradycardia (less common), other dysrhythmias, palpitations
- Hypotension, feeling faint, incontinence, shock
- Cardiac arrest

Central nervous system

- Feeling of impending doom, uneasiness, headache (pre-adrenaline), altered mental status or confusion owing to hypoxia, dizziness or tunnel vision owing to hypotension, loss of consciousness

Other

- Metallic taste in the mouth

*This can occur in patients with coronary artery disease and (owing to vasospasm) in those with normal coronary arteries.

BOX 4 DIFFERENTIAL DIAGNOSIS OF ANAPHYLAXIS[1][2][8][14][15][18]

- Common diagnostic dilemmas*: acute asthma, acute generalised urticaria†, acute angio-oedema‡, syncope or fainting, panic attack, acute anxiety attack
- Postprandial syndromes, such as food poisoning, scombroidosis, pollen-food allergy syndrome (oral allergy syndrome), monosodium glutamate reaction, sulphite reaction
- Flush syndromes, such as menopause, carcinoid syndrome
- Excess endogenous histamine syndromes, such as mastocytosis
- Upper airway obstruction as a result of non-allergic angio-oedema‡
- Shock (other forms), such as hypovolaemic, septic, or cardiogenic shock
- Non-organic diseases, such as vocal cord dysfunction, hyperventilation, psychosomatic episode, Munchausen's stridor
- Other: certain tumours, system capillary leak syndrome (rare)

*The differential diagnosis is, to some extent, age dependent—for example, in infants, consider choking and foreign body aspiration, breath holding, and food protein induced enterocolitis. In middle aged or older patients, consider myocardial infarction or stroke.
†Acute urticaria can occur with intercurrent or subclinical infection.
‡May be due to hereditary angio-oedema types I, II, and III; use of angiotensin converting enzyme inhibitors; or cancer. Non-allergic angio-oedema is typically not associated with itching or urticaria.

BOX 5 DISCHARGE MANAGEMENT OF ANAPHYLAXIS AND LONG TERM RISK REDUCTION[1][2][3][10][11][14][36][37]

Discharge management*

- Equip with an adrenaline autoinjector or a prescription for one†
- Give the patient an anaphylaxis emergency action plan (personalised, written)
- Provide medical identification (such as bracelet, wallet card)
- Arrange for a medical record electronic flag or chart sticker
- Make a follow-up appointment with a doctor (see below)

Long term risk reduction: investigations for sensitisation to allergen(s)‡

- Skin tests or measurement of allergen specific IgE concentrations
- Challenge or provocation tests conducted by trained and experienced staff in a well equipped medical setting using incremental amounts of the relevant allergen, such as a food or drug

Long term risk reduction: avoidance and immune modulation‡

- Food triggered anaphylaxis: strict avoidance of relevant food(s)
- Drug triggered anaphylaxis: avoidance of relevant drugs and use of safe substitutes; if indicated, conduct desensitisation in a medical setting
- Stinging insect triggered anaphylaxis: avoidance of stinging insects; subcutaneous venom immunotherapy
- Idiopathic anaphylaxis: consider the possibility of a novel or atypical trigger§; examine the skin and measure a baseline serum tryptase concentration to rule out mastocytosis
- Optimal management of asthma and other concomitant diseases*

*All doctors play an important role in preparing patients for self treatment of anaphylaxis by teaching them how to recognise the common symptoms and signs and how to inject adrenaline safely using an autoinjector. In addition, all doctors play a role in optimal management of asthma, cardiovascular disease, and other comorbidities that contribute to the severity of anaphylaxis and death.
†No adrenaline autoinjectors contain an ideal dose for infants weighing <10-12 kg.
‡Allergy and immunology specialists play an important role in ascertaining the trigger(s) of an anaphylaxis episode, providing written information about avoidance of specific triggers, and, where relevant, preventing anaphylaxis by desensitisation to a drug or initiating and monitoring stinging insect venom immunotherapy.
§See examples in box 1 footnotes.

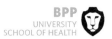

When given promptly, it reduces the release of mast cell mediators[34] and the possibility of escalation of symptoms.

The transient anxiety, pallor, palpitations, and tremor experienced after administration of a relatively low first aid dose of exogenous adrenaline are caused by its intrinsic pharmacological effects. These symptoms are uncommon after an intramuscular injection of the correct adrenaline dose.[14 33] They are similar to the symptoms caused by increased endogenous adrenaline during the "fight or flight" response to an acute stressful situation.[31]

Serious adverse effects such as hypertension or pulmonary oedema can occur after adrenaline overdose by any route of administration. They are most commonly reported after an intravenous bolus dose, overly rapid intravenous infusion, or intravenous infusion of a concentrated adrenaline solution 1 mg/mL (1:1000) instead of a solution that is appropriately diluted for intravenous use. Hypoxia, acidosis, and the direct effects of the inflammatory mediators released during anaphylaxis can contribute to cardiovascular complications.[1 2 33 35]

Do not allow patients with anaphylaxis to stand or sit suddenly. They should be placed on their back (or in a semi-reclining position if dyspnoeic or vomiting) with their lower extremities elevated.[14]

What additional treatment might be indicated for an acute episode of anaphylaxis?

At any time during the episode, when indicated, additional important steps include giving high flow supplemental oxygen and maintaining the airway, establishing intravenous access and administering high volumes of fluid, and initiating cardiopulmonary resuscitation with chest compressions before starting rescue breathing.[1 2 3 10 11 36 37] As soon as possible, start continuous monitoring of blood pressure, heart rate and function, respiratory rate, and oxygenation using pulse oximetry to titrate oxygen therapy (fig 2).[1 10 11]

Do not delay prompt intramuscular injection of adrenaline—the first line drug—by taking time to draw up and give a second line drug such as an H1 antihistamine or a glucocorticoid.[1 2 3 10 38 39] H1 antihistamines relieve skin and nasal symptoms and glucocorticoids might prevent biphasic or protracted symptoms, but these drugs fail to prevent release of the inflammatory mediators that escalate the response; fail to relieve life threatening upper or lower airway obstruction, hypotension, or shock; and fail to prevent death.[38 39]

Promptly transfer patients who are refractory to initial treatment of anaphylaxis to the care of specialists in emergency medicine, critical care medicine, or anaesthesiology. Such specialists and their teams are trained, experienced, and equipped to provide skilled management of the airway and mechanical ventilation, and to manage shock by administering adrenaline or other vasopressors through an infusion pump. The absence of established dosing regimens for intravenous vasopressors necessitates frequent dose titrations based on continuous monitoring of vital signs, cardiac function, and oxygenation.[1 2 3 10 36 37]

After treatment and resolution of anaphylaxis, keep patients under observation in a healthcare facility for at least four to six hours.[1 2 3] Observe those who have experienced respiratory or circulatory compromise for eight to 10 hours, or even longer.[1]

How should patients be equipped for self treatment of anaphylaxis in the community?

Tell patients that they have experienced a potentially life threatening medical emergency. If possible, they should be discharged with an adrenaline autoinjector, or at a minimum, a prescription for one, and taught why, when, and how to inject adrenaline (box 5).[1 2 3 8 10 11 14 36] They should also be equipped with a personalised emergency action plan that lists common anaphylaxis symptoms to help them recognise a recurrence and reminds them to inject adrenaline promptly using an autoinjector and seek prompt medical help.[36] Such plans typically also list patients' confirmed anaphylaxis trigger(s), their relevant comorbidities (such as asthma or cardiovascular disease), and relevant concurrent drugs. In addition, patients should wear medical identification (bracelet or card) that states their diagnosis of anaphylaxis, its causes, and any relevant diseases or drugs.

Beyond the acute episode: how should anaphylaxis be investigated?

The natural course of anaphylaxis is one of recurrent acute episodes, unless the patient's specific triggers are identified and consistently avoided. Appropriate investigation and follow-up after recovery from an episode may protect against recurrences.[14] Confirm triggers suggested by a meticulous history of previous episodes by measuring allergen specific IgE in serum or by performing allergen skin tests (or both), because self identification of food, drug, and stinging insect triggers by patients may be non-specific or incorrect and prevention of recurrence must be trigger specific. Avoid testing with large numbers of allergens because sensitisation to allergens is common even without a history of symptoms or signs after exposure to the specific allergen. Skin tests are optimally performed about four weeks after the acute episode, rather than immediately after, when test results may be falsely negative. Patients with a convincing history of anaphylaxis who have negative skin tests within a few weeks after an episode should be retested later.[1]

Some patients will need additional investigations to rule out other diseases in the differential diagnosis. Patients with idiopathic anaphylaxis need additional tests to investigate any unusual or novel triggers and to rule out mastocytosis.[40] Other patients might need additional tests to distinguish asymptomatic sensitisation to an allergen, such as a food or venom, from risk of subsequent clinical reaction to this allergen.[1 2 3 36] Allergen component tests, such as microassay based immunoassays, might help to distinguish patients who are sensitised to an allergen and at increased risk of anaphylaxis after exposure to the allergen from those who are sensitised but clinically tolerant (remain asymptomatic after exposure to the allergen).[41]

Most doctors will want their patients with anaphylaxis to be investigated by a qualified allergy specialist, although ready access to such specialists and to basic tests for sensitisation to allergens is a problem in many parts of the world.[1 2 3 10 11 29 36 42] In the United Kingdom, an evidence and consensus based national care pathway has been designed to improve assessment and management of infants, children, and young people who have experienced anaphylaxis.[43]

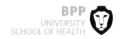
How can recurrences of acute anaphylaxis be prevented?

Personalised written instructions about avoidance of confirmed relevant trigger(s) and safe alternatives should be provided for patients at risk, who should also be directed to reliable, up to date information resources. In healthcare settings, flag medical records with "anaphylaxis" and list relevant triggers.[1 2 3 14]

For anaphylaxis to foods, strict avoidance of the relevant foods, even in trace amounts, is currently the only recommended approach for prevention of recurrence. Long term avoidance of food triggers can be stressful because of the threat of hidden crossreactive or cross contaminating allergens. New immune modulation strategies to achieve clinical and immunological tolerance to implicated foods and prevent recurrences of food triggered anaphylaxis are within reach, as demonstrated in randomised controlled trials, although they are not yet recommended for clinical implementation because of high adverse event rates.[1 2 3 22 36 44 45 46]

For anaphylaxis to a drug, prevention of recurrence involves substitution of a safe effective non-crossreacting agent, preferably from a different pharmacological class. If such an agent is not available, desensitisation to the implicated agent is indicated to induce temporary clinical tolerance for one uninterrupted course of treatment with that agent. Desensitisation to antimicrobials, antifungals, antivirals, chemotherapeutics, monoclonal antibodies, and other agents is carried out in specialised hospital units.[1 2 3 47 48]

For anaphylaxis to stinging insect venoms, recurrences can be prevented by a three to five year course of subcutaneous immunotherapy with the relevant standardised specific venom(s). This approach, which is based on high quality randomised controlled trials, should be initiated and monitored by an allergist. It leads to clinical and immunological tolerance, and in about 90% of adults and 98% of children, to longlasting protection against recurrence.[1 49 50]

For exercise induced anaphylaxis and food dependent exercise induced anaphylaxis, recurrence can be prevented by avoiding relevant co-triggers such as foods, non-steroidal anti-inflammatory drugs, or alcohol and avoiding exercise under adverse environmental conditions (extreme cold or heat, high humidity, or high pollen counts). Patients should not exercise alone and should carry an adrenaline autoinjector and a mobile phone. If an episode occurs despite preventive measures, treatment involves discontinuing exertion immediately on recognition of initial symptoms, calling for help, and self injecting adrenaline promptly.[1]

Pharmacological approaches are commonly used in the prevention of anaphylaxis. As an example, patients at high risk of anaphylaxis from infusion of radiocontrast medium during diagnostic procedures, or those with frequent episodes of idiopathic anaphylaxis, are often treated prophylactically with an H1 antihistamine, glucocorticoid, or other drug. Most prophylactic regimens are based on clinical experience rather than on randomised controlled trials.[1]

Do patients with a history of anaphylaxis need long term follow-up?

Patients at risk for anaphylaxis in the community should be monitored regularly—for example, at yearly intervals—by their doctor. Such visits provide the opportunity for personalised education on how to prevent recurrences, recognise anaphylaxis symptoms, and self inject adrenaline correctly. An important aspect of follow-up is to help patients (and carers of at risk children) control asthma or other comorbid disease that potentially increase the risk of severe or fatal anaphylaxis episodes.[1 2 3 11 36]

TIPS FOR NON-SPECIALISTS

- Be prepared to diagnose anaphylaxis on the basis of clinical criteria and to provide fast, effective, and safe treatment by injecting adrenaline 0.01 mg/kg (using a 1 mg/mL (1:1000) solution, to a maximum adult dose of 0.5 mg) intramuscularly in the mid-outer thigh
- Specialist referral is suggested for all patients to confirm specific triggers, discuss allergen avoidance, and if relevant, receive immunomodulation (for example, to prevent recurrence of anaphylaxis triggered by stinging insect venom) or investigate idiopathic anaphylaxis
- Specialist referral is strongly suggested for patients who are at increased risk of severe or fatal anaphylaxis because of concomitant asthma, cardiovascular disease, or mastocytosis

---

ADDITIONAL EDUCATIONAL RESOURCES

Resources for healthcare professionals

- World Allergy Organization (www.worldallergy.org)—Federation of 89 national and regional allergy and clinical immunology organisations; developed the World Allergy Organization Guidelines for the assessment and management of anaphylaxis
- Resuscitation Council UK (www.resus.org.uk)—Produced the Resuscitation Council (UK) guidelines for the emergency treatment of anaphylactic reactions

Resources for patients

- Anaphylaxis Campaign (www.anaphylaxis.org.uk)—This UK charity provides information, support, and a helpline for people with anaphylaxis
- Anaphylaxis Canada (www.anaphylaxis.ca)—This not for profit organisation supports, educates, and advocates for people with anaphylaxis and their families; it also supports anaphylaxis research
- Australasian Society of Clinical Immunology and Allergy (www.allergy.org.au)—ASCIA has developed anaphylaxis guidelines, action plans, a list of frequently asked questions about adrenaline autoinjectors, and e-training for first aid (community) treatment of anaphylaxis
- Food Allergy Research and Education (www.foodallergy. org)—This not for profit organisation (formerly the Food Allergy and Anaphylaxis Network) is dedicated to food allergy research and education, with the mission of ensuring the safety and inclusion of people with food allergies, while seeking a cure

---

AREAS OF ONGOING RESEARCH

- Development of rapid in vitro tests to confirm the clinical diagnosis at the time of the episode
- Development of additional in vitro tests to distinguish patients at risk of anaphylaxis from those with asymptomatic sensitisation
- Observational studies of adrenaline in anaphylaxis and randomised controlled clinical pharmacology studies (with or without placebo) of different doses and routes of administration in people not experiencing anaphylaxis at the time of study
- Randomised placebo controlled trials (listing clinical trial registration numbers) of second line drugs, such as systemic glucocorticoids, in patients with anaphylaxis
- Randomised controlled trial (clinical trial registration number ISRCTN29793562) of access to a 24 hour helpline providing expert management advice for the emergency management of anaphylaxis in infants, children, and young people
- Randomised placebo controlled trials of immune modulation to prevent anaphylaxis from food (listing clinical trial registration numbers)

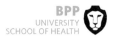

The authors sincerely appreciate the help of Lori McNiven, and Jacqueline Schaffer, who prepared the figures. We thank the editors and reviewers for their constructive feedback.

Contributors: FERS conceived the review, interpreted the literature, extracted the evidence, and drafted the manuscript. AS commented critically on drafts of the manuscript. Both authors approved the final version. FERS is guarantor.

Competing interests: We have read and understood the BMJ Group policy on declaration of interests and declare the following interests: FERS serves on the Food Allergy Research and Education Medical Advisory Board, and on ALK, Mylan, and Sanofi medical advisory boards for anaphylaxis; she also served on the NIH/NIAID food allergy expert panel; she is a contributing editor to *The Medical Letter* and the editor of the anaphylaxis section in *UpToDate*; she chairs the World Allergy Organization special committee on anaphylaxis; she is a past president of the American Academy of Allergy Asthma and Immunology, and a past president of the Canadian Society of Allergy and Clinical Immunology. AS has undertaken advisory work for ALK-Abello, Lincoln Medical, Meda, and Thermo Fisher Scientific; he was a member of the Royal College of Paediatrics and Child Health's care pathway for children at risk of anaphylaxis, a member of the UK Resuscitation Council's anaphylaxis guidelines committee, the World Allergy Organization's special committee on anaphylaxis, the European Academy of Allergy and Clinical Immunology's steering committee of the food allergy and anaphylaxis guidelines, and the scientific committee of the Anaphylaxis Campaign; he is also the Royal College of General Practitioners' clinical champion for allergy.

Provenance and peer review: Commissioned; externally peer reviewed.

1   Simons FER, Ardusso LRF, Bilo MB, El-Gamal YM, Ledford DK, Ring J, et al. World Allergy Organization guidelines for the assessment and management of anaphylaxis. *J Allergy Clin Immunol* 2011;127:593. e1-22.
2   Soar J, Pumphrey R, Cant A, Clarke S, Corbett A, Dawson P, et al. Emergency treatment of anaphylactic reactions—guidelines for healthcare providers. *Resuscitation* 2008;77:157-69.
3   Sampson HA, Munoz-Furlong A, Campbell RL, Adkinson NF Jr, Bock SA, Branum A, et al. Second symposium on the definition and management of anaphylaxis: summary report—second National Institute of Allergy and Infectious Disease/Food Allergy and Anaphylaxis Network symposium. *J Allergy Clin Immunol* 2006;117:391-7.
4   Lieberman P, Camargo CA Jr, Bohlke K, Jick H, Miller RL, Sheikh A, et al. Epidemiology of anaphylaxis: findings of the American College of Allergy, Asthma and Immunology Epidemiology of Anaphylaxis Working Group. *Ann Allergy Asthma Immunol* 2006;97:596-602.
5   Sheikh A, Hippisley-Cox J, Newton J, Fenty J. Trends in national incidence, lifetime prevalence and adrenaline prescribing for anaphylaxis in England. *J R Soc Med* 2008;101:139-43.
6   Gupta R, Sheikh A, Strachan DP, Anderson HR. Time trends in allergic disorders in the UK. *Thorax* 2007;62:91-6.
7   Gibbison B, Sheikh A, McShane P, Haddow C, Soar J. Anaphylaxis admissions to UK critical care units between 2005 and 2009. *Anaesthesia* 2012;67:833-8.
8   Simons FER. Anaphylaxis. *J Allergy Clin Immunol* 2010;125:S161-81.
9   Tanno LK, Ganem F, Demoly P, Toscano CM, Bierrenbach AL. Undernotification of anaphylaxis deaths in Brazil due to difficult coding under the ICD-10. *Allergy* 2012;67:783-9.
10 Soar J, Perkins GD, Abbas G, Alfonzo A, Barelli A, Bierens JJLM, et al. European Resuscitation Council guidelines for resuscitation 2010 section 8. Cardiac arrest in special circumstances: electrolyte abnormalities, poisoning, drowning, accidental hypothermia, hyperthermia, asthma, anaphylaxis, cardiac surgery, trauma, pregnancy, electrocution. *Resuscitation* 2010;81:1400-33.
11 Simons FER, Ardusso LRF, Bilo MB, Dimov V, Ebisawa M, El-Gamal YM, et al. 2012 update: World Allergy Organization guidelines for the assessment and management of anaphylaxis. *Curr Opin Allergy Clin Immunol* 2012;12:389-99.
12 Campbell RL, Hagan JB, Manivannan V, Decker WW, Kanthala AR, Bellolio MF, et al. Evaluation of National Institute of Allergy and Infectious Diseases/Food Allergy and Anaphylaxis Network criteria for the diagnosis of anaphylaxis in emergency department patients. *J Allergy Clin Immunol* 2012;129:748-52.
13 Harduar-Morano L, Simon MR, Watkins S, Blackmore C. Algorithm for the diagnosis of anaphylaxis and its validation using population-based data on emergency department visits for anaphylaxis in Florida. *J Allergy Clin Immunol* 2010;126:98-104.
14 Pumphrey R. Anaphylaxis: can we tell who is at risk of a fatal reaction? *Curr Opin Allergy Clin Immunol* 2004;4:285-90.
15 Simons FER. Anaphylaxis in infants: can recognition and management be improved? *J Allergy Clin Immunol* 2007;120:537-40.
16 Gallagher M, Worth A, Cunningham-Burley S, Sheikh A. Strategies for living with the risk of anaphylaxis in adolescence: qualitative study of young people and their parents. *Prim Care Respir J* 2012;21:392-7.
17 Simons FER, Schatz M. Anaphylaxis during pregnancy. *J Allergy Clin Immunol* 2012;130:597-606.
18 Campbell RL, Hagan JB, Li JTC, Vukov SC, Kanthala AR, Smith VD, et al. Anaphylaxis in emergency department patients 50 or 65 years or older. *Ann Allergy Asthma Immunol* 2011;106:401-6.
19 Gonzalez-Perez A, Aponte Z, Vidaurre CF, Rodriguez LAG. Anaphylaxis epidemiology in patients with and patients without asthma: a United Kingdom database review. *J Allergy Clin Immunol* 2010;125:1098-104. e1.
20 Rueff F, Przybilla B, Bilo MB, Muller U, Scheipl F, Aberer W, et al. Predictors of severe systemic anaphylactic reactions in patients with Hymenoptera venom allergy: importance of baseline serum tryptase—a study of the European Academy of Allergology and Clinical Immunology interest group on insect venom hypersensitivity. *J Allergy Clin Immunol* 2009;124:1047-54.
21 Hompes S, Kohli A, Nemat K, Scherer K, Lange L, Rueff F, et al. Provoking allergens and treatment of anaphylaxis in children and adolescents—data from the anaphylaxis registry of German-speaking countries. *Pediatr Allergy Immunol* 2011;22:568-74.
22 Keet CA, Frischmeyer-Guerrerio PA, Thyagarajan A, Schroeder JT, Hamilton RG, Boden S, et al. The safety and efficacy of sublingual and oral immunotherapy for milk allergy. *J Allergy Clin Immunol* 2012;129:448-55.e5.
23 Pumphrey RSH. Lessons for management of anaphylaxis from a study of fatal reactions. *Clin Exp Allergy* 2000;30:1144-50.
24 Ellis AK, Day JH. Incidence and characteristics of biphasic anaphylaxis: a prospective evaluation of 103 patients. *Ann Allergy Asthma Immunol* 2007;98:64-9.
25 Brown SGA, Stone SF. Laboratory diagnosis of acute anaphylaxis. *Clin Exp Allergy* 2011;41:1660-2.
26 Schwartz LB. Diagnostic value of tryptase in anaphylaxis and mastocytosis. *Immunol Allergy Clin North Am* 2006;26:461-3.
27 Simons FER, Frew AJ, Ansotegui IJ, Bochner BS, Finkelman F, Golden DBK, et al. Risk assessment in anaphylaxis: current and future approaches. *J Allergy Clin Immunol* 2007;120(suppl):S2-24.
28 Arroabarren E, Lasa EM, Olaciregui I, Sarasqueta C, Munoz JA, Perez-Yarza EG. Improving anaphylaxis management in a pediatric emergency department. *Pediatr Allergy Immunol* 2011;22:708-14.
29 Simons FER; for the World Allergy Organization. World Allergy Organization survey on global assessment and management of anaphylaxis by allergy/immunology specialists in healthcare settings. *Ann Allergy Asthma Immunol* 2010;104:405-12.
30 Phillips JF, Lockey RF, Fox RW, Ledford DK, Glaum MC. Systemic reactions to subcutaneous allergen immunotherapy and the response to epinephrine. *Allergy Asthma Proc* 2011;32:288-94.
31 Simons KJ, Simons FER. Epinephrine and its use in anaphylaxis: current issues. *Curr Opin Allergy Clin Immunol* 2010;10:354-61.
32 Sheikh A, Shehata YA, Brown SGA, Simons FER. Adrenaline auto-injectors for the treatment of anaphylaxis with and without cardiovascular collapse in the community. *Cochrane Database Syst Rev* 2012;8:CD008935.
33 McLean-Tooke APC, Bethune CA, Fay AC, Spickett GP. Adrenaline in the treatment of anaphylaxis: what is the evidence? *BMJ* 2003;327:1332-5.
34 Vadas P, Perelman B. Effect of epinephrine on platelet-activating factor-stimulated human vascular smooth muscle cells. *J Allergy Clin Immunol* 2012;129:1329-33.
35 Triggiani M, Patella V, Staiano RI, Granata F, Marone G. Allergy and the cardiovascular system. *Clin Exp Immunol* 2008;153(suppl 1):7-11.
36 Boyce JA, Assa'ad A, Burks AW, Jones SM, Sampson HA, Wood RA, et al. Guidelines for the diagnosis and management of food allergy in the United States: summary of the NIAID-sponsored expert panel report. *J Allergy Clin Immunol* 2010;126:1105-18.
37 Field JM, Hazinski MF, Sayre MR, Chameides L, Schexnayder SM, Hemphill R, et al. Part 1: executive summary: 2010 American Heart Association guidelines for cardiopulmonary resuscitation and emergency cardiovascular care. *Circulation* 2010;122:S640-56.
38 Sheikh A, Ten Broek V, Brown SGA, Simons FER. H1-antihistamines for the treatment of anaphylaxis: Cochrane systematic review. *Allergy* 2007;62:830-7.
39 Choo KJL, Simons FER, Sheikh A. Glucocorticoids for the treatment of anaphylaxis. *Cochrane Database Syst Rev* 2012;4:CD007596.
40 Akin C. Anaphylaxis and mast cell disease: what is the risk? *Curr Allergy Asthma Rep* 2010;10:34-8.
41 Shreffler WG. Microarrayed recombinant allergens for diagnostic testing. *J Allergy Clin Immunol* 2011;127:843-9.
42 Lowe G, Kirkwood E, Harkness S. Survey of anaphylaxis management by general practitioners in Scotland. *Scott Med J* 2010;55:11-4.
43 Clark A, Lloyd K, Sheikh A, Alfaham M, East M, Ewan P, et al. The RCPCH care pathway for children at risk of anaphylaxis: an evidence and consensus based national approach to caring for children with life-threatening allergies. *Arch Dis Child* 2011;96(suppl 2):i6-9.
44 Nowak-Wegrzyn A, Sampson HA. Future therapies for food allergies. *J Allergy Clin Immunol* 2011;127:558-73.
45 Varshney P, Jones SM, Scurlock AM, Perry TT, Kemper A, Steele P, et al. A randomized controlled study of peanut oral immunotherapy: clinical desensitization and modulation of the allergic response. *J Allergy Clin Immunol* 2011;127:654-60.
46 Burks AW, Jones SM, Wood RA, Fleischer DM, Sicherer SH, Lindblad RW, et al. Oral immunotherapy for treatment of egg allergy in children. *N Engl J Med* 2012;367:233-43.
47 Khan DA, Solensky R. Drug allergy: an updated practice parameter. *J Allergy Clin Immunol* 2010;125: S126-37.

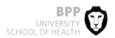

48 Liu A, Fanning L, Chong H, Fernandez J, Sloane D, Sancho-Serra M, et al. Desensitization regimens for drug allergy: state of the art in the 21st century. *Clin Exp Allergy* 2011;41:1679-89.

49 Golden DBK, Moffitt J, Nicklas RA, Freeman T, Graft DF, Reisman RE, et al. Stinging insect hypersensitivity: a practice parameter update 2011. *J Allergy Clin Immunol* 2011;127: 852-4.e23.

50 Bilo MB. Anaphylaxis caused by Hymenoptera stings: from epidemiology to treatment. *Allergy* 2011;66:35-7.

Related links

bmj.com/archive

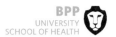

Emergency and early management of burns and scalds

Stuart Enoch, specialty registrar in burns and plastic surgery[1],
Amit Roshan, specialty registrar in burns and plastic surgery[2],
Mamta Shah, consultant burns and plastic surgeon[3]

[1]University Hospitals of Manchester, Manchester M23 9LT

[2]Cambridge University Hospitals, Addenbrooke's Hospital, Cambridge CB2 8QE

[3]Central Manchester and Manchester Children's Hospitals NHS Trust, Manchester

Correspondence to: M Shah, Regional Paediatric Burns Unit, Booth Hall Children's Hospital, Manchester M9 7AA
mamta.shah@cmmc.nhs.uk

Cite this as: BMJ 2009;338:b1037

DOI: 10.1136/bmj.b1037

http://www.bmj.com/content/338/bmj.b1037

Burn injuries are an important global health problem. Most simple burns can be managed by general practitioners in primary care, but complex burns and all major burns warrant a specialist and skilled multidisciplinary approach for a successful clinical outcome. This article discusses the principles behind managing major burns and scalds using an evidence based approach and provides a framework for managing simple burns in the community.

What is the burden of burns injuries?

Annually in the United Kingdom, around 175 000 people attend accident and emergency departments with burns from various causes (box 1).[1] This represents 1% of all emergency department attendances, and about 10% of these patients need inpatient management in a specialist unit.[2] A further 250 000 patients are managed in the community by general practitioners and allied professionals. Of patients referred to hospital, some 16 000 are admitted, and about 1000 patients need active fluid resuscitation. The number of burns related deaths average 300 a year.[1]

Globally, the World Health Organization estimates that 322 000 people die each year from fire related burns.[3] This could be an underestimate, however, because we have no valid comprehensive statistics from developing countries, where >95% of these deaths occur.[3] [4] High population density, illiteracy, poverty, and unsafe cooking methods contribute to the higher incidence in developing countries.[4]

How is the area of a burn estimated?

In adults, Wallace's "rule of nines" is useful for estimating the total body surface area—18% each for chest, back, and legs apiece, 9% each for head and arms apiece, and 1% for the perineum. It is quick to apply and easily remembered, although it tends to overestimate the area by about 3%.[5] The Lund and Browder chart takes into account changes in body surface area with age (and growth). It is useful across all age groups and has good interobserver agreement.[5] Another useful, but rather subjective, guide is to use the surface area of the patient's palm and fingers, which is just under 1% of the total body surface area. This method is useful for estimating small burns (<15%) or large burns (>85%). In large burns, the burnt area can be quickly calculated by estimating the area

SOURCES AND SELECTION CRITERIA

We searched Medline, Ovid, Burns, and the Cochrane Library until June 2008 for randomised controlled trials, systematic reviews, evidence reports, and recent evidence based guidelines from international burn associations.

of uninjured skin and subtracting it from 100.[6] A common mistake is to include erythema—only de-epithelialised areas should be included in these calculations.

How is the depth of a burn assessed?

Clinical estimation of burn depth (fig 1) is often subjective—an independent blinded comparison among experienced surgeons showed only 60-80% concurrence.[7] Burn wounds are dynamic and need reassessment in the first 24-72 hours, because depth can increase after injury as a result of inadequate treatment or superadded infection.[8] Burn wounds can be superficial in some parts but deeper in other areas (fig 2). The table shows some characteristic features of burns of varying depth.

A blinded rater comparison of laser Doppler imaging, which assesses skin blood flow, with clinical assessment and histopathology found that imaging was 90-100% sensitive and 92-96% specific for estimating burn depth.[7] However, the high outlay costs for this equipment preclude its use outside specialist burns units. Other methods such as transcutaneous videomicroscopy (direct visualisation of dermal capillary integrity) and infrared thermography (temperature gradient between burnt and intact skin) remain largely experimental.[9] [10]

The terms "partial thickness" or "full thickness" burns describe the level of burn injury and indicate the likelihood and estimated duration for healing to occur. Superficial burns usually heal (by epithelialisation) within two weeks without surgery, whereas deeper burns probably need excision and closure of the area, often with skin grafts. Hypertrophic scarring is more common in deeper burns treated by surgery and skin grafting than in superficial burns.[11]

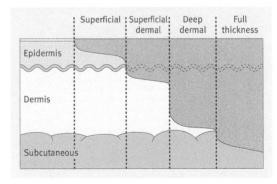

Fig 1 Burn depth nomenclature

SUMMARY POINTS

- Most minor burns can be managed in primary care
- Appropriate first aid limits progression of burn depth and influences outcome
- Assessment of area and depth is crucial to formulating a management plan
- Burn depth may progress with time, so re-evaluation is essential
- All major burns require fluid resuscitation, which should be guided by monitoring of the physiological parameters
- A multidisciplinary approach is crucial for a successful clinical outcome

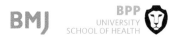

What factors influence outcome?

Logistic regression analysis of survival data from 1665 burns patients from the Massachusetts General Hospital identified three risk factors for death: age over 60 years, more than 40% of body surface area injured, and inhalation injury.[12] As survival outcomes have improved (mortality about 5-6% in resourced centres),[13] however, assessment of outcome has shifted from mortality to quality of life measures.[14] Thus, the current focus in burns patients is the preservation of function, reconstruction, and rehabilitation.[13]

How are minor burns managed?

Flowchart 1 (web fig 1 on bmj.com) provides a guideline for managing a "minor" burn in the community. The European working party of burns specialists recommends cleaning burns with soap and water (or a dilute water based disinfectant) to remove loose skin, including open blisters.[15] Although the clinical evidence for "deroofing" of blisters is poor, without deroofing burn depth cannot be assessed. All blisters should therefore be deroofed, apart from isolated lax blisters <1 cm² in area, which can be left alone.[16] A simple non-adhesive dressing, such as soft silicone (for example, Mepitel), padded by gauze is effective in most superficial and superficial dermal burns. However, biological dressings such as Biobrane are better,

especially for children, because they reduce pain, and the wound bed can be inspected through the translucent sheet.[17] New non-animal derived synthetic polymers such as Suprathel look promising for treating partial thickness burns, but further studies are needed. Silver sulfadiazine can be used for deep dermal burns. Dressings should be examined at 48 hours to reassess depth and the wound in general, and dressings on superficial partial thickness burns can be changed after three to five days in the absence of infection. If evidence of infection exists, daily wound inspection and dressing change is indicated. Deep dermal burns need daily dressings until the eschar has lifted and re-epithelialisation is under way, after which dressings can be changed more often.

When is referral to a specialist burns unit needed?

Box 2 shows the criteria for referring a "complex" burn to the specialist burns unit. Small area burns that take more than 14 days to heal; become infected; or are likely to lead to considerable aesthetic, functional, or psychological impairment (face, hands, feet, across flexures, genitalia) may also need to be referred.[1]

How should major burns be managed?

All major burns should be managed initially according to trauma resuscitation guidelines.[8] Box 3 shows a consensus summary on first aid management (prehospital care) for burns,[18] and box 4 shows the principles for managing any large burns.

Prompt irrigation with running cool tap water for 20 minutes provides optimal intradermal cooling.[19] Ice and very cold water should be avoided because they cause vasoconstriction and worsen tissue ischaemia and local oedema.[20] Hypothermia should be avoided, especially in children. Patients with chemical burns may need longer periods of irrigation (up to 24 hours), and specific antidote information should be obtained from the regional or national toxicology unit.

The prehospital consensus guidelines emphasise that dressings help relieve pain from exposed nerve endings and keep the area clean.[18] Polyvinylchloride film (such as clingfilm) is useful, but remember that circumferential wrapping can cause constriction. Cellophane films can worsen chemical burns, so the area should be irrigated thoroughly until pain has decreased and only wet dressings should be applied. Intravenous opiates or intranasal diamorphine should be used for analgesia.

All patients with facial burns or burns in an enclosed area should be assessed by an anaesthetist and the need for early intubation ascertained before transfer to a specialist unit. In full thickness circumferential burns—especially to the neck, chest, abdomen, or limbs—escharotomy may be needed to avert respiratory distress or vascular compromise of the limbs from constriction. Flowcharts 2 and 3 (web figs 2 and 3 on bmj.com) show the management of patients in the emergency department or the specialist burns unit.

What is the role of fluid resuscitation?

Effective fluid resuscitation remains the cornerstone of management in major burns. If more than 25% of the body is burnt, intravenous fluids should be given "on scene," although transfer should not be delayed by more than two attempts at cannulation.[18] The aims are to maintain vital organ perfusion and tissue perfusion to the zone of stasis (around the burn) to prevent extension of the thermal necrosis.[15] In the UK, expert consensus recommends that

---

BOX 1 SOME IMPORTANT CAUSES OF BURNS AND SCALDS

- Flame burns
- Scalds (hot liquids)
- Contact burns (hot solid)
- Chemicals (acids or alkalis)
- Electrical burns (high and low voltage)
- Flash burns (burns resulting from brief exposure to intense radiation)
- Sunburns
- Friction burns
- Radiation burns
- Burns from lightning strike

BOX 2 NATIONAL BURN INJURY GUIDELINES FOR REFERRAL TO A BURNS UNIT

All complex injuries should be referred. Such injuries are likely to be associated with:

- Extremes of age (<5 or >60 years)
- Site of injury
- Face, hands, or perineum
- Any flexure including neck or axilla
- Circumferential dermal burns or full thickness burn of the limb, torso, or neck
- Inhalation injury (excluding pure carbon monoxide poisoning)
- Mechanism of injury
- Chemical burns >5% total body surface area (except for hydrofluoric acid when >1% area needs referral)
- Exposure to ionising radiation
- High pressure steam injury
- High tension electrical injury
- Hydrofluoric acid burns >1%
- Suspected non-accidental injury in a child (if delayed presentation, unusual pattern of injury, inconsistent history, discrepancy between history and clinical findings, multiple injuries, or old scars in unusual anatomical locations)
- Large size
- Child (<16 years old) >5% total body surface area
- Adult (≥16 years) >10% total body surface area
- Coexisting conditions
- Serious medical conditions (such as immunosuppression)
- Pregnancy
- Associated injuries (fractures, head injury, or crush injuries)

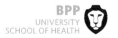

fluid resuscitation be initiated in all children with 10% burns and adults with 15% burns; children who had early (within two hours) fluid resuscitation had a lower incidence of sepsis, renal failure, and overall mortality.[8][21]

How much fluid?

Several formulae, based on body weight and area burnt, estimate volume requirements for the first 24 hours. Although none is ideal, the Parkland formula (3-4 ml/kg/% burn of crystalloid solution in the first 24 hours, with half given in the first eight hours) and its variations are the most commonly used. Resuscitation starts from the time of injury, and thus any delays in presentation or transfer to the hospital or specialist unit should be taken into account and fluid requirement calculated accordingly. Resuscitation

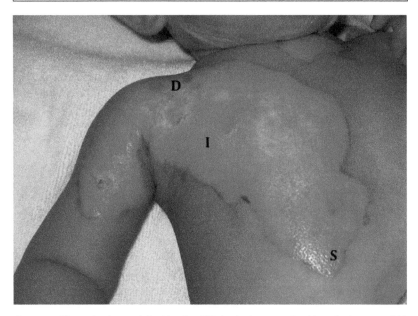

Fig 2 Tea scald over the chest and shoulder of a child showing heterogeneity of burn depth. S=superficial, I=intermediate, D=deep

Characteristic features of burns of different depths

Burn type	Feature			
	Appearance	Blisters	Capillary refill	Sensation
Epidermal	Red, glistening	None	Brisk	Painful
Superficial dermal	Pale pink	Small	Brisk	Painful
Deep dermal	Dry, blotchy cherry red	May be present	Absent	Dull or absent
Full thickness	Dry, white or black	None	Absent	Absent

formulae are only guidelines, and the volume must be adjusted against monitored physiological parameters.

Historically, under-resuscitation was an important cause of death from major burns, but reports suggest that the pendulum may have swung towards over-resuscitation. Resuscitation volumes greater than two to three times the estimated requirements have been used, with associated complications of volume overload, such as pulmonary oedema.[w1] Volume overload, also known as "fluid creep,"[w2] may be made worse by the relative unresponsiveness of fluids during the first 24 hours. Studies using invasive monitoring in burns resuscitation have shown that the rate of intravascular volume replacement is independent of the volume of crystalloid infused.[w3] Studies have therefore looked at using smaller volumes as long as resuscitation is early and suitably monitored—an approach termed permissive hypovolaemia.[w4] Although early studies have been encouraging, randomised controlled trials (RCTs) are lacking.

Which fluid?

The preferred resuscitation fluid varies greatly. Currently, the most popular one is crystalloid Hartmann's solution, which effectively treats hypovolaemia and extracellular sodium deficits. Sodium chloride solution (0.9%) should be avoided because it causes hyperchloraemic metabolic acidosis.

The early phase after burn injury is characterised by increased capillary permeability, so large volume crystalloid resuscitation may lead to a decrease in the plasma protein concentration and egression of the fluid into the extravascular space. Capillary integrity may be sufficiently restored by about 12-24 hours, however, and many burns units manipulate the intravascular oncotic pressure by adding a colloid (albumin or plasma) after the first 12 hours in large area burns.[22]

A recent Cochrane meta-analysis of 67 RCTs of trauma, burns, and post-surgery patients found no evidence that colloid resuscitation reduces mortality more effectively than crystalloids.[23] Although the addition of colloids in burn resuscitation may decrease total volume requirements, RCTs are needed to evaluate its other benefits.[24]

How should resuscitation be monitored?

The use of urine output alone to assess adequate fluid resuscitation in burns has been challenged.[5][w1] Invasive haemodynamic monitoring with central venous pressure or pulmonary artery catheters are not recommended for routine monitoring of fluid replacement in burns because of the risk of infection. Less invasive monitoring using thermodilution methods to measure intrathoracic blood volume, cardiac output, and cardiac index have recently received attention. Although preliminary studies have suggested that this may aid resuscitation, one RCT failed to support these findings in burns.[w6]

What is the role of nutrition?

The role of nutritional support in major burns has shifted from one of preventing malnutrition to one of disease modulation.[w6] Nutritional requirements are dynamic, and early debridement and skin cover result in a 50-75% increase in energy expenditure. Thus, a nutritional plan—that takes account of factors such as the extent and depth of the burn, the need for repeated surgical interventions, the appropriateness of the enteral or parenteral route, and the pre-injury health status of the patient—should be implemented within 12 hours.

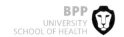

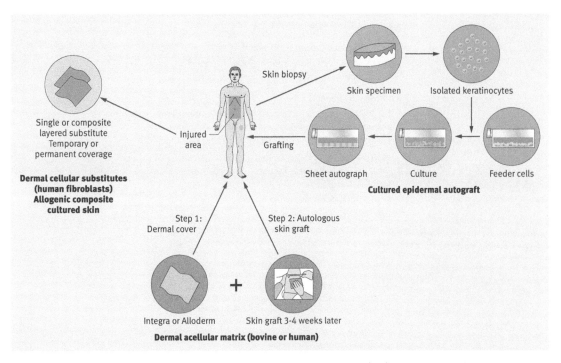

Fig 3 Newer tissue engineering directions in burns management. Cultured epidermal autografts (right), staged dermal acellular substitutes (bottom), single application dermal cellular substitutes or allogenic composites (left)

BOX 4 EMERGENCY MANAGEMENT OF SEVERE BURNS APPROACH (ADAPTED FROM THE AUSTRALIAN AND NEW ZEALAND BURNS ASSOCIATION)

Order of management priority in patients with severe burns
- A. Airway with cervical spine control
- B. Breathing and ventilation
- C. Circulation with haemorrhage control
- D. Disability—neurological status
- E. Exposure preventing hypothermia
- F. Fluid resuscitation

Adults
Resuscitation fluid alone (first 24 hours):
- Give 3-4 ml (3 ml in superficial or partial thickness burns, 4 ml in full thickness burns or those with associated inhalation injury) Hartmann's solution/kg body weight/% total body surface area. Half of this calculated volume is given in the first eight hours after injury. The remaining half is given in the second 16 hour period

Children
Resuscitation fluid as above plus maintenance (0.45% saline with 5% dextrose, the volume should be titrated against nasogastric feeds or oral intake):
- Give 100 ml/kg for first 10 kg body weight plus 50 ml/kg for the next 10 kg body weight plus 20 ml/kg for each extra kg

---

Psychosocial aspects
The psychological requirements of patients and their carers change over the early resuscitative phase, acute phase, and rehabilitation phase. The prevalence of depression is estimated to be high (up to 60%) in burns inpatients, and up to 30% have some degree of post-traumatic stress disorder.[w7] All burns centres offer specialist advice on long term psychosocial adjustment in burns patients. Changing faces in the UK and the Phoenix society in the United States provide excellent support for burns survivors.

How are scar and burn areas managed after healing?
A retrospective cohort study of 337 children with up to a five year follow-up found hypertrophic scarring in less than 20% of superficial scalds that healed within 21 days but in up to 90% of burns that took 30 days or more to heal.[11]

Appropriate treatment must therefore be instituted early and infection prevented to encourage rapid healing. Healed burns do not have adnexal structures, and are therefore dry, sensitive, and irregularly pigmented. Hence the area should be moisturised and massaged to reduce dryness and to keep the healed area supple. A sun cream, with a sun protection factor of 30, is advised to prevent further thermal damage and pigmentation changes.

New directions in burn wound management
Although autografting is the gold standard for skin replacement in burns, limited availability of donor skin precludes this option in large area burns. Hence, various tissue engineered skin substitutes (fig 3) have been developed to provide temporary or permanent wound coverage.

Autologous keratinocyte grafts (obtained after biopsy and culture of the patient's own keratinocytes) and or allogenic keratinocyte grafts have been developed for large area superficial burns. Other developments include a keratinocyte suspension in a fibrin sealant matrix aimed at increasing the adherence of keratinocytes to the wound bed (keratinocyte-fibrin glue suspension) and a total lysate of cultured human keratinocytes made up of growth factors, cytokines, and matrix molecules in a hydrophilic gel.[w8]

Processed skin from human cadavers—in which the cells are removed to leave a non-antigenic dermal scaffold—is used as a dermal replacement for treating deeper burns. Allogeneic fibroblasts, obtained from neonatal human foreskin and cultured in vitro, seeded on a biologically absorbable scaffold or on a nylon mesh, have also been developed. The proliferating fibroblasts secrete collagen, matrix proteins, and growth factors and aid healing. Composite skin substitutes comprising allogeneic keratinocytes (epidermal equivalent) and fibroblasts (dermal equivalent) are also available.[w9]

Although a recent meta-analysis of 20 RCTs has shown these substitutes to be safe, their efficacy could not be determined on the basis of current evidence.[w9]

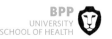

ADDITIONAL EDUCATIONAL RESOURCES

Resources for healthcare professionals

- Burn Surgery (www.burnsurgery.org)—Good resource for health professionals regarding all aspects of burns

Resources for patients

- Fire Safety in the Home (www.firekills.gov.uk)—Government website with burn prevention and fire safety information
- Changing Faces (www.changingfaces.org.uk)—UK charity that supports and represents people who have disfigurements of the face or body from any cause
- Salamanders (www.kernoweb.myby.co.uk/salamanders)—Provides networking and education opportunities for young burns survivors
- Phoenix Society (www.phoenix-society.org/resources)—Patient resource directed at burns survivors and families

---

Contributors: SE and AR designed the paper, carried out the literature search, collated the up to date evidence, and prepared the manuscript. SE created the flow charts and AR created fig 3. Both authors contributed equally in the development and completion of this article. MS is the senior author who proofread the article, provided invaluable suggestions, did the necessary corrections and amendments, and provided the expert advice. SE is guarantor.

Competing interests: None declared.

Provenance and peer review: Commissioned; externally peer reviewed.

1   National Burn Care Review. National burn injury referral guidelines. In: *Standards and strategy for burn care* . London: NBCR, 2001:68-9.
2   Wilkinson E. The epidemiology of burns in secondary care, in a population of 2.6 million people. *Burns* 1998;24:139-43.
3   WHO. *Facts about injuries: burns.* www.who.int/violence_injury_prevention/publications/other_injury/en/burns_factsheet.pdf.
4   Peck MD, Kruger GE, van der Merwe AE, Godakumbura W, Ahuja RB. Burns and fires from non-electric domestic appliances in low and middle-income countries. Part I. The scope of the problem. *Burns* 2008;34:303-11.
5   Wachtel TL, Berry CC, Wachtel EE, Frank HA. The inter-rater reliability of estimating the size of burns from various burn area chart drawings. *Burns* 2000;26:156-70.
6   Hettiaratchy S, Papini R. Initial management of a major burn: II—assessment and resuscitation. *BMJ* 2004;329:101-3.
7   La Hei ER, Holland AJA, Martin HCO. Laser Doppler imaging of paediatric burns: burn wound outcome can be predicted independent of clinical examination. *Burns* 2006;32:550-3.
8   British Burn Association. *Emergency management of severe burns course manual , UK version* . Manchester: Wythenshawe Hospital, 2008.
9   McGill DJ, Sørensen K, MacKay IR, Taggart I, Watson SB. Assessment of burn depth: a prospective, blinded comparison of laser Doppler imaging and videomicroscopy. *Burns* 2007;33:833-42.
10 Renkielska A, Nowakowski A, Kaczmarek M, Ruminski J. Burn depths evaluation based on active dynamic IR thermal imaging—a preliminary study. *Burns* 2006;32:867-75.
11 Cubison TCS, Pape SA, Parkhouse N. Evidence for the link between healing time and the development of hypertrophic scars (HTS) in paediatric burns due to scald. *Burns* 2006;32:992-9.
12 Ryan CM, Schoenfield DA, Thorpe WP, Sheriden RL, Cassem EH, Tompkins RG. Objective estimates of the probability of death from burn injuries. *N Engl J Med* 1998;338:362-6.
13 Bloemsma GC, Doktera J, Boxmaa H, Oen IMMH. Mortality and causes of death in a burn centre. *Burns* 2008;34:1103-7.
14 Pereira C, Murphy K, Herndon D. Outcome measures in burn care: is mortality dead? *Burns* 2004;30:761-71.
15 Alsbjörn B, Gilbert P, Hartmann B, Kazmierski M, Monstrey S, Palao R, et al. Guidelines for the management of partial-thickness burns in a general hospital or community setting—recommendations of a European working party. *Burns* 2007;33:155-60.
16 Hudspith J, Rayatt S. First aid and treatment of minor burns. *BMJ* 2004;328:1487-9.
17 Whitaker IS, Prowse S, Potokar TS. A critical evaluation of the use of Biobrane as a biologic skin substitute: a versatile tool for the plastic and reconstructive surgeon. *Ann Plast Surg* 2008;60:333-7.
18 Allison K, Porter K. Consensus on the pre-hospital approach to burns patient management. *Emerg Med J* 2004;21:112-4.
19 Yuan J, Wu C, Holland AJA, Harvey JG, Martin HCO, La Hei ER, et al. Assessment of cooling on an acute scald burn injury in a porcine model. *J Burn Care Res* 2007;28:514-20.
20 Sawadal Y, Urushidate S, Yotsuyanagil T, Ishita K. Is prolonged and excessive cooling of a scalded wound effective? *Burns* 1997;23:55-8.
21 Barrow RE, Jeschke MG, Herndon DN. Early fluid resuscitation improves outcomes in severely burned children. *Resuscitation* 2000;45:91-6.
22 Wharton SM, Khanna A. Current attitudes to burns resuscitation in the UK. *Burns* 2001;27:183-4.
23 Perel P, Roberts I. Colloids versus crystalloids for fluid resuscitation in critically ill patients. *Cochrane Database Syst Rev* 2007;(4):CD000567.
24 Pham TN, Cancio LC, Gibran NS. American Burn Association practice guidelines burn shock resuscitation. *J Burn Care Res* 2008;29:257-66.

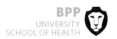
Early fluid resuscitation in severe trauma

Tim Harris, professor of emergency medicine[12],
G O Rhys Thomas, Lieutenant Colonel and honorary consultant [342],
Karim Brohi, professor of trauma sciences and consultant trauma and vascular surgeon [12]

[1]Barts and the London School of Medicine and Dentistry, Queen Mary University of London, London, UK

[2]Barts Health NHS Trust, London

[3]16 Air Assault Medical Regiment

[4]Royal London and Queen Victoria, East Grinstead, UK

Correspondence to: T Harris, Department of Emergency Medicine, Royal London Hospital, Whitechapel, London E11BB
tim.harris@bartshealth.nhs.uk

Cite this as: *BMJ* 2012;345:e5752

DOI: 10.1136/bmj.e5752

http://www.bmj.com/content/345/bmj.e5752

Trauma is a global health problem that affects patients in both rich and poor countries and accounts for 10 000 deaths each day.[1][2] Trauma is the second leading cause of death after HIV/AIDS in the 5-45 year old age group.[w1][w2] Early triage and resuscitation decisions affect outcome in trauma situations.[w3][w4] The two leading causes of mortality in trauma are neurological injury and blood loss.[3][4w5][w6] There has been considerable improvement in our understanding of trauma resuscitation in the past 20 years, and data from databases and observational trials suggests outcomes are improving.[w7] For patients with severe traumatic injuries (defined as >15 by the injury severity score, an anatomical scoring system), the high volume fluid resuscitation promoted by early advanced trauma life support manuals,[5] followed by definitive surgical care, has given way to a damage control resuscitation (DCR) strategy (box).

This DCR approach has seen a fall in the volume of crystalloid delivered in the emergency department and an associated fall in mortality.[6w8] In this review, we summarise the evidence guiding the initial period of resuscitation from arrival in the emergency department to transfer to intensive care or operating theatre, focusing on trauma in critically injured adults. This article emphasises newer developments in trauma care. There is debate on whether patients with brain injury should be resuscitated to higher blood pressures, which is briefly discussed later in the text.

KEY COMPONENTS OF DCR

- Permissive hypovolaemia (hypotension) (see summary points)
- Haemostatic transfusion (resuscitation)—that is, fresh frozen plasma, platelets, or packed red blood cells, and tranexamic acid. Avoidance of crystalloids (normal saline, Hartmann's, Ringer's lactate solutions), colloids (a substance microscopically dispersed evenly throughout another substance; with resuscitation fluids, this term refers to larger molecules dispersed most usually in normal saline, such as gelofusion, haemaccel, or volulyte), and vasopressors
- Damage control surgery or angiography to treat the cause of bleeding
- Restore organ perfusion and oxygen delivery with definitive resuscitation

SUMMARY POINTS

- Critically injured trauma patients may have normal cardiovascular and respiratory parameters (pulse, blood pressure, respiratory rate), and no single physiological or metabolic factor accurately identifies all patients in this group
- Initial resuscitation for severely injured patients is based on a strategy of permissive hypovolaemia (hypotension) (that is, fluid resuscitation delivered to increase blood pressure without reaching normotension, aiming for cerebration in the awake patient, or 70-80 mm Hg in penetrating trauma and 90 mm Hg in blunt trauma) and blood product based resuscitation
- This period of hypovolaemia (hypotension) should be kept to a minimum, with rapid transfer to the operating theatre for definitive care
- Crystalloid or colloid based resuscitation in severely injured patients is associated with worse outcome
- Once haemostasis has been achieved, resuscitation targeted to measures of cardiac output or oxygen delivery or use improves outcome
- Tranexamic acid administered intravenously within 3 h of injury improves mortality in patients who are thought to be bleeding

SOURCES AND SELECTION CRITERIA

We searched Medline, Embase, the Cochrane database, and Google for randomised controlled trials, meta-analyses, and peer reviewed articles, limiting the search to adults. The search was performed once by the lead author (TH) and once by a professional librarian. All articles were shared and supplemented by the author's own libraries. The main search terms used were "trauma," "resuscitation," "fluid," and "goal directed therapy." Ongoing studies were identified from www.clinicaltrials.gov.

How can patients who need DCR be identified?

A DCR strategy applies to patients who present with suspected major haemorrhage. While many definitions exist, the most practical in the acute trauma setting is for estimated blood transfusion volumes of over four units in the initial 2-4 h. Identifying these patients can be a challenge because they are often young with good physiological reserve and may have no physiological evidence of hypovolaemic shock.[7] A number of tools have been developed to identify this group of patients; however, physician decision and experience have been found to be just as accurate.[w9][w10][w11][w12][w13] Failure to identify these patients early and to apply DCR is associated with excess mortality.[8]

How can trauma patients in shock be identified?

Shock may be defined as a life threatening condition characterised by inadequate delivery of oxygen to vital organs in relation to their metabolic requirements.[9] A systolic blood pressure of 90 mm Hg is commonly used to define both hypotension and shock; however, oxygen delivery depends on cardiac output rather than blood pressure. Homeostasis with peripheral vasoconstriction acts to preserve blood pressure even as circulating volume is lost. In patients who have had trauma, adequate cardiac output cannot be inferred from blood pressure. Only when blood loss approaches half the circulating volume or occurs rapidly is there a relation between the cardiac output and blood pressure.[10] Patients presenting with hypotension, tachycardia, and obvious blood loss are readily identified as being in a state of haemorrhagic shock. However, many patients will maintain their pulse and blood pressure even after massive blood loss and tissue hypoxia. This condition is termed cryptic shock and is associated with increased mortality.[w14]

The role of basic physiological parameters to estimate the severity of blood loss has been popularised in the advanced trauma life support courses and manuals.[5] These materials describe physiological deterioration with increasing volumes of blood loss, and categorise four stages of shock. But data from a 1989-2007 analysis of the United Kingdom Trauma Audit Research Network database suggest that this model is not reflected in practice. Patients with progressive levels of blood loss to stage 4 haemorrhagic shock (equating to >2 L blood loss) were found to increase their pulse rates from 82 to 95 beats per minute, not to change respiratory

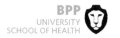

rates or Glasgow coma scale, and maintain systolic blood pressures above 120 mm Hg.[11] Although an important part of the initial assessment, physiological derangement alone is neither sensitive nor specific as a tool to identify shock in trauma patients.[7]

There is observational evidence from large datasets in the UK and United States that mortality increases in trauma patients in both blunt and penetrating trauma, while systolic blood pressure falls below 110 mm Hg.[12W15 W16 W17 W18 W19] A US review of 870 634 sets of trauma records identified that for every 10 mm Hg below 110 mm Hg, mortality increased by 4.8%.[12] Shock index does not improve after risk stratification of trauma patients.[W20]

Metabolic assessment with lactate[W21 W22] and base excess[W23 W24] also predicts blood loss and mortality. Furthermore, these parameters may be increased from exercise around the time of injury (running, fighting) or may be (falsely) low if the hypoxic tissues are not being perfused sufficiently to wash anaerobic products into the circulation (for example, when a tourniquet is applied). For patients in whom central access is obtained, mixed venous oxygen saturation is also a good indicator of blood loss, with levels below 70% suggesting inadequate oxygen delivery.[W25]

Estimated injuries and associated blood loss are an important part of the initial trauma assessment. Clinical examination is augmented by focused ultrasound assessment of the chest, pericardium, and peritoneal cavity (extended focused assessment with sonography in trauma (eFAST), a specific but insensitive test for blood loss); and computed tomography (a sensitive and specific test for blood loss).

What is permissive hypotension (hypovolaemic) resuscitation?

Permissive (hypotension) hypovolaemic resuscitation is used to describe a process that minimises administration of fluid resuscitation until haemorrhage control has been achieved, or is deemed unnecessary on definitive imaging. Resuscitation is the restoration of oxygen delivery and organ perfusion to match requirements. In the 1960s and 1970s, a strategy of high volume crystalloid resuscitation in a ratio of 3 mL per 1 mL of blood loss was promoted, which was thought to replace intravascular and interstitial losses and reduce the risk of organ failure.[13] However, vigorous fluid resuscitation increases blood pressure, the effect of which increases hydrostatic forces on newly formed clot, dilutes clotting factors and haemoglobin, and reduces body temperature. These effects could promote further bleeding. In permissive

hypotension, definitive resuscitation is deferred until haemostasis is obtained. It is now recognised that aggressive crystalloid resuscitation also impairs organ perfusion.[14W26]

What evidence do we have for hypovolaemic resuscitation?

Considerable animal work has informed our understanding of hypovolaemic resuscitation. In summary, this research found that withholding fluid resuscitation from animals with critical blood loss (about half their circulating volume) was associated with death, whereas animals with less severe blood loss had a lower mortality with no fluid resuscitation.[15]

The table summarises three randomised controlled trials exploring the risks and benefits of hypovolaemic resuscitation.[16 17W27] These trials provide evidence of a mortality advantage in favour of this resuscitation strategy for truncal penetrating trauma and evidence of no harm in blunt trauma.

The National Institute for Health and Clinical Excellence has recommended that in older children and adults with blunt trauma, no fluid be administered in the prehospital resuscitation phase if a radial pulse can be felt, or for penetrating trauma if a central pulse is palpable.[18] In the absence of this, 250 mL crystalloid fluid boluses are administered and the patient is reassessed until these pulses, as described, return.

Much of the evidence for hypovolaemic resuscitation was developed before the advent of haemostatic resuscitation, as described below. This period of hypovolaemic resuscitation is maintained for as short a period as possible, until the injury complex is defined and any sites of blood loss treated surgically or embolised.

Untreated hypovolaemic shock leads to microvascular hypoperfusion and hypoxia, leading to multiorgan failure.[19] Hypovolaemic resuscitation sacrifices perfusion for coagulation and haemorrhage control. The trauma team carefully balances the resuscitation process to maintain organ perfusion but at lower than normal blood pressure to regulate bleeding. Based on the evidence available, we suggest that fluid resuscitation before haemorrhage control should aim to maintain a systolic blood pressure of 80 mm Hg or a palpable radial pulse or cerebration by using small volume boluses of 250 mL. This value is arbitrary with little evidence to support it. The 250 mL boluses are able to increase blood pressure, since the circulation is highly constricted with a small volume of distribution. In practice, achieving target blood pressures is challenging. Patients

Randomised trials of permissive hypotension in trauma

Trial	Intervention	Patient group	Setting	Findings	Comments
Pseudo-randomised controlled trial[16]	No fluid resuscitation before surgical intervention in operating theatre v crystalloid based resuscitation	Penetrating truncal trauma and systolic blood pressure >90 mm Hg (n=598)	Prehospital and in emergency department	Lower mortality in group with no fluid resuscitation than in group with crystalloid based resuscitation (survival 70% v 62%, P=0.04)	Short transport distances, mortality benefit predominantly vascular injuries, young cohort (mean age 31 years), 8% in no fluid group received fluids
Randomised controlled trial[17]	Resuscitation to target systolic blood pressure 100 mm Hg v 70 mm Hg	Blunt or penetrating trauma and systolic blood pressure <90 mm Hg in first hour (n=110)	Urban trauma centre resuscitation room	No mortality difference, low mortality of four (7.3%) patients in each group	Low mortality, study underpowered to show mortality difference, observed systolic blood pressures were 114 mm Hg and 100 mm Hg despite targets
Randomised controlled trial: interim analysis[W27]	Intraoperative resuscitation to mean arterial pressure 50 mm Hg v 65 mm Hg	Traumatic injuries excluding traumatic brain injury with at least one episode of systolic blood pressure <90 mm Hg (n=90)	Operating theatre	No mortality difference	Observed blood pressures did not differ significantly despite targets; results may not translate to preoperative environment[W28]

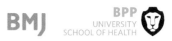

with severe injuries will probably need blood product based resuscitation, as described below.

Fluid resuscitation in traumatic brain injury

This review does not deal in detail with the complexities of resuscitation in brain injury; however, retrospective observational data for patients with traumatic brain injury suggest that any single reduction in mean arterial blood pressure below 90 mm Hg is associated with a doubling in mortality.[w28] [w29] Guidelines published by the Brain Trauma Foundation advocate maintaining a systolic blood pressure above 90 mm Hg but do not specifically state whether this is during active haemorrhage.[w30] Currently, there is controversy about whether the guidelines for permissive hypotension should be changed in the presence of head injury because there is no human evidence from prospective studies.

What is the role of blood products in trauma resuscitation?

Severe bleeding in trauma patients can result in disordered blood clotting. Until recently, this effect was thought to be a late phenomenon arising primarily from loss of coagulation factors during haemorrhage and dilution from resuscitation fluids. However, it is now recognised that trauma induced coagulopathy occurs within minutes of injury, and is associated with a fourfold increase in mortality.[20] The process is multifactorial[21] but is partly due to an endogenous coagulopathy that occurs as a result of tissue damage in severe shock.[w31] This understanding has led to changes in the management of trauma haemorrhage.

Haemostatic resuscitation

Haemostatic resuscitation is a combination of strategies targeting trauma induced coagulopathy to reduce bleeding and improve outcomes.[w32] [w33]

How do blood products aid in resuscitation?

The main strategy to treat trauma induced coagulopathy is to provide volume replacement that augments coagulation. This replacement has been achieved by the transfusion of fresh frozen plasma, platelets, and packed red blood cells. A retrospective observational study performed on military personnel with similar injuries but differing resuscitation fluid strategies suggested that the use of higher ratios of fresh frozen plasma to packed red blood cells may improve outcomes.[22] Similar results have been seen in other retrospective studies and a few small prospective cohort studies,[23] although the retrospective studies are subject to survival bias.

It is also unclear whether the benefit from these strategies comes from the coagulation factors present in fresh frozen plasma or from reducing the amount of crystalloid and colloid administered. Nevertheless, it seems clear that the usual 1-2 units of plasma previously administered after massive transfusions was insufficient to prevent dilutional coagulopathy. Current consensus is that plasma should be given from the beginning of the resuscitation, alongside transfusions of packed red blood cells, in a ratio of 1 "unit" of plasma for each 1-2 units of packed red blood cells.[24] Very little is known about platelet function in trauma induced coagulopathy or the effectiveness of platelet transfusions.[w34] [w35] Although these early strategies of blood product in high doses seem effective, they are based on limited evidence. These regimens also place substantial resource demands on blood banks and are logistically difficult to implement owing to the requirements for rapid thawing and delivery.

Research is also being undertaken to look at alternatives to blood component therapy for the management of trauma induced coagulopathy. Fibrinogen is the central substrate of blood clotting, and levels are low in this patient group.[w36] Some retrospective evidence suggests that patients who receive more fibrinogen replacement (in the form of cryoprecipitate and plasma) have better outcomes in terms of total use of packed red blood cells and mortality.[w37] Fibrinogen is also available as a powdered concentrate and could be a replacement therapy that can be easily administered in trauma induced coagulopathy.[w38] [w39]

How do I identify patients with trauma induced coagulopathy?

Standard clotting tests from laboratories such as the prothrombin time do not show any of the key derangements in trauma induced coagulopathy, such as reduced clot strength and fibrinolysis.[25] Furthermore, in a trauma setting, it is impractical to wait for tests that can take up 1 h to process. The point of care versions of these tests (such as the prothrombin time) are prone to be under-read in the presence of low haematocrits. These difficulties have led to a renewed interest in the use of thromboelastography—a point of care assessment of clot generation, strength, and breakdown. This procedure has the potential to provide a rapid assessment of the whole clotting process, but it has not yet been validated in the acute setting.[25] In the absence of a validated diagnostic test at the point of care, management is therefore blind to the status of the coagulation system and relies on clinical judgment and empiric therapy.

What fluids should be used to resuscitate trauma patients who do not need DCR?

Patients who do not need DCR need no immediate resuscitation until definitive imaging has identified the underlying injuries. These patients should be observed carefully for signs of physiological and metabolic deterioration, consequent on disease progression with blood loss, visceral injury, and pericardial or pleural tamponade. Debate continues on the relative merits of colloid or crystalloid based resuscitation strategies, with a recent Cochrane review concluding that there was no evidence that survival was better with one or the other solution.[26]

However, a subgroup analysis of 460 patients with traumatic brain injury (Glasgow coma scale ≤13) from a large randomised controlled trial comparing the safety of albumin in normal saline with normal saline identified a survival advantage in the crystalloid group (33.2% v 20.4%, P=0.003).[27]

Hypertonic solutions have been proposed to improve cerebral perfusion and reduce cerebral oedema, and have been advocated for resuscitation of patients with traumatic brain injury.[w40] A meta-analysis of eight randomised trials identified a survival advantage in this group,[w41] but a randomised controlled trial of 229 patients with hypotension and severe traumatic brain injury (Glasgow coma scale <9) who received prehospital resuscitation with hypertonic or normal saline had almost identical survival and neurological function six months after injury.[28] Furthermore, a recent randomised controlled trial of prehospital use of hypertonic solutions was terminated by the data and safety monitoring board after randomisation of 1331 patients, having met prespecified futility criteria. Among patients with severe

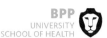

 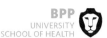

TIPS FOR NON-SPECIALISTS

- Doctors and nurses who care for trauma patients who are severely injured need to be familiar with the principles of resuscitation strategies for damage control, as outlined in this review
- A clearly written protocol for massive transfusion facilitates rapid access to and delivery of blood product based resuscitation
- Transfer patients with severe traumatic injuries to a dedicated trauma unit
- Trauma teams bring together doctors and nurses from a range of disciplines, and scenario based practice is likely to facilitate smooth teamwork

---

ADDITIONAL EDUCATIONAL RESOURCES

Resources for healthcare professionals

- Trauma.org (www.trauma.org/)—an independent, non-profit organisation providing global education and information for professionals involved in trauma care
- Eastern Association for Surgery of Trauma guidelines (www.east.org/research/treatment-guideline)—provides a series of evidence based guidelines for trauma care
- Online lectures from massive transfusion and coagulopathy state of the art symposium at the London Trauma Conference in 2008 (www.trauma.org/index.php/main/articles/)—provides a series of lectures on blood transfusion, resuscitation, and trauma induced coagulopathy

Resources for patients

- Patient.co.uk website (www.patient.co.uk/)—UK patient website providing wide range of information and discussing a variety of injuries
- Cohen D. Code red: repairing blood in the emergency room. *New Scientist* 2011. www.newscientist.com/article/mg21228352.900-code-red-repairing-blood-in-the-emergency-room.html
- Trauma information pages (www.trauma-pages.com/)—provides simply worded information specifically for non-healthcare professionals concerning traumatic injuries
- National Institute of Neurological Disorders and Stroke. Information page on traumatic brain injury. 2012. www.ninds.nih.gov/disorders/tbi/tbi.htm—provides clearly written information directed at members of the public and healthcare professionals on a variety of neurological insults, including traumatic brain injuries

---

traumatic brain injury not in hypovolaemic shock, initial resuscitation with either hypertonic saline or hypertonic saline and dextran, compared with normal saline, did not result in improved neurological outcome or survival at six months.[29] Thus, we suggest the use of crystalloid based fluid administration in this cohort of patients who are less severely injured.

Once haemostasis is achieved, what should be done to ensure adequate resuscitation in severe trauma?

Once haemostasis has been achieved with surgical intervention, fracture splintage or angiography, or the requirement for these interventions identified as not necessary, then definitive resuscitation is required. If patients are resuscitated to normal blood pressure and pulse without further parameters being used to evaluate for tissue hypoxia, over half of patients would be inadequately resuscitated, with increased morbidity and mortality.[30 w42] Resuscitation to targets of oxygen delivery or use is termed goal directed therapy, and good quality evidence from randomised trials indicates that this approach should be used in trauma; indeed, the original evidence for this approach came from trauma studies.[w43 w44 w45 w46 w47 31 32]

What other agents should be used in the initial resuscitation period?

Hyperfibrinolysis is common after trauma, owing to associated hypovolaemic shock and tissue injury.[w48] In a recent, large, multinational randomised controlled trial researchers targeted a specific component of trauma induced coagulopathy—hyperfibrinolysis. They showed a reduction in mortality with the use of tranexamic acid, which has antifibrinolytic properties (1 g delivered over 15 min, then 1 g over 4 h, commenced within 3 h of injury).[33]

ONGOING RESEARCH

- PROPPR (pragmatic, randomised optional platelets and plasma ratios): randomised controlled trial of 1:1:1 v 1:1:2 of red blood cells to platelets to plasma in patients requiring massive transfusion, seeking to better define the ratio of plasma to packed red blood cells for damage control resuscitation (NCT01545232)
- MP4OX phase IIb trial for ischaemia rescue (lactate clearance): trial exploring the use of an oxygen carrying colloid in trauma resuscitation (NCT01262196)
- VITRIS (vasopressin for therapy of persistent traumatic hemorrhagic shock): multicentre randomised controlled trial further exploring the role of vasopressin in fluid resistant shock (NCT00379522)
- CIST (colloids in severe trauma): multicentre pilot study of volume resuscitation based on crystalloid only versus crystalloid-colloid (starch based) in trauma; this randomised controlled trial has just been completed, looking particularly at the incidence of intra-abdominal hypertension (NCT00890383)
- HypoResus (field trial of hypotensive v standard resuscitation for hemorrhagic shock after trauma): randomised controlled trial comparing standard resuscitation with hypotensive resuscitation prehospital and in the first 2 h in the emergency department (NCT01411852)

QUESTIONS FOR FUTURE RESEARCH

- How do we balance the risks of impaired organ perfusion consequent on hypovolaemic resuscitation with clot preservation?
- How do we identify and target trauma induced coagulopathy in the acute phase?
- What is the most effective combination of blood products for initial trauma resuscitation?
- Should patients with traumatic brain injury be subject to different initial resuscitation strategies?
- Does therapeutic hypothermia have a role in trauma resuscitation or traumatic brain injury in the acute phase?

Contributors: TH conceived the review and wrote the introduction, sections of permissive hypovolaemia, resuscitation endpoints, and fluid resuscitation. RT wrote the sections contrasting colloids and crystalloids with hypertonic saline. KB wrote the sections on blood product use and trauma induced coagulopathy. The contributions were correlated by TH, and all authors reviewed the paper. TH is guarantor.

Competing interests: All authors have completed the Unified Competing Interest form at www.icmje.org/coi_disclosure.pdf (available on request from the corresponding author) and declare: no support from any organisation for the submitted work; KB has received unrestricted research funding from Octapharma and Thromboelastometry and has consulted for Haemonetics and Sangart; no other relationships or activities that could appear to have influenced the submitted work.

Provenance and peer review: Commissioned; externally peer reviewed.

1 Roberts I, Shakur H, Edwards P, Yates D, Sandercock P. Trauma care research and the war on uncertainty. *BMJ* 2005;331:1094-6.
2 Kauvar DS, Lefering R, Wade CE. Impact of haemorrhage on trauma outcome: an overview of epidemiology, clinical presentations and therapeutic considerations. *J Trauma* 2006;60:S3-11.
3 Chesnut RM, Marshall LF, Klauber MR, Blunt BA, Baldwin N, Eisenberg HM, et al. The role of secondary brain injury in determining outcome from severe head injury. *J Trauma* 1993;34:216-22.
4 Bratton SL, Chestnut RM, Ghajar J, McConnell Hammond FF, Harris OA, Hartl R, et al. Guidelines for the management of severe traumatic brain injury. I. Blood pressure and oxygenation. *J Neurotrauma* 2007;24(suppl 1):S7-13.
5 American College of Surgeons Committee on Trauma. Advanced trauma life support for doctors. American College of Surgeons Committee on Trauma, 1997.

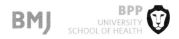

6   Ley EJ, Clond MA, Srour MK, Barnajian M, Mirocha J, Margulies DR, et al. Emergency department crystalloid resuscitation of 1.5 L or more is associated with increased mortality in elderly and nonelderly trauma patients. *J Trauma* 2011;70:398-400.

7   Stanworth SJ, Morris TP, Gaarder C, Goslings JC, Maegele M, Cohen MJ, et al. Reappraising the concept of massive transfusion in trauma. *Crit Care Med* 2010;14:R239.

8   Larson CR, White CE, Spinella PC, Jones JA, Holcomb JB, Blackbourne LH, et al. Association of shock, coagulopathy, and initial vital signs with massive transfusion in combat casualties. *J Trauma* 2010;69:S26-32.

9   Strehlow MC. Early identification of shock in critically ill patients. *Emerg Med Clin N Am* 2010;28:57-66.

10 Wo CJ, Shoemaker WC, Appel PL, Bishop MH, Kram HB, Hardin E. Unreliability of blood pressure and heart rate to evaluate cardiac output in emergency resuscitation and critical illness. *Crit Care Med* 1993;21:218-23.

11 Guly HR, Bouamra O, Spiers M, Dark P, Coats T, Lecky F. Vital signs and estimated blood loss in patients with major trauma: testing the validity of the ATLS classification of hypovolaemic shock. *Resuscitation* 2011;82:556-9.

12 Eastridge BJ, Salinas J, McManus JG, Blackburn L, Bugler EM, Cooke WH, et al. Hypotension begins at 110 mm Hg: redefining 'hypotension' with data. *J Trauma* 2007;63:291-9.

13 Shires GT, Canizaro PC. Fluid resuscitation in the severely injured. *Clin Surg N Am* 1973;53:1341-66.

14 Cotton BA, Guy JS, Morris JA Jr, Abumrad NN. The cellular, metabolic, and systemic consequences of aggressive fluid resuscitation strategies. *Shock* 2006;26:115-21.

15 Mapstone J, Roberts I, Evans P. Fluid resuscitation strategies: a systematic review of animal trials. *J Trauma* 2003;55:571-89.

16 Bickell WH, Wall MJ, Pepe PE, Martin RR, Ginger VF, Allen MK, et al. Immediate versus delayed fluid resuscitation for hypotensive patients with penetrating torso injuries. *N Engl J Med* 1994;331:1105-9.

17 Dutton RP, Mackenzie CF, Scalae TM. Hypotensive resuscitation during active haemorrhage: impact on hospital mortality. *J Trauma* 2002;52:1141-6.

18 National Institute for Health and Clinical Excellence. Pre-hospital initiation of fluid replacement therapy in trauma. Technology appraisal 74. January 2004. www.nice.org.uk/nicemedia/live/11526/32820/32820.pdf.

19 Santry HP, Alam HB. Fluid resuscitation: past, present and the future. *Shock* 2010;33:229-41.

20 Floccard B, Rugeri L, Faure A, Saint Denis M, Boyle EM, Peguet O, et al. Early coagulopathy in trauma patients: an on-scene and hospital admission study. *Injury* 2012;43:26-32.

21 Hess JR, Brohi K, Dutton RP, Hauser CJ, Holcomb JB, Kluger Y, et al. The coagulopathy of trauma: a review of mechanisms. *J Trauma* 2008;65:748-54.

22 Borgman MA, Spinella PC, Perkins JG, Grathwohl KW, Repine T, Beekley AC, et al. The ratio of blood products transfused affects mortality in patients receiving massive transfusions at a combat support hospital. *J Trauma* 2007;63:805-13.

23 Rajasekhar A, Gowing R, Zarychanski R, Arnold DM, Lim W, Crowther MA,et al. Survival of trauma patients after massive red blood cell transfusion using a high or low red blood cell to plasma transfusion ratio. *Crit Care Med* 2011;39:1507-13.

24 Davenport R, Curry N, Manson J, De'Ath H, Coates A, Rourke C, et al. Hemostatic effects of fresh frozen plasma may be maximal at red cell ratios of 1:2. *J Trauma* 2011;70:90-5.

25 Davenport R, Manson J, De'Ath H, Platton S, Coates A, Allard S, et al. Functional definition and characterization of acute traumatic coagulopathy. *Crit Care Med* 2011;39:2652-8.

26 Perel P, Roberts I. Colloids versus crystalloids for fluid resuscitation in critically ill patients. *Cochrane Database Syst Rev* 2011;3:CD000567.

27 SAFE Study Investigators; Australian and New Zealand Intensive Care Society Clinical Trials Group; Australian Red Cross Blood Service; George Institute for International Health, Myburgh J, Cooper DJ, et al. Saline or albumin for fluid resuscitation in patients with traumatic brain injury. *N Engl J Med* 2007;357:874-84.

28 Cooper JD, Myles PS, McDermott FT, Murray LJ, Laidlaw J, Cooper G, et al. Pre-hospital hypertonic saline resuscitation of patients with hypotension and severe traumatic brain injury: a randomized controlled trial. *JAMA* 2004;291:1350-7.

29 Bulger EM, May S. Out-of-hospital hypertonic resuscitation following severe traumatic brain injury: a randomized controlled trial. *JAMA* 2010;304:1455-64.

30 Claridge JA, Crabtree TD, Pelletier SJ, Butler K, Sawyer RG, Young JS. Persistent occult hypoperfusion is associated with a significant infection rate and mortality in major trauma patients. *J Trauma* 2000;48:8-13.

31 McKinley BA, Valdivia A, Moore FA. Goal-orientated shock resuscitation for major torso trauma: what are we learning? *Curr Opin Critical Care* 2003;9:292-9.

32 Chytra I, Pradl R, Bosman R, Pelnár P, Kasal E, Zidková A. Esophageal Doppler-guided fluid management decreases blood lactate levels in multiple-trauma patients: a randomized controlled trial. *Critical Care* 2007;11:R24.

33 CRASH-2 Collaborators, Shakur H, Roberts I, Bautista R, Caballero J, Coats T, et al. Effects of tranexamic acid on death, vascular occlusive events, and blood transfusion in trauma patients with significant haemorrhage (CRASH-2): a randomised, placebo-controlled trial. *Lancet* 2010;376:23-32.

Related links

bmj.com/archive
Previous articles in this series

- Irritable bowel syndrome (2012;345:e5836)
- Management of renal colic (2012;345:e5499)
- Diagnosis and management of peripheral arterial disease (2012;345:e5208)
- Diagnosis and management of cellulitis (2012;345:e4955)
- Management of osteoarthritis of the knee (2012;345:e4934)

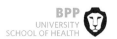

Cardiopulmonary resuscitation

Jerry P Nolan, consultant in anaesthesia and intensive care medicine[1],
Jasmeet Soar, consultant in anaesthesia and intensive care medicine[2],
Gavin D Perkins, professor of critical care medicine[3]

[1]Royal United Hospital NHS Trust, Bath BA1 3NG, UK

[2]Southmead Hospital, North Bristol NHS Trust, Bristol, UK

[3]University of Warwick, Warwick Medical School, Warwick, UK

Correspondence to: J P Nolan jerry.nolan@nhs.net

Cite this as: BMJ 2012;345:e6122

DOI: 10.1136/bmj.e6122

http://www.bmj.com/content/345/bmj.e6122

Cardiorespiratory arrest is the most extreme medical emergency—death or permanent brain injury will ensue unless cardiopulmonary resuscitation (CPR) is started within minutes. Four key interventions—known collectively as the chain of survival and comprising early recognition of cardiac arrest, high quality CPR, prompt defibrillation, and effective post-resuscitation care—improve outcomes.[w1] This review covers recent developments in CPR and the evidence supporting them.

What is the incidence and outcome of sudden cardiac arrest?

The global incidence of out of hospital cardiac arrest in adults treated by emergency medical services is 62 cases per 100 000 person years; 75-85% of these arrests have a primary cardiac cause.[1] The reported incidence of out of hospital cardiac arrest and its outcome vary considerably. In Europe, the estimated survival to hospital discharge for such cardiac arrests is 8%.[1] Evidence suggests that survival rates are increasing,[w2-w4] mainly because CPR is being attempted more often. The improvement is modest, however, because of the decreasing incidence of ventricular fibrillation and pulseless ventricular tachycardia (25-30% of out of hospital cardiac arrests), which have a better prognosis. A recent high quality observational study from the Netherlands has shown that implantable cardioverter defibrillators account for about a third of this decline.[2] The decline in these rhythms has also been attributed to increased use of β blockers.[w5]

Patients having an in hospital cardiac arrest often have multiple comorbidities and the cause of the cardiac arrest is often multifactorial (table 1). According to American registry data, about 200 000 cardiac arrests occur in hospital each year (67 cases per 100 000 person years), with 17.6% of patients surviving to hospital discharge.[3][4] A quarter of patients present with ventricular fibrillation or pulseless ventricular tachycardia. These patients have better survival to discharge (37.2%) than those with pulseless electrical activity or asystole (survival 11.3%). Early data

SOURCES AND SELECTION CRITERIA

The 2010 Consensus on Cardiopulmonary Resuscitation Science with Treatment recommendations published by the International Liaison Committee on Resuscitation summarised the findings from 277 systematic reviews based on PICO (population, intervention, comparison, outcome) format questions. We continuously screen the scientific literature for resuscitation studies and have supplemented our findings and the contents of the 2010 recommendations with PubMed searches to identify other relevant resuscitation studies published since 2010.

(unpublished) from the UK National Cardiac Arrest Audit show similar outcomes.[w6] Outcomes of in hospital cardiac arrest are probably better than those of out of hospital arrests because the arrests are witnessed and CPR and advanced life support are started promptly.

How are CPR guidelines developed?

Since the 1990s, the International Liaison Committee on Resuscitation has facilitated systematic reviews of CPR science. In 2005 and 2010, the committee published an International Consensus on CPR Science with Treatment Recommendations.[5][6] The 2010 recommendations involved experts from more than 30 countries who evaluated the findings from 277 systematic reviews based on PICO (population, intervention, comparison, outcome) format questions that had been undertaken over three years. The summary treatment recommendations that came from this rigorous process were used to formulate more detailed practical resuscitation guidelines globally.[7][8] It has not been possible to produce a single set of global guidelines because of regional variations driven by cultural and economic differences. Nevertheless, the guidelines are sufficiently similar to enable international application of the core interventions. The CPR science review and guideline cycle occurs every five years. The remainder of this review will cover key aspects of the 2010 CPR guidelines and will also highlight new research that may influence future guidelines.

Is cardiac arrest preventable?

The vital signs of patients about to have a cardiac arrest in hospital often deteriorate in the hours preceding the event. A meta-analysis concluded that rapid response systems (that incorporate "tracking" of vital signs and criteria for "triggering" a clinical response) reduce the incidence of cardiac arrests outside of the intensive care unit but do not reduce hospital mortality rates.[9][w7] This might be explained by an increase in the number of do not attempt CPR (DNACPR) decisions.

When should a do not attempt CPR (DNACPR) decision be considered?

CPR has undoubtedly saved many thousands of lives over the years. Successful CPR was first described in groups of patients considered to have "hearts too young to die."

SUMMARY POINTS

- About 8% of resuscitation attempts after out of hospital cardiac arrest result in survival to hospital discharge
- Give chest compressions to a depth of 5-6 cm at 100-120 per minute; fully release between each compression and minimise interruptions; untrained bystanders should use compression only cardiopulmonary resuscitation (CPR)
- CPR prompt and feedback devices improve the quality of CPR but have yet to be shown to improve survival
- Undertake defibrillation with minimal interruption in chest compressions
- The optimal method for managing the airway during cardiac arrest is unknown
- Mechanical CPR devices may have a role during transport and in the cardiac catheterisation laboratory
- Although adrenaline is recommended and used routinely, its effect on long term neurological outcome is unclear

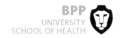

However cardiac arrest (cessation of heart beat) is also part of the natural dying process. Different countries' laws and ethics relating to resuscitation, end of life care, and advance decisions (living wills) vary greatly. In the United Kingdom, CPR may be withheld when clinical judgment concludes that CPR will not be able to restart the patient's heart and breathing and restore circulation; the benefits of CPR are agreed to be outweighed by the burdens and risks after careful discussion with the patient (or those close to the patient); a patient has an advanced decision (living will) or makes an informed decision to refuse CPR.[w8]

A recent National Confidential Enquiry into Patient Outcome and Death reviewed more than 700 in hospital cardiac arrests in the UK. The report found that most patients receiving CPR were elderly, frail, and had multiple comorbidities.[w9] Of the 230 cases for which assessors could form an opinion, they considered resuscitation on clinical grounds would be futile in 196 (85%). The report rightly calls for increased involvement of consultants in decisions on CPR among patients admitted to hospital. Better linkage with community DNACPR decisions is also needed.

How is cardiac arrest recognised?

People with cardiac arrest are unconscious, unresponsive, and not breathing or breathing abnormally—laypeople and healthcare professionals are taught to recognise these signs of cardiac arrest (fig 1). A short seizure or gasping (agonal breathing) is common immediately after cardiac arrest.[w10] Agonal breathing is a sign of cardiac arrest and should prompt initiation of CPR.[10] Palpating for a carotid pulse is an unreliable and time consuming method to detect cardiac arrest and should be attempted only by those who are experienced in clinical assessment. Electrocardiography or other advanced monitoring, if available, may confirm the diagnosis, but its absence should not delay treatment.

How is CPR started?

In adults, CPR is started with 30 chest compressions followed by two ventilations (see table 2 for summary of resuscitation interventions based on age). Continue to alternate chest compressions and ventilations (30:2) until a tracheal tube or a supraglottic airway device (see below) has been inserted, then continue ventilation at 10 breaths per minute while compressing the chest continually.

Animal data and evidence from observational clinical studies indicate that the quality of CPR strongly influences blood flow and outcome. The European Resuscitation Council currently recommends 100-120 chest compressions of 5-6 cm depth per minute ("push hard and fast"); pressure should be fully released between chest compressions and interruptions minimised.[11]

A recent observational clinical study found that the highest rates of return of spontaneous circulation were associated with chest compression rates of about 125 per minute[12]; however, other studies have shown that compression depth becomes too shallow at rates of more than 120 per minute.[13w11] On the basis of all the available data, the optimal compression rate is 120 per minute.[w12]

The proportion of time during which chest compressions are performed in each minute of CPR (the chest compression fraction) is independently associated with better survival after out of hospital cardiac arrest caused by ventricular fibrillation: in one observational study a chest compression fraction of 61-80% was associated with the highest survival rate.[14]

Does compression only cardiopulmonary resuscitation have a role?

Standard CPR, which includes mouth to mouth ventilation, is more difficult to learn and remember than chest compression only CPR,[w13] and it interrupts chest compressions.[w14]

At the onset of sudden (non-asphyxial) cardiac arrest, the patient's lungs and great vessels contain enough oxygen to supply the tissues for several minutes if an adequate amount of blood can be circulated. A meta-analysis of several observational studies reported similar survival rates in people who received bystander compression only CPR compared with those resuscitated with standard CPR.[15w15-w21] After introducing a programme of bystander compression only CPR throughout Arizona, lay rescuer CPR increased from 28% to 40% (P<0.001) and overall survival increased from 3.7% to 9.8% (P<0.001).[16] By contrast, the most recent and largest observational study showed that, compared with compression only CPR, standard CPR was associated with increased neurologically favourable survival at one month. This was particularly true for young people with a non-cardiac cause of cardiac arrest or if the start of CPR was delayed in witnessed cases of cardiac arrest of a non-cardiac cause.[17] Most (about 70%) out of hospital cardiac arrests in children have a non-cardiac cause, and, in a Japanese nationwide prospective observational study, outcome in children was better when laypeople performed standard CPR rather than compression only CPR.[18]

Reliable data support dispatcher assisted bystander CPR, which occurs when the dispatcher instructs the caller to perform CPR while awaiting arrival of the emergency medical services. A meta-analysis of three prospective randomised trials found a 22% increase in the rate of survival to hospital discharge when the dispatcher gave telephone instructions for compression only CPR instead of standard CPR.[15w22-w24]

The 2010 European Resuscitation Council (ERC) guidelines recommend teaching standard CPR to laypeople and healthcare providers, but compression only CPR is encouraged for those who are untrained or unable or unwilling to perform mouth to mouth ventilation.[11]

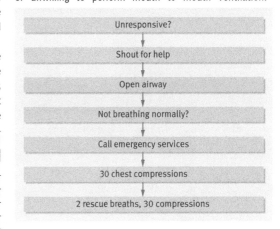

Fig 1 Adult basic life support algorithm; reproduced with permission from the Resuscitation Council (UK)

Table 1   Immediate factors (present within 1 hour) related to 51 919 in hospital cardiac arrests*

Factor	No (%)
Acute respiratory insufficiency	18 948 (37)
Hypotension	20 410 (39)
Acute myocardial infarction or ischaemia	4989 (10)
Metabolic or electrolyte disturbance	5240 (10)
Acute pulmonary oedema	991 (2)
Acute pulmonary embolism	978 (2)

Data from the United States National Registry of Cardiopulmonary Resuscitation.[4]

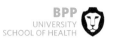
Compression only CPR is clearly better than no CPR, and this was the primary message in high profile media campaigns in the UK and the United States that target people untrained in CPR.[w25 w26]

Can the quality of CPR be improved?

The quality of CPR can be improved with the use of CPR prompt and feedback devices. These vary in sophistication—from simple metronomes that guide compression rate, to modified defibrillators that monitor compression depth and rate from an accelerometer placed on the chest and ventilation volume and rate by measuring changes in transthoracic impedance. Audio and visual feedback to rescuers are given in real time and data can be stored for later review during debriefing.[w27] A systematic review of prompt and feedback devices concluded that during training they improve the acquisition and retention of skills, and that they improve the quality of CPR in clinical practice, but there is no evidence that they improve patient outcomes.[19] A prospective cluster randomised study showed that real time visual and audible feedback resulted in CPR that more closely matched the guidelines, but patient outcomes were not affected.[20]

Mechanical chest compression devices deliver consistent high quality CPR, but meta-analyses have failed to show that they improve patient outcomes.[w28 w29] The two main devices are the load distributing band (ZOLL Medical Corporation), which comprises a backboard and a disposable chest band that is tightened and loosened 80 times a minute, and a mechanical compression-decompression device (Physio-Control), which incorporates a suction cup that is pushed up and down on the chest by a battery powered piston.

A large multicentre randomised study of the load distributing band (Circulation Improving Resuscitation Care (CIRC) trial) showed that it did not improve survival to hospital discharge compared with high quality manual CPR (presented by L Wik at the Resuscitation Science Symposium, Orlando, Florida, 12-13 Nov 2011). Two ongoing large randomised studies (LINC and PARAMEDIC trials) are evaluating the prehospital use of the mechanical compression-decompression device.

Although existing data do not support the routine use of mechanical devices, they are used in many parts of the world and may have a role in specific circumstances, such as during transport or when access to the patient is limited, such as CPR during percutaneous coronary intervention.[21]

What is the role of impedance threshold devices in CPR?

The impedance threshold device augments the negative intrathoracic pressure generated during the decompression phase of chest compression; this increases the return of venous blood, thereby increasing blood flow with the subsequent chest compression. Animal and human studies show that use of these devices improves haemodynamic values compared with standard CPR.[w30] The devices have a greater haemodynamic effect when used together with active compression-decompression CPR. In an unblinded randomised trial in out of hospital cardiac arrests, the impedance threshold device combined with active compression-decompression CPR improved survival to hospital discharge with good neurological function compared with conventional CPR.[w31] When compared with a sham valve during standard CPR, use of the impedance threshold device produced no benefit.[w32] Given these conflicting data and the cost of the single use valve, routine use of these devices is not recommended.

Are manual or automated defibrillators more effective?

Defibrillation using a manual defibrillator or an automated external defibrillator is the only effective treatment for ventricular fibrillation or pulseless ventricular tachycardia cardiac arrest. Current guidelines recommend an energy level of 150 J for the first shock, with subsequent shocks at the same or higher values (up to 360 J) depending on the specific defibrillator. Use of an automated defibrillator does not require specific training (the rescuer simply follows the audiovisual instructions when the device is switched on). Two high quality population based cohort studies show that use of these devices by bystanders doubles survival after out of hospital cardiac arrest.[w33 w34]

Despite one study showing that shocks from a defibrillator can be delivered without injury to a gloved rescuer who maintains contact with the patient's chest,[22] expert consensus and current guidelines recommend that manual chest compressions are interrupted to enable safe defibrillation.[w35] When chest compressions are paused the right ventricle dilates and encroaches on the left ventricle—this may prevent the myocardium from contracting effectively even if defibrillation restores coordinated electrical activity.[w36] One observational study of in hospital cardiac arrest found increased shock success with shorter pre-shock pauses (the interval between stopping compressions and shock delivery; adjusted odds ratio 1.86 for every five second decrease in pre-shock pause).[23] In an observational out of hospital cardiac arrest study, survival to hospital discharge decreased by 18% for every five second increase in pre-shock pause up to 40 seconds.[24] It should be possible to deliver a shock with a manual defibrillator with no more than a five second interruption to chest compression.[25] A strategy to do this safely includes the continuation of chest compressions while the defibrillator is charging, and this is now taught in advanced life support courses (fig 2).

Table 2 Summary of resuscitation interventions by patient age group

Intervention	Age group			
	Adults	Children (1 year to puberty)	Infants (<1 year)	Newborns
Compression: ventilation ratio (compressions at 100-120/min)	30:2	15:2	15:2	3:1
Starting with	Compressions first	5 breaths first	5 breaths first	5 breaths first
Chest compression landmark	Middle of lower half sternum	1 finger breadth above xiphisternum (lower third of chest)		Just below inter-nipple line (lower third of chest)
Compression depth	5-6 cm	At least 1/3 anteriorposterior diameter of chest (4 cm infants, 5 cm children)		
Defibrillation energy	According to manufacturer or maximum setting	4 J/kg	4 J/kg	4 J/kg
Adrenaline dose (intravenous or intraosseous)	1 mg	10 µg/kg	10 µg/kg	10 µg/kg
Amiodarone dose (intravenous or intraosseous)	300 mg	5 mg/kg	5 mg/kg	5 mg/kg

Adapted from Nolan and Soar.[w40]

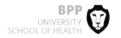

What is the best way to manage the airway during CPR?

The optimal method for managing the airway during CPR is unknown. Attempting to intubate the trachea can cause serious interruption to chest compressions —longer than one minute in 30% of cases in one high quality observational study of intubation by paramedics.[26] Attempted intubation has a high failure rate unless undertaken by highly experienced workers, and it may result in unrecognised oesophageal intubation.[w37] The routine use of waveform capnography (a monitor that displays exhaled carbon dioxide as a waveform and not just a numerical value or colour) reduces the incidence of unrecognised oesophageal intubation (pulmonary blood flow during CPR is usually sufficient to generate detectable exhaled carbon dioxide). It also provides an early indication of return of spontaneous circulation (sudden increase in end tidal carbon dioxide).[27] Some observational studies have documented an association between tracheal intubation and worse survival after out of hospital cardiac arrest.[w38] Supraglottic airway devices (such as the laryngeal mask airway, i-gel (airway device with a non-inflatable laryngeal cuff, integral bite block, and gastric drain tube, made by Intersurgical), and laryngeal tube) are increasingly being used for resuscitation. Although they are easier to insert, no prospective controlled trials are available to provide data on clinical outcomes compared with intubation. Two recent observational studies found

Table 3 Post-cardiac arrest care

Problem	Intervention	Rationale
Post-cardiac arrest brain injury, which is the cause of death in two thirds of patients with out of hospital cardiac arrest and in a quarter of those with in hospital cardiac arrest admitted to the intensive care unit[w51]	Controlled reoxygenation aimed at 94-98% oxygen saturation of arterial blood	Animal studies show worse neurological outcome with hyperoxaemia during the first hour after return of spontaneous circulation.[w52] Two adult observational studies based on the same dataset and a paediatric observational study show worse outcomes associated with hyperoxaemia.[w53- w55] However, another observational study in adults failed to show an association between hyperoxaemia and death once severity of illness had been included in the analysis[w56]
	In patients who need mechanical ventilation, control arterial carbon dioxide—aim for a normal value	Hypocapnia is harmful to the injured brain because of cerebral vasoconstriction and decreased cerebral blood flow.[w57] The resultant cerebrospinal fluid alkalosis is neurotoxic because of increased release of excitatory amino acids
	Blood glucose control—aim for blood glucose concentration of 4-10 mmol/L*	Both hypoglycaemia and hyperglycaemia are associated with worse outcome.[w58-w60] Therapeutic hypothermia increases insulin requirements and blood glucose variability[w61]
	Control seizures—treat with benzodiazepines, phenytoin, sodium valproate, propofol, or a barbiturate; clonazepam may be the most effective treatment for myoclonus[w62]	Seizures occur in about a quarter of comatose patients after return of spontaneous circulation and increase mortality fourfold, but 17% of those developing seizures can still achieve a good neurological outcome.[w63] In a sedated mechanically ventilated patient who is receiving neuromuscular drugs, electroencephalographic monitoring is needed to recognise seizure activity
	Targeted temperature management (therapeutic hypothermia)—cool patients to 32-34°C, maintain for 24 hours, and rewarm at 0.25°C/h	Animal data indicate that hyperthermia worsens outcome.[w64] Two randomised controlled trials also showed better neurological outcome in comatose patients who had experienced out of hospital ventricular fibrillation cardiac arrest and were cooled to 32-34°C for 12-24 hours.[w65 w66] Observational data indicate that mild hypothermia may also improve neurological outcome after non-ventricular fibrillation or pulseless ventricular tachycardia cardiac arrest[w67]
	Optimise sedation with short acting drugs (such as propofol, alfentanil, remifentanil)	Sedation helps facilitate cooling during treatment with therapeutic hypothermia. Short acting drugs enable earlier neurological assessment. Sedation reduces oxygen consumption and helps prevent shivering.[w68] Hypothermia reduces clearance of many drugs by at least a third.[w69] Ensure that drugs have been cleared before considering withdrawal in a comatose patient[w70]
	Control shivering with adequate sedation, bolus doses of a neuromuscular blocker, and magnesium[w62]	Shivering will increase oxygen consumption and reduce cooling rate[w71]
Post-cardiac arrest myocardial dysfunction; this problem is common and usually resolves after 72 hours[w72]	Fluid resuscitation	This can be guided by blood pressure, heart rate, urine output, and rate of plasma lactate clearance, central venous oxygen saturation or cardiac output monitoring[w62]
	Inotropes and vasopressors	
	Mechanical circulatory support	An intra-aortic balloon pump or extracorporeal support may be needed in those with severe cardiogenic shock[w73]
Ischaemia-reperfusion injury	Supportive treatments in the intensive care unit	Ischaemia-reperfusion may be associated with a marked systemic inflammatory response[w74]
Persistent precipitating pathology	Coronary reperfusion after myocardial infarction	Consider urgent coronary angiography and percutaneous coronary intervention in all those with a primary out of hospital cardiac arrest, especially, but not exclusively, if the 12 lead electrocardiograph shows ST elevation myocardial infarction[w75]
Prognostication	Identify comatose patients who have no chance of a neurological recovery	It is not in the patient's best interests to continue active treatment after resuscitation if the patient is comatose and there is no chance of a good neurological outcome. Use of therapeutic hypothermia (along with the additional sedation usually needed) makes existing guidelines[w76] on prognostication unreliable.[w77] [w78] Outcome is most reliably predicted by clinical examination 3 days after return to normothermia combined, if possible, with electrophysiological testing[w79]

*1 mmol/L=18 mg/dL.

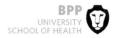

worse survival rates with the use of such devices than with tracheal intubation during resuscitation after out of hospital cardiac arrest.[28] [29] Until data from prospective controlled trials are available, European Resuscitation Council consensus guidelines recommend that tracheal intubation is attempted only by highly skilled people and that other rescuers manage the airway with a facemask or a supraglottic airway device.

What is the role of adrenaline during resuscitation?

When injected during cardiac arrest, adrenaline (epinephrine) increases aortic relaxation (diastolic) pressure and, in animal studies, thereby augments coronary and cerebral blood flow. Two randomised controlled trials evaluated the use of 1 mg doses of adrenaline in out of hospital cardiac arrest.[30] [31] The first trial randomised patients to intravenous

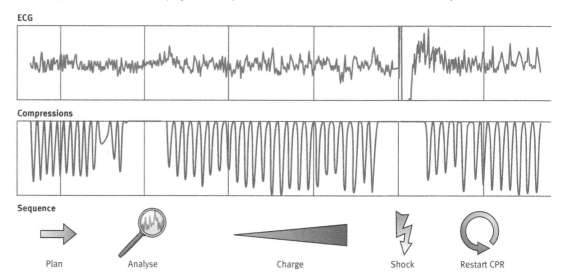

ECG

Compressions

Sequence

Plan   Analyse   Charge   Shock   Restart CPR

Fig 2 Defibrillation sequence: plan; pause chest compressions briefly; check rhythm, and confirm shockable rhythm (ventricular fibrillation or pulseless ventricular tachycardia). Restart chest compressions. Charge defibrillator while chest compressions are ongoing; once defibrillator is charged stop chest compressions; give shock—no one should touch the patient during shock delivery; resume chest compressions immediately after shock delivery. CPR=cardiopulmonary resuscitation; ECG=electrocardiograph

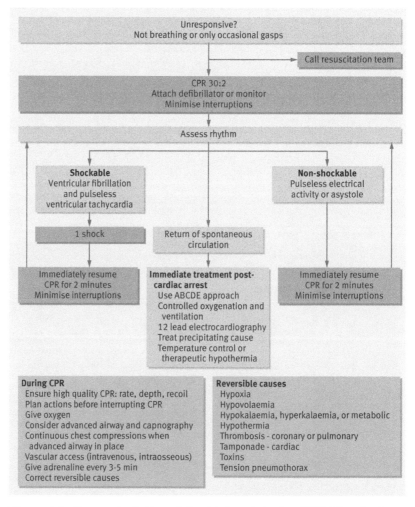

Fig 3 Advanced life support algorithm; reproduced with permission of the Resuscitation Council (UK). CPR=cardiopulmonary resuscitation

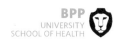

QUESTIONS FOR FUTURE RESEARCH

Key research studies currently recruiting

- Continuous chest compressions (CCC; ClinicalTrials.gov NCT01372748)
- Randomised comparison of the effectiveness of the Laryngeal Mask Airway Supreme, i-gel, and current practice in the initial airway management of prehospital cardiac arrest: a feasibility study (REVIVE-Airways; ISRCTN18528625)
- Comparison of conventional adult out of hospital cardiopulmonary resuscitation against a concept with mechanical chest compressions and simultaneous defibrillation—LINC study (ClinicalTrials.gov NCT00609778)
- Prehospital randomised assessment of a mechanical compression device in cardiac arrest (PaRAMeDIC; ISRCTN08233942) www.warwick.ac.uk/go/paramedic
- Amiodarone, lidocaine, or neither for out of hospital cardiac arrest caused by ventricular fibrillation or tachycardia (ALPS; ClinicalTrial.gov NCT01401647)
- Therapeutic hypothermia to improve survival after cardiac arrest in paediatric patients—THAPCA-OH (out of hospital) trial (ClinicalTrials.gov NCT00878644)
- Therapeutic hypothermia to improve survival after cardiac arrest in paediatric patients—THAPCA-IH (in hospital) trial (ClinicalTrials.gov NCT00880087)
- Target temperature management after cardiac arrest (TTM; ClinicalTrials.gov NCT01020916)
- Prehospital resuscitation intranasal cooling effectiveness survival study (PRINCESS; ClinicalTrials.gov NCT01400373)

OTHER AREAS FOR FUTURE RESEARCH

- What are the optimal methods for acquisition and retention of cardiopulmonary resuscitation skills?
- Does the use of adrenaline in cardiac arrest improve long term neurological outcome? The definitive answer will come only with a large placebo controlled randomised trial
- After the return of spontaneous circulation, does the use of controlled reoxygenation (targeting a specific arterial blood oxygen saturation) improve neurological outcome?

TIPS FOR NON-SPECIALISTS

If someone collapses, is unconscious, unresponsive, and not breathing (or taking occasional gasps)*:

- 1 Call for help—ensure that an ambulance is coming, and if available an automated external defibrillator
- 2 Start chest compressions—push hard (5-6 cm in an adult) and fast (100-120 times per minute)
- 3 If you are trained, willing, and able to do so, give two ventilations after every 30 compressions
- 4 Do not stop unless the person shows signs of regaining consciousness—such as coughing, opening of the eyes, speaking, or moving purposefully—and starts to breathe normally
- 5. If an automated external defibrillator is available switch on and follow the audiovisual prompts

Do not check for a pulse because this sign is unreliable for confirming cardiac arrest

ADDITIONAL EDUCATIONAL RESOURCES

Resources for healthcare professionals

- Resuscitation Council (UK) (www.resus.org.uk)—Information on courses, guidelines, and conferences
- National Cardiac Arrest Audit (https://ncaa.icnarc.org)—Information about the audit, including instructions on how to enrol a hospital in the scheme
- International Liaison Committee on Resuscitation (www.ilcor.org)—Provides access to the International Consensus on Cardiopulmonary Resuscitation (CPR) Science
- European Resuscitation Council (ERC) (www.erc.edu)—Information on CPR courses and training opportunities in Europe; includes access to the full ERC guidelines
- American Heart Association CPR and Emergency Cardiovascular Care (http://www.heart.org/HEARTORG/CPRAndECC/CPR_UCM_001118_SubHomePage.jsp)—Information for healthcare professionals and lay people on all aspects of CPR

Resources for patients

- British Heart Foundation (www.bhf.org.uk/heart-health/life-saving-skills/hands-only-cpr.aspx)—Information on a hands only CPR campaign
- Citizen CPR Foundation (www.citizencpr.org/)—Information for lay people interested in CPR
- American Heart Association (http://handsonlycpr.org)—Information on a hands only CPR campaign
- Resuscitation Council (UK) (www.resus.org.uk/pages/pub_AED.htm)—CPR training material
- Resuscitation Council (UK) (www.youtube.com/user/ResusCouncilUK)—Link to public information videos on CPR

cannulation with injection of drugs (including adrenaline) versus neither until return of spontaneous circulation.[30] The other study compared adrenaline with placebo.[31] Both studies found increased rates of return of spontaneous circulation with adrenaline but no difference in survival to hospital discharge. Post hoc analysis of one of these trials showed that patients who received adrenaline had better short term outcomes but an overall decrease in survival to discharge (odds ratio 0.52, 95% confidence interval 0.29 to 0.92; P=0.024) and worse neurological outcomes.[w39] In an observational study of 417 188 out of hospital cardiac arrests in Japan, after adjustment for potential confounders, use of adrenaline was associated with a return of spontaneous circulation rate 2.5 times higher but a one month survival rate roughly half of that in those not given adrenaline.[32] Similar findings have been seen in North American and Swedish registry data.[w40 w41] Animal data indicate that, although adrenaline improves global cerebral blood flow during CPR, flow in the microcirculation is reduced.[w42] This might account for the failure of adrenaline to convert the higher return of spontaneous circulation rates into better long term survival. The uncertainty should be resolved through a large randomised placebo controlled trial. Until such a trial is completed, current guidelines recommend that adrenaline is given every three to five minutes during cardiac arrest (adults 1 mg; children 10 µg/kg; fig 3).

Does echocardiography have a role during CPR?

Focused echocardiography used during the brief pause for a rhythm check may enable identification of potentially reversible causes of cardiac arrest: pericardial tamponade, pulmonary embolism, and hypovolaemia.[w43] A prospective observational study found that the finding of pseudo-pulseless electrical activity (cardiac wall motion seen on echocardiography in a pulseless patient) alters management and is associated with increased survival.[w44]

What happens after successful CPR?

Once return of spontaneous circulation is achieved, unless the duration of cardiac arrest has been very short, patients will be comatose for variable periods and most will develop the post-cardiac arrest syndrome, which comprises post-cardiac arrest brain injury, post-cardiac arrest myocardial dysfunction, the systemic ischaemia-reperfusion response, and any persistent precipitating pathology.[33w45] Coronary artery disease is the most common cause of out of hospital cardiac arrest, and many of these patients will require urgent coronary angiography and percutaneous coronary intervention.[34] The increasing use of urgent percutaneous coronary intervention in this situation is driving the treatment of these patients in regional cardiac arrest centres.[35] Table 3 describes interventions to optimise outcome.

A systematic review of nine prospective studies, three follow-up of untreated control groups in randomised controlled trials, 11 retrospective cohort studies, and 47 cases series concluded that the quality of life in survivors who leave hospital is generally good, although they may have psychological and cognitive problems.[36] The wide range in the type and timing of the neurological assessments used in the studies make it impossible to provide specific summary data. It is generally accepted that long term assessments should not be made until at least six months, and preferably one year, after cardiac arrest. Studies documenting these long term neurological

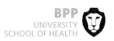

outcomes generally report that more than 85% of patients have a "good" outcome defined by a cerebral performance category of 1 or 2 (online appendix).[w46 w47] Category 2 is described broadly as "disabled but independent" and includes patients with hemiplegia, seizures, and permanent memory changes. This system provides only a crude measurement of neurological outcome; studies that use much more sensitive tests of memory and cognition generally show subtle cognitive deficits in most survivors of cardiac arrest.[w48 w49]

How should we teach CPR?

The ability to recognise cardiac arrest and deliver CPR is an essential skill for all healthcare professionals. Knowledge and skills in this area can deteriorate within three to six months after training. Frequent assessments and, when needed, refresher training, are recommended to maintain knowledge and skills. Properly validated short video and online self instruction courses with hands on practice are an effective alternative to instructor led basic life support skills.[w50] A large randomised controlled trial showed that the costs of training can be reduced if courses that combine e-learning and face to face training are used.[37]

Contributors: All authors helped plan and write this review. JPN is guarantor.

Competing interests: All authors have completed the ICMJE uniform disclosure form at www.icmje.org/coi_disclosure.pdf (available on request from the corresponding author) and declare: no support from any organisation for the submitted work; no financial relationships with any organisations that might have an interest in the submitted work in the previous three years; JPN is editor in chief of *Resuscitation* (honorarium received), a board member of the European Resuscitation Council (unpaid), and a member of the executive committee of the Resuscitation Committee (UK) (unpaid), and the immediate past co-chair of the International Liaison Committee on Resuscitation (unpaid); JS is vice chair of the Resuscitation Council (UK) (unpaid), chair of the advanced life support working group of the European Resuscitation Council (unpaid), co-chair of the advanced life support task force of the International Liaison Committee on Resuscitation (unpaid), and an editor of *Resuscitation* (honorarium received); GDP is chair of the Resuscitation Council (UK) advanced life support committee (unpaid), chair of the basic life support and automated external defibrillation working group of the European Resuscitation Council (unpaid), co-chair of the basic life support and automated external defibrillation task force of the International Liaison Committee on Resuscitation (unpaid), and an editor of *Resuscitation* (honorarium received); GDP holds research funding from the National Institute for Health Research to investigate mechanical chest compression and CPR feedback and prompt devices. All authors have been involved in local, national, and international resuscitation guideline development processes and in producing learning materials.

Provenance and peer review: Commissioned; externally peer reviewed.

1   Berdowski J, Berg RA, Tijssen JG, Koster RW. Global incidences of out-of-hospital cardiac arrest and survival rates: systematic review of 67 prospective studies. *Resuscitation* 2010;81:1479-87.
2   Hulleman M, Berdowski J, de Groot JR, van Dessel PF, Borleffs CJ, Blom MT, et al. Implantable cardioverter-defibrillators have reduced the incidence of resuscitation for out-of-hospital cardiac arrest caused by lethal arrhythmias. *Circulation* 2012;126:815-21.
3   Merchant RM, Yang L, Becker LB, Berg RA, Nadkarni V, Nichol G, et al. Incidence of treated cardiac arrest in hospitalized patients in the United States. *Crit Care Med* 2011;39:2401-6.
4   Meaney PA, Nadkarni VM, Kern KB, Indik JH, Halperin HR, Berg RA. Rhythms and outcomes of adult in-hospital cardiac arrest. *Crit Care Med* 2010;38:101-8.
5   Nolan JP, Hazinski MF, Billi JE, Böttiger BW, Bossaert L, de Caen AR, et al. 2010 international consensus on cardiopulmonary resuscitation and emergency cardiovascular care science with treatment recommendations. Part 1: Executive summary. *Resuscitation* 2010;81:e1-25.
6   Nolan JP, Nadkarni VM, Billi JE, Bossaert L, Boettiger BW, Chamberlain D, et al. Part 2: International collaboration in resuscitation science: 2010 International consensus on cardiopulmonary resuscitation and emergency cardiovascular care science with treatment recommendations. *Resuscitation* 2010;81(suppl 1):e26-31.
7   Nolan JP, Soar J, Zideman DA, Biarent D, Bossaert LL, Deakin C, et al. European Resuscitation Council guidelines for resuscitation 2010 section 1. Executive summary. *Resuscitation* 2010;81:1219-76.
8   Field JM, Hazinski MF, Sayre MR, Chameides L, Schexnayder SM, Hemphill R, et al. Part 1: executive summary: 2010 American Heart Association guidelines for cardiopulmonary resuscitation and emergency cardiovascular care. *Circulation* 2010;122:S640-56.
9   Jones DA, DeVita MA, Bellomo R. Rapid-response teams. *N Engl J Med* 2011;365:139-46.
10   Perkins GD, Walker G, Christensen K, Hulme J, Monsieurs KG. Teaching recognition of agonal breathing improves accuracy of diagnosing cardiac arrest. *Resuscitation* 2006;70:432-7.
11   Koster RW, Baubin MA, Bossaert LL, Caballero A, Cassan P, Castren M, et al. European Resuscitation Council guidelines for resuscitation 2010 section 2. Adult basic life support and use of automated external defibrillators. *Resuscitation* 2010;81:1277-92.
12   Idris AH, Guffey D, Aufderheide TP, Brown S, Morrison LJ, Nichols P, et al. Relationship between chest compression rates and outcomes from cardiac arrest. *Circulation* 2012;125:3004-12.
13   Stiell IG, Brown SP, Christenson J, Cheskes S, Nichol G, Powell J, et al. What is the role of chest compression depth during out-of-hospital cardiac arrest resuscitation? *Crit Care Med* 2012;40:1192-8.
14   Christenson J, Andrusiek D, Everson-Stewart S, Kudenchuk P, Hostler D, Powell J, et al. Chest compression fraction determines survival in patients with out-of-hospital ventricular fibrillation. *Circulation* 2009;120:1241-7.
15   Hupfl M, Selig HF, Nagele P. Chest-compression-only versus standard cardiopulmonary resuscitation: a meta-analysis. *Lancet* 2010;376:1552-7.
16   Bobrow BJ, Spaite DW, Berg RA, Stolz U, Sanders AB, Kern KB, et al. Chest compression-only CPR by lay rescuers and survival from out-of-hospital cardiac arrest. *JAMA* 2010;304:1447-54.
17   Ogawa T, Akahane M, Koike S, Tanabe S, Mizoguchi T, Imamura T. Outcomes of chest compression only CPR versus conventional CPR conducted by lay people in patients with out of hospital cardiopulmonary arrest witnessed by bystanders: nationwide population based observational study. *BMJ* 2011;342:c7106.
18   Kitamura T, Iwami T, Kawamura T, Nagao K, Tanaka H, Nadkarni VM, et al. Conventional and chest-compression-only cardiopulmonary resuscitation by bystanders for children who have out-of-hospital cardiac arrests: a prospective, nationwide, population-based cohort study. *Lancet* 2010;375:1347-54.
19   Yeung J, Meeks R, Edelson D, Gao F, Soar J, Perkins GD. The use of CPR feedback/prompt devices during training and CPR performance: a systematic review. *Resuscitation* 2009;80:743-51.
20   Hostler D, Everson-Stewart S, Rea TD, Stiell IG, Callaway CW, Kudenchuk PJ, et al. Effect of real-time feedback during cardiopulmonary resuscitation outside hospital: prospective, cluster-randomised trial. *BMJ* 2011;342:d512.
21   Perkins GD, Brace S, Gates S. Mechanical chest-compression devices: current and future roles. *Curr Opin Crit Care* 2010;16:203-10.
22   Lloyd MS, Heeke B, Walter PF, Langberg JJ. Hands-on defibrillation: an analysis of electrical current flow through rescuers in direct contact with patients during biphasic external defibrillation. *Circulation* 2008;117:2510-4.
23   Edelson DP, Abella BS, Kramer-Johansen J, Wik L, Myklebust H, Barry AM, et al. Effects of compression depth and pre-shock pauses predict defibrillation failure during cardiac arrest. *Resuscitation* 2006;71:137-45.
24   Cheskes S, Schmicker RH, Christenson J, Salcido DD, Rea T, Powell J, et al. Perishock pause: an independent predictor of survival from out-of-hospital shockable cardiac arrest. *Circulation* 2011;124:58-66.
25   Deakin CD, Nolan JP, Sunde K, Koster RW. European Resuscitation Council guidelines for resuscitation 2010 section 3. Electrical therapies: automated external defibrillators, defibrillation, cardioversion and pacing. *Resuscitation* 2010;81:1293-304.
26   Wang HE, Simeone SJ, Weaver MD, Callaway CW. Interruptions in cardiopulmonary resuscitation from paramedic endotracheal intubation. *Ann Emerg Med* 2009;54:645-52 e1.
27   Heradstveit BE, Sunde K, Sunde GA, Wentzel-Larsen T, Heltne JK. Factors complicating interpretation of capnography during advanced life support in cardiac arrest—a clinical retrospective study in 575 patients. *Resuscitation* 2012;83:813-8.
28   Wang HE, Szydlo D, Stouffer J, Lin S, Carlson J, Vaillancourt C, et al. Endotracheal intubation versus supraglottic airway insertion in out-of-hospital cardiac arrest. *Resuscitation* 2012;83:1061-6.
29   Tanabe S, Ogawa T, Akahane M, Koike S, Horiguchi H, Yasunaga H, et al. Comparison of neurological outcome between tracheal intubation and supraglottic airway device insertion of out-of-hospital cardiac arrest patients: a nationwide, population-based, observational study. *J Emerg Med* 2012; published online 26 April.
30   Olasveengen TM, Sunde K, Brunborg C, Thowsen J, Steen PA, Wik L. Intravenous drug administration during out-of-hospital cardiac arrest: a randomized trial. *JAMA* 2009;302:2222-9.
31   Jacobs IG, Finn JC, Jelinek GA, Oxer HF, Thompson PL. Effect of adrenaline on survival in out-of-hospital cardiac arrest: a randomised double-blind placebo-controlled trial. *Resuscitation* 2011;82:1138-43.
32   Hagihara A, Hasegawa M, Abe T, Nagata T, Wakata Y, Miyazaki S. Prehospital epinephrine use and survival among patients with out-of-hospital cardiac arrest. *JAMA* 2012;307:1161-8.

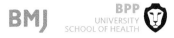

33 Nolan JP, Neumar RW, Adrie C, Aibiki M, Berg RA, Bottiger BW, et al. Post-cardiac arrest syndrome: epidemiology, pathophysiology, treatment, and prognostication. A scientific statement from the International Liaison Committee on Resuscitation; the American Heart Association Emergency Cardiovascular Care Committee; the Council on Cardiovascular Surgery and Anesthesia; the Council on Cardiopulmonary, Perioperative, and Critical Care; the Council on Clinical Cardiology; the Council on Stroke. *Resuscitation* 2008;79:350-79.

34 Dumas F, Cariou A, Manzo-Silberman S, Grimaldi D, Vivien B, Rosencher J, et al. Immediate percutaneous coronary intervention is associated with better survival after out-of-hospital cardiac arrest: insights from the PROCAT (Parisian Region Out of hospital Cardiac ArresT) registry. *Circ Cardiovasc Interv* 2010;3:200-7.

35 Nichol G, Aufderheide TP, Eigel B, Neumar RW, Lurie KG, Bufalino VJ, et al. Regional systems of care for out-of-hospital cardiac arrest: a policy statement from the American Heart Association. *Circulation* 2010;121:709-29.

36 Elliott VJ, Rodgers DL, Brett SJ. Systematic review of quality of life and other patient-centred outcomes after cardiac arrest survival. *Resuscitation* 2011;82:247-56.

37 Perkins GD, Kimani PK, Bullock I, Clutton-Brock T, Davies RP, Gale M, et al. Improving the efficiency of advanced life support training: a randomized, controlled trial. *Ann Intern Med* 2012;157:19-28.

Related links

bmj.com
- Cardiology updates from BMJ Group
- Get Cleveland Clinic CME points for this articlebmj.com/archive
- Weight faltering and failure to thrive in infancy and early childhood (2012;345:e5931)
- Preimplantation genetic testing (2012;345:e5908)
- Early fluid resuscitation in severe trauma (2012;345:e5752)
- Irritable bowel syndrome (2012;345:e5836)
- Management of renal colic (2012;345:e5499)
- Facial basal cell carcinoma (2012;345:e5342)

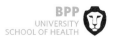

Prehospital management of severe traumatic brain injury

Clare L Hammell, specialist registrar anaesthesia and intensive care medicine[1] [3],
J D Henning, consultant anaesthesia and intensive care[2] [3]

[1]Royal Liverpool University Hospital, Liverpool L7 8XP

[2]James Cook University Hospital, Middlesbrough TS4 3BW

[3]Great North Air Ambulance Service, Darlington DL1 5NQ

Correspondence to: C Hammell cham37uk@yahoo.com

Cite this as: BMJ 2009;338:b1683

DOI: 10.1136/bmj.b1683

http://www.bmj.com/content/338/bmj.b1683

Traumatic brain injury is a substantial cause of morbidity and mortality in the UK. An estimated 11 000 people per year sustain a severe traumatic brain injury, mostly between ages 15 and 29 years.[1] Patients with severe traumatic brain injury have a high mortality rate (30-50%) and many survivors will have persistent severe neurological disability.[2] Prompt identification and appropriate early management of traumatic brain injury is essential to optimise outcome, however, few guidelines are available for clinicians on management in the challenging prehospital environment. The 2007 report by the national enquiry into patient outcome and death on the provision of trauma services in the UK[3] highlighted concerns about prehospital management of airways and ventilation in 15% of patients with severe head injuries. Doctors from various hospital specialties or general practice may be involved in providing prehospital care, so this review aims to provide a generic overview of available evidence on management of severe traumatic brain injury in adults in this environment.

What is the pathophysiology of severe traumatic brain injury?

Severe traumatic brain injury is defined as a head injury resulting in a Glasgow coma score of less than 9.[4] Primary brain injuries that can occur at the time of impact include extradural and subdural haematomata, intracerebral contusions, and diffuse axonal injuries. Additional insults such as hypoxaemia, hypotension, or hyperpyrexia result in further cerebral damage and secondary brain injury. Modern management of head injuries focus on the identification and treatment of such potential secondary insults.

SOURCES AND SELECTION CRITERIA

We searched Medline 1980-2008, Pubmed and the Cochrane library for clinical trials and reviews. The medical subject headings "head injury", "brain injury", "trauma", "prehospital", and combinations thereof were used. Individual therapeutic options (such as "mannitol") were also searched for. Search results were individually reviewed and manually cross referenced. Reference lists were searched for additional works. Priority was given to review articles, meta analyses, and well designed large trials. The websites www.braintraumafoundation.org, www.trauma.org, and www.east.org were also searched for additional information.

SUMMARY POINTS

- Management of severe traumatic brain injury is focused on rapid transfer to secondary care while preventing secondary brain injury
- Airway compromise and inadequate ventilation are common and should be addressed immediately
- Prehospital endotracheal intubation should be undertaken with the assistance of anaesthetic drugs by appropriately trained physicians
- Hypotension is an independent risk factor for mortality; small boluses of isotonic crystalloid fluids should be given if it occurs
- Patients may be best managed in a neurosurgical centre where they should receive definitive neurosurgical treatment within 4 hours of injury
- There is no role for the routine use of corticosteroids in patients with head injury

What are the priorities in prehospital management of severe traumatic brain injury?

Time from injury to definitive neurosurgical care can affect outcome for patients with severe traumatic brain injury. Patients with mass lesions have a better outcome if they receive neurosurgical treatment within four hours of injury.[5] Rapid patient transfer to an appropriate secondary care facility is essential, in addition to the implementation of measures to prevent secondary brain injury. Epidemiological studies show that a third of patients with severe traumatic brain injury already have a documented secondary brain insult on hospital admission.[w1] Prehospital management of these patients focuses on provision of an adequate airway, effective oxygenation and ventilation, maintenance of an adequate cerebral perfusion pressure and avoidance of further increases in intracranial pressure. Two retrospective reviews found improved outcomes in patients with severe head injuries when these parameters were specifically targeted in the prehospital setting.[w2] [w3] Box 1 lists problems that may be encountered during extrication of the patient from a vehicle (figure).

What are the options for airway management?

Airway compromise is common after severe traumatic brain injury and has an important contribution to the development of secondary brain injury. Basic airway adjuncts are used initially and high flow oxygen is administered. Controlled trials of simulated prehospital scenarios[6] have shown that laryngeal mask airways have a greater success rate for establishing an airway than endotracheal intubation, particularly with inexperienced clinicians. Laryngeal mask airways are becoming increasingly popular in prehospital care for airway maintenance, particularly in situations where access to the patient is limited. The devices are easy to insert, usually provide a good seal within the oropharynx, and provide airway protection from upper airway secretions. Regurgitation and aspiration of gastric contents remains a risk, but may be reduced with the use of alternative laryngeal masks such as LMA Pro-Seal.

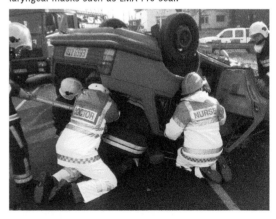

Scene from a road traffic collision demonstrating multiple difficulties encountered during extrication

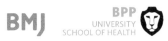
Endotracheal intubation is inevitably required in almost all patients with severe traumatic brain injury, although evidence for its benefit in the prehospital environment is controversial. Most studies are retrospective and study paramedics performing endotracheal intubation with minimal use of sedative agents and muscle relaxants. Several large retrospective reviews have, however, shown that this approach results in a high risk of complications, such as failed intubation and hypoxaemia.[7][8] Laryngoscopy without the use of anaesthetic agents is particularly damaging in patients with traumatic brain injury because increases in intracranial pressure are not attenuated; this may explain the association between prehospital endotracheal intubation and increased mortality and poor neurological outcome in patients with severe traumatic brain injury, which was reported in two retrospective analyses of trauma registries.[9][10]

Data about true rapid sequence induction of anaesthesia performed by physicians are more promising. A recent retrospective analysis of prehospital rapid sequence induction procedures in the UK reported low incidences of complications,[11] and similar studies have reported intubation success rates of 94-97%, in addition to low complication rates for prehospital drug assisted intubation.[w4] These data suggest that prehospital rapid sequence induction is beneficial if done by an appropriately trained physician; this finding is in line with recommendations from the recent trauma report from the national enquiry into patient outcome and death (box 2). With few doctors present at the scene of emergency situations, only a few patients with severe traumatic brain injury are intubated before hospital transfer in the UK, although at least half of all these patients need intubation within 30 minutes of arrival at the hospital.[3] A few patients, for example, those with severe facial trauma, may however require a primary surgical airway.

Which anaesthetic agents should be used to facilitate intubation?

Administering anaesthetic and neuromuscular blocking drugs to facilitate intubation leads to improved outcomes in patients with head injuries.[12] Ideal agents should have minimal effects on heart rate and blood pressure and reduce intracranial pressure while maintaining cerebral perfusion. Etomidate results in a low incidence of hypotension when used to facilitate intubation in patients with head injury and is perhaps the most widely used drug despite concerns

about inhibition of steroid synthesis after a single dose.[13][w5] Ketamine has usually been avoided in patients with head injuries, but a review of randomised clinical trials concluded that with controlled normocapnic ventilation, ketamine has minimal or favourable effects on intracranial pressure in sedated patients with head injury.[14] Ketamine has also been associated with maintenance of better cerebral perfusion pressure compared with other sedative agents.[w6] After intubation, adequate sedation and neuromuscular blockade must be provided for all patients during transfer to avoid rises in intracranial pressure associated with coughing.

How should patients with severe traumatic brain injury be ventilated?

Hypoxaemia is common after severe traumatic brain injury and prospective studies show an association with increased mortality rate and poorer neurological outcome.[w7] Hypoxaemia is usually multifactorial in patients with such injury and the presence of serious chest injuries—for example, haemopneumothorax or pulmonary contusions—needs to be considered. Hypercapnia is a common consequence of respiratory depression leading to cerebral vasodilatation, increased cerebral blood flow, and a rise in intracranial pressure. One argument in favour of performing rapid sequence induction before transfer to hospital is that this approach allows carbon dioxide levels to be controlled. Hyperventilation leads to cerebral vasoconstriction and ischaemia and should be avoided in patients with head injuries. A large retrospective review reported that 18% of head injured patients were hypocapnic after prehospital intubation with a worse outcome in the group that had a $PaCO_2$ of less than 4 KPa on admission to the emergency department.[15] A well conducted prospective randomised study showed that monitoring end-tidal carbon dioxide reduced the incidence of hyperventilation by more than 50%.[16] End tidal monitoring of carbon dioxide is now considered a routine standard of monitoring for all mechanically ventilated patients during transfer.[17] Box 3 describes additional monitoring standards.

How should circulatory complications be managed?

Patients with severe traumatic brain injury who are hypotensive have a doubled risk of mortality compared with normotensive patients.[3] Hypotension results in reduced cerebral perfusion and neuronal ischaemia and is often multifactorial in origin in trauma patients. It is best to assume that hypotension is due to hypovolaemia until proven otherwise. Cerebral perfusion pressure (CPP) is calculated by subtracting intracranial pressure from the mean arterial pressure. Maintaining a CPP of 60-70 mm Hg is an essential foundation of hospital management of severe traumatic brain injury. However, measuring an accurate mean arterial pressure is difficult in the prehospital environment so most guidelines use the systolic value as a target during the resuscitation phase.

The Brain Trauma Foundation recommends a minimum systolic pressure of 90 mm Hg in adults with severe head injuries.[4] This target is based on prospectively collected large datasets showing that a systolic blood pressure of less than 90 mm Hg is an independent risk factor for mortality after severe traumatic brain injury.[19] No studies have been done to assess the effects of aiming for values higher than 90 mm Hg, although this approach is probably desirable in patients with isolated severe traumatic brain injury. In patients with multiple injuries and hypovolaemia a conflict exists

---

BOX 1 PROBLEMS ENCOUNTERED DURING EXTRICATION FROM A VEHICLE

- Multiple hazards in and around the vehicle
- Difficulty with patient assessment due to noise level
- Physical entrapment of patient
- Limited access for interventions
- Poor communication between various agencies involved
- Time pressure

BOX 2 INDICATIONS FOR PREHOSPITAL RAPID SEQUENCE INDUCTION OF ANAESTHESIA (GREAT NORTH AIR AMBULANCE STANDARD OPERATING PROTOCOL)

- Airway problems that cannot reliably be managed by simple manoeuvres, such as severe facial injury
- Respiratory insufficiency (SpO2 <92%) despite 15 l/min oxygen or impending respiratory collapse due to exhaustion or pathology
- Glasgow coma scale <9 or rapidly falling
- Patients at risk of respiratory deterioration when access is difficult during transfer to definitive care (for example, those with facial burns)
- Patients needing sedation before transfer to hospital because they present a danger to themselves or attending staff, or for humanitarian reasons (for example, to provide complete analgesia)

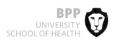

BOX 3 GUIDELINES FOR MONITORING PATIENTS WITH SEVERE TRAUMATIC BRAIN INJURY IN THE PREHOSPITAL ENVIRONMENT[4]

- Patients with suspected severe traumatic brain injury should be monitored in the prehospital setting for hypoxaemia (arterial desaturation <90%) or hypotension (systolic blood pressure <90 mm Hg)
- Blood oxygen saturation should be monitored continuously in the field with a pulse oximeter
- Systolic blood pressure and diastolic blood pressure should be measured with the most accurate method available
- Oxygenation and blood pressure should be measured as often as possible and should be monitored continuously if possible
- End-tidal carbon dioxide monitoring is essential for the transfer of ventilated patients[18]

BOX 4 RECOMMENDATIONS FOR MANAGEMENT OF HEAD INJURY[3]

- Prehospital assessment of neurological status should be done in all cases where head injury is apparent or suspected, using the Glasgow coma scale. Pupil size and reactivity should also be recorded
- A pre-alert should be made for all trauma patients with a Glasgow coma scale less than or equal to 8, to ensure appropriately experienced professionals are available and to prepare for imaging
- Patients with severe head injury need early definitive airway control and rapid delivery to a centre with onsite neurosurgical service. This requires regional planning of trauma services, including prehospital physician involvement
- Patients with severe head injury should have a CT scan as soon as possible after admission and within an hour of arrival at hospital
- All patients with severe head injury should be transferred to a neurosurgical or critical care centre irrespective of need for surgical intervention

---

between "permissive hypotension" resuscitative strategies to minimise blood loss and the need to maintain an adequate cerebral perfusion pressure to prevent secondary brain injury. The ideal resuscitation fluid is unknown for patients with severe traumatic brain injury. A well conducted large multicentre randomised controlled trial found a relative risk of death of 1.8 in patients with such injuries in intensive care who were resuscitated with albumin compared with 0.9% saline.[20] This finding has led guidelines to recommend use of small boluses of isotonic crystalloid to correct hypotension in patients with severe traumatic brain injury.[18] Hypertonic crystalloid solutions may have a future clinical role in this subgroup. A meta-analysis of randomised, double-blinded controlled trials,[21] found improved survival rates in patients with head injury who were resuscitated with hypertonic saline and dextran solutions compared with those who received standard care. Currently the use of hypertonic solutions is not widespread in prehospital care in the UK.

What treatments can be used to reduce intracranial pressure?

Intracranial pressure is often raised in patients with severe traumatic brain injury and specific treatment should be given to lower it if clinical signs are present (for example, pupillary dilatation) and if transfer time allows. Hypoxaemia, hypotension, hypercapnia, and inadequate sedation (in an intubated patient) should all be addressed before specific treatment. Little data is available about strategies to reduce intracranial pressure in the prehospital environment. A recent Cochrane review reported a relative risk of death of 0.8 when mannitol was used to reduce intracranial pressure compared with standard care in hospital, but it concluded that there was insufficient data to support prehospital administration of the drug.[22] Hypertonic saline can be used as an alternative to mannitol; studies directly comparing the drugs' capacity to lower intracranial pressure have yielded conflicting results. A large randomised prehospital trial of hypertonic saline in traumatic brain injury is about to begin recruiting.

What is the role of corticosteroids in patients with severe traumatic brain injury?

Owing to the findings of a large randomised controlled trial published in 2004, which showed a significant increase in the risk of death in patients randomised to receive corticosteroids, routine use of corticosteroids is no longer recommended for patients with head injury.[23]

How should patients with severe traumatic brain injury be immobilised?

The presence of a head injury is the strongest independent risk factor for injury of the cervical spine. In patients with severe traumatic brain injury, an assumption of spinal injury should be made and full spinal immobilisation should be implemented as early as practically possible in the field. Early assessment of the cervical spine should be done after transfer to hospital to avoid the risk of intracranial hypertension associated with hard cervical collars.[w8] In sedated and paralysed patients the use of sandbags and tape may achieve better immobilisation than rigid cervical collar.

Is hypothermia beneficial?

There is little doubt that hyperpyrexia is detrimental to outcome after severe traumatic brain injury, but the role of induced hypothermia in severe head injury is unclear. Early randomised controlled trials showed benefits in outcome for hypothermia as a treatment for refractory intracranial hypertension in patients with severe traumatic brain injury, but subsequent meta analyses have not confirmed this benefit.[24] One randomised trial[w9] showed improved neurological outcome at six months in younger patients (younger than age 45 years) who arrived at hospital with a low body temperature, which was then maintained, suggesting that patients with severe traumatic brain injury who are cold should not be actively rewarmed. This observation must be considered in relation to the fact that hypothermia is a key factor in the development of traumatic coagulopathy in patients with multiple injuries.

Should patients with traumatic brain injury be transferred directly to a neurosurgical centre?

A recent retrospective analysis showed a reduction in mortality in patients with head injuries managed in neurosurgical centres and concluded that all patients with severe traumatic brain injury should be managed in such centres (box 4).[25] Although this review was large, it only included data from about two thirds of institutions in the UK and may have been subjected to a triage bias because patients with very severe injuries are not usually accepted for treatment in neurosurgical centres. Currently, in the UK, neurointensive care beds are insufficient to manage all patients with severe traumatic brain injury and so a substantial proportion will still be treated in non-specialist centres. The presence of other injuries to the patient, mode of transport and proximity to institutions should all be considered when deciding which secondary care facility is appropriate.

Conclusion

Severe traumatic brain injury is common and often results in a poor neurological outcome. Outcomes can be improved if patients receive definitive treatment for their head injury as soon as possible after injury, preferably in a neurosurgical centre. Hypoxaemia and hypotension are common in these patients and together result in a mortality rate of more than 75%.[3] Careful identification and treatment of these factors can reduce the development of secondary brain injury.

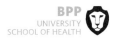
TIPS FOR NON-SPECIALISTS
• Airway obstruction is common in these patients but can usually be managed initially with simple maneouvres and adjuncts
• Focus on the basics, ensuring adequate oxygenation and ventilation
• Do not delay patient extrication by performing unnecessary interventions
• Transfer rapidly to secondary care

ADDITIONAL EDUCATIONAL RESOURCES
• Trauma.org (www.trauma.org)—education and resources for all involved in care of trauma patients
• Eastern Association for the Surgery of Trauma (www.east.org)
• Brain Trauma Foundation (www.braintrauma.org)—evidence based guidelines on management of traumatic brain injury
• Association of Anaesthetists of Great Britain and Ireland. Transfer of patients with brain injury. www.aagbi.org

Contributors: CH searched the literature and drafted the manuscript. JH conceived the idea for the review and reviewed and revised the manuscript. CH is the guarantor.

Competing interests: None declared.

Provenance and peer review: Not commissioned; externally peer reviewed.

1. The British Society of Rehabilitation Medicine. Rehabilitation after traumatic brain injury. London: British Society of Rehabilitation Medicine, 1998.
2. Royal College of Surgeons of England. Report of the working party on the management of patients with head injuries. London: Royal College of Surgeons of England, 1999.
3. Findlay G, Martin IC, Smith M, Wayman D, Carter S, Mason M. Trauma: who cares? National confidential enquiry into patient outcome and death, 2007. www.ncepod.org.uk (accessed 8 June 2008).
4. Brain Trauma Foundation. Guidelines for prehospital management of traumatic brain injury, 2nd edn. www.braintraumafoundation.org (accessed 9 June 2008).
5. Poon WS, Li AKC. Comparison of management outcome of primary and secondary referred patients with traumatic extradural haematoma in a neurosurgical unit. Injury 1991;22:323.
6. Hoyle JD, Jones JS, Deibel M, Lock DT, Reischmann D. Comparative study of airway management techniques with restricted access to patient airway. Prehosp Emerg Care 2007;11:330-6.
7. Wang HE, Sweeney TA, O'Connor RE, Rubinstein H. Failed prehospital intubations: an analysis of emergency department courses and outcomes. Prehosp Emerg Care 2001;5:134-41.
8. Davis DP, Stern J, Sise MJ, Hoyt DB. A follow up analysis of factors associated with head injury mortality after paramedic rapid sequence intubation. J Trauma 2005;59:486-90.
9. Davis DP, Peay J, Sise MJ, Vilke GM, Kennedy F, Eastman AB, et al. The impact of prehospital endotracheal intubation on outcome in moderate-severe traumatic brain injury. J Trauma 2005;58:933-9.
10. Wang HE, Peitzman AB, Cassidy LD, Adelson PD, Yealy DM. Out of hospital endotracheal intubation and outcome after traumatic brain injury. Ann Emerg Med 2004;44:439-50.
11. Newton A, Ratchford A, Khan I. Incidence of adverse events during prehospital rapid sequence intubation: a review of one year on the London Emergency Helicopter Service. J Trauma 2008;64:487-92.
12. Bulger EM, Copass MK, Sabath DR, Maier RV, Jurkovich GJ. The use of neuromuscular blocking agents to facilitate prehospital intubation does not impair outcome after traumatic brain injury. J Trauma 2005;58:718-23.
13. Deitch S, Davis DP, Schatteman J, Chan TC, Vilke GM. The use of etomidate for prehospital rapid sequence intubation. Prehosp Emerg Care 2003;7:380-3.
14. Himmelseher S, Durieux ME. Revising a dogma: ketamine for patients with neurological injury? Anesth Analg 2005;101:524-34.
15. Warner KJ, Cuschieri J, Copass MK, Jurkovich GJ, Bulger EM. The impact of prehospital ventilation on outcome after severe traumatic brain injury. J Trauma 2007;62:1330-6.
16. Helm M, Schuster R, Hauke J, Lampl L. Tight control of prehospital ventilation by capnography in major trauma victims. Br J Anaesth 2003;90:327-32.
17. Association of Anaesthetists of Great Britain and Ireland. Transfer of patients with brain injury. 2006. www.aagbi.org.
18. National Institute for Health and Clinical Excellence. The clinical and cost effectiveness of prehospital intravenous fluid therapy in trauma. 2004. www.nice.org.uk/nicemedia/pdf/ta074guidance.pdf.
19. Marmarou A, Anderson RL, Ward JD. Impact of ICP stability and hypotension on outcome in patients with severe head trauma. J Neurosurg 1991;75:S159-66.
20. The SAFE Study Investigators. A comparison of albumin and saline for fluid resuscitation in the intensive care unit. N Engl J Med 2004;350:2247-56.
21. Wade CE, Grady JJ, Kramer JC, Younes RN, Gehlsen K, Holcroft JW. Individual patient cohort analysis of the efficacy of hypertonic saline/dextran in patients with traumatic brain injury and hypotension. J Trauma 1997;42:61-5.
22. Wakai A, Roberts I, Schierhout G. Mannitol for acute traumatic brain injury. Cochrane Database Syst Rev 2007;1:CD001049.
23. Roberts I, Yates D, Sandercock P, Farrell B, Waserberg G, Lomax J, et al. Effect of intravenous corticosteroids on death within 14 days in 10 008 adults with clinically significant head injury. Lancet 2004;364:1321-8.
24. Alderson P, Gadkary C, Signorini DF. Therapeutic hypothermia for head injury. Cochrane Database Syst Rev 2004;18:CD001048.
25. Patel HC, Bouamra M, Woodford M, King AT, Yates DW, Lecky FE. Trends in head injury outcome from 1989 to 2003 and the effect of neurosurgical care: an observational study. Lancet 2005;366:1538-44.

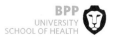
Management of the effects of exposure to tear gas

Pierre-Nicolas Carron, specialist in internal and emergency medicine,
Bertrand Yersin, professor of emergency medicine

¹Service of Emergency Medicine,
University Hospital Center and
University of Lausanne, 1011
Lausanne CHUV, Switzerland

Correspondence to: P-N Carron
Pierre-Nicolas.Carron@chuv.ch

Cite this as: BMJ 2009;338:b2283

DOI: 10.1136/bmj.b2283

http://www.bmj.com/content/338/
bmj.b2283

Despite the frequent use of riot control agents by European law enforcement agencies, limited information exists on this subject in the medical literature. The effects of these agents are typically limited to minor and transient cutaneous inflammation, but serious complications and even deaths have been reported. During the 1999 World Trade Organisation meeting and at the 2001 Summit of the Americas in Quebec, exposure to tear gas was the most common reason for medical consultations.[1] [2] Primary and emergency care physicians play a role in the first line management of patients as well as in the identification of those at risk of complications from exposure to riot control agents. In 1997 the National Poisons Information Service in England received 597 inquiries from doctors seeking advice about problems related to crowd control.[3] Our article reviews the different riot control agents, including the most common tear gases and pepper sprays, and provides an up to date overview of related medical sequelae.

Sources and selection criteria

We searched the following resources for relevant information on the medical toxicity and management of acute exposure to tear gas and pepper spray: Medline, PreMedline, Embase, CINAHL, SCIRUS, the Cochrane Library, ISI Web of Knowledge, Toxnet, Google Scholar, and personal archives. We used the subject headings "riot control agents", "pepper spray", "lacrimator", "tear gas", "irritants", "incapacitating agents", as well as the toxicological terms "chlorobenzylidene-malononitrile", "chloroacetophenone", "dibenzoxazepine", "chlorodiphenylarsine" and "capsaicin". We also searched the reference lists for additional articles. The overall evidence supporting the current therapeutic approach to patients exposed to tear gas or pepper spray is of poor quality.

What is a tear gas?

Tear gases (along with pepper sprays, toxic emetics, and some sedative substances) are among the so called riot control agents.[4] A tear gas is actually not a gas at all, but a toxic chemical irritant in the form of powder or drops mixed to variable concentrations (1%-5%) in a solvent, and delivered with a dispersion vehicle (a pyrotechnically delivered aerosol or spray solution).[4] [5] Tear gases are not currently considered as chemical weapons by Western countries. Since the 1950s, they have been mainly used

by law enforcement agencies for crowd control purposes in most European countries, including the United Kingdom, France, Germany, and Switzerland. Tear gases are also used in military training exercises to test the rapidity or efficacy of protective measures in the event of a chemical attack.

Of the known disabling chemical irritants (of which there are more than a dozen), the five that are traditionally used in the European Union are chlorobenzylidene-malononitrile (also known as CS, after the chemists Corson and Stoughton who first synthesised it), chloroacetophenone (CN or "Mace"), dibenzoxazepine (CR), oleoresin capsicum (OC), and pelargonic acid vanillylamide (PAVA) (fig 1).[6] Diphenylaminochloroarsine (DM or adamsite) is an irritating and harassing arsenic based agent used in some countries outside the EU. Oleoresin capsicum is a mixture of cayenne pepper extracts, of which capsaicin is the main active ingredient.[4] [7] Its concentration varies from 1% to 15% depending on the mixture.[7] Pepper strength is measured in Scoville heat units, ranging from zero for green pepper to 15 million units for pure capsaicin.[8] Pelargonic acid vanillylamide is a new standardised synthetic variant of oleoresin capsicum used mainly in Switzerland, Austria, and Germany.[6] [7]

How do riot control agents work?

The irritant effects of crowd control agents probably result from the action of chlorine or cyanide groups in addition to alkalising compounds (fig 1). These agents interact with muco-cutaneous sensory nerve receptors such as TRPA1 cation channels.[9] The effect of oleoresin capsicum is linked to a direct stimulation of type C and Aδ sensory nerve endings, provoking an immediate release of the inflammatory P substance.[7] [8]

A toxic effect of the solvent methyl-isobutyl-ketone or of certain metabolites has also been documented in animal experimental studies, in particular for chlorobenzylidene-malononitrile (formation of cyanide and thiosulfate derivatives) and chloroacetophenone (formation of hydrogen chloride).[7] [10] [11]

Assessments of the effects of riot control agents must take into account the weather (wind, rain, and ambient temperature) in addition to the characteristics of the site of deployment (open or closed space) as the effects of tear gas are enhanced by heat and by high ambient humidity.[4] Characteristics common to all agents include a rapid onset time and a short duration of effects, as well as a wide margin of safety between the incapacitating dose (ICt 50, the concentration (C) that causes incapacitation (I) in 50% of individuals after one minute (t=time)) and the lethal dose (LCt 50, the concentration that causes death (L) in 50% of individuals after one minute).[4] The agents differ from one another by their duration of action, their toxicity (chloroacetophenone and diphenylaminochloroarsine are more toxic than chlorobenzylidene-malononitrile or dibenzoxazepine), and their physical and chemical characteristics (table 1). Current information on toxicity is largely based on in vitro and animal studies.[4]

SUMMARY POINTS

- Tear gas and pepper spray used for crowd control are not without risks, particularly for people with pre-existing respiratory conditions
- Pulmonary, cutaneous, and ocular problems can result from exposure to these agents
- Treatment for the effects of exposure to tear gas requires chemical decontamination, including protective measures for healthcare staff
- Some people are at risk of delayed complications that can be severe enough to warrant admission to hospital and even ventilation support

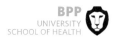

What are the medical consequences of acute exposure to tear gas and pepper spray?

There is limited human research on the risks of tear gas in terms of inducing disability or death. The irritant effect of tear gases affects exposed cutaneous and mucous membrane surfaces.[4] [5] Table 2 summarises the medical complications. Clinical experience and retrospective case studies suggest that the cutaneous effect is by far the most serious symptom, including first and second degree burns.[12] [13] Even in minor cases, skin erythema can last several hours. Direct contact with the flame or a hot canister increases the risk of severe lesions.[14] [15] Delayed contact allergy, leukodermia, or exacerbation of pre-existing dermatitis have also been described in case reports.[16]

In experimental studies, transient conjunctivitis and blepharospasm occurred a few seconds after exposure and varied with the concentration of the agent and the duration of exposure.[5] Corneal damage, hyphema, or vitreous haemorrhage have been described in isolated cases.[5] [17]

Case studies indicate that shortness of breath, sore throat, and chest pain are the most common pulmonary complaints, and these typically resolve within 30 minutes.[5] [11] Some authors have also reported bronchospasm and laryngospasm.[18] Delayed pulmonary oedema has been described in recent case studies, but permanent long term lung damage seems improbable.[19] [20] Several cases of death have been attributed to the use of chloroacetophenone in confined spaces. Some of the deaths in the 1993 siege on the Branch Davidians in Waco, Texas, were attributed to the use of large amounts of chlorobenzylidene-malononitrile in a confined space.[5] [7]

With pepper sprays, the irritant effect is immediate and lasts 30 minutes on average, mainly affecting the eyes, skin, and respiratory tract.[17] [21] Minor side effects (corneal erosion, respiratory irritability) are described in many case reports.[22] The rare deaths that have been documented were caused by bronchospasm, pulmonary oedema, or respiratory arrest and occurred mainly in patients with asthma.[6] [7] [17] Capsaicin also has neurotoxic and skin desensitising effects (hence its use in treating refractory pain) and animal studies indicate it may play a role as a procarcinogen after repeated cutaneous or digestive system contact.[6]

Avoidance of exposure and initial management of people exposed to tear gas

The best way for people (including medical staff) to avoid exposure to crowd control agents is obviously not to enter areas that pose a risk of exposure and to move away from these areas quickly if such agents are used. However, emergency medical staff do often have to go near or into such areas to treat affected people, so they must protect themselves by avoiding gaseous areas and by staying on higher ground whenever possible. As tear gases are heavier than air, the patient should be lifted off the ground as quickly as possible and the emergency medical vehicles should be parked in higher areas.

In clinical experience, tear gas or pepper spray has caused secondary contamination of healthcare staff as a result of contact with contaminated patients.[23] [24] Therefore, experts recommend that the initial medical management of patients exposed to tear gases should be symptomatic and consist primarily of non-specific chemical decontamination.[25] Identification of affected people and appropriate personal protection (such as clothes gathered at the wrists and neck; gloves; and surgical masks) can prevent secondary contamination of medical staff.[23]

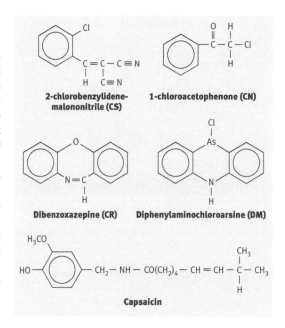

Fig 1 Chemical structure of riot control agents

An initial triage allows for identification of at-risk patients, including those with loss of consciousness or with dyspnoea, those of advanced age, those with comorbidities, and those who have had prolonged exposure to the tear gas or pepper spray (box).[4] Medical staff should be aware that there may be particularly serious consequences of exposure, such as respiratory symptoms, bronchospasm, and blepharospasm. Staff should move patients away quickly from the toxic vapours and undress them in a well ventilated area. If contamination is severe, pullovers and T shirts must be removed by cutting and should not be pulled over the patient's head. Contaminated clothes must be sealed hermetically in a double plastic bag.[4] [26]

What is the treatment for people with symptoms of exposure?

How to best manage symptomatic patients is still a matter of debate and is currently based on case series or limited human studies. Eyes should be rinsed for 10-15 minutes

---

FACTORS INFLUENCING THE EFFECT OF EXPOSURE TO TEAR GAS[4] [7]

Pre-existing conditions and characteristics of the affected person

- Asthma
- Chronic obstructive pulmonary disease
- Cardiovascular disease
- Severe hypertension
- Young children
- Patients over 60 years
- Ocular diseases
- Contact lenses

Environmental factors

- Confined space
- Poor ventilation

Amount and potency of exposure

- High concentration
- Prolonged exposure
- Repeated exposure
- Potent toxicity of the product (chloroacetophenone is more toxic than chlorobenzylidene-malononitrile)

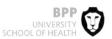

Table 1 Physical and chemical characteristics of tear gases and pepper spray [4 7]

Name	Characteristics	Time to activation	Duration of action (minutes)	Relative potency*	ICt 50 (mg/min per m³)†	LCt 50‡ (mg/min per m³)
Chloroacetophenone	Apple odour; powder or emulsion; aerosol	3-10 seconds	10-20	1	20-50	8500-25 000
Chlorobenzylidene malononitrile	Pepper odour; microparticles; dispersing effect (grenades)	10-60 seconds	10-30	5	4-20	25 000-100 000
Dibenzoxazepine	Odourless; aerosol; persists for prolonged periods in the environment or on clothes	Instantaneous	15-60	20-50	0.2-1	>100 000
Diphenylaminochloroarsine	Odourless or slightly bitter almond odour; emetic	Rapid	>60	0.5-2	50-100	10 000-35 000
Oleoresin capsicum	Pepper odour; persists for prolonged periods in the environment or on clothes; short distance spray	Rapid	30-60	Not applicable	Not applicable	>100 000

*Refers to the irritant effect.
†ICt 50=the concentration that causes incapacitation in 50% of individuals after one minute.
*LCt 50=the concentration that causes death in 50% of individuals after one minute.

Table 2 Clinical manifestations and potential complications [4 6 7]

Area affected	Clinical manifestations	Potential complications	Potential sequelae
Eyes	Tearing, burning sensation; blepharospasm; photophobia; corneal oedema (OC)	Keratitis (CN); corneal erosion (OC); intraocular haemorrhage	Cataract; glaucoma
Respiratory tract	Severe rhinorrhoea (CS); sneeze, cough, dyspnoea (CS); pharyngitis; tracheal bronchitis	Bronchospasm, hypoxaemia (CN); delayed pulmonary oedema (CS)	Reactive airways dysfunction syndrome; asthma (possibly)
Cardiovascular system	Hypertension (CS)	Heart failure; cerebral haemorrhage	Not described
Skin	Rash; oedema; erythema; blistering (CS)	Irritant dermatitis (CN); facial oedema (CN); aggravation of dermatitis	Allergic dermatitis (CN)
Digestive tract*	Buccal irritation, salivation (CS); odynodysphagia; abdominal pain; diarrhoea; nausea; vomiting (DM)	Liver toxicity (CS)	Not described
Nervous system	Trembling (DM)Agitation, anxiety	Hysterical reaction	Not described

Some tear gases are more likely to induce specific complications (as noted by abbreviations):CN = chloracetophenone; CS = o-chlorobenzylidene malononitrile; CR= dibenzoxazepine; DM = diphenylaminochloroarsine; OC = oleoresin capsicum.
*In rare cases the digestive tract may be affected by ingestion.

TIPS FOR NON-SPECIALISTS

- Medical teams should wear protection for their own safety and to prevent secondary contamination
- Contaminated clothes must be removed; eyes and affected skin surfaces should be cleaned with water
- For persistent ocular symptoms, ophthalmological assessment is recommended
- For severe pulmonary symptoms, oxygen therapy, β2-mimetics and ipratropium aerosols may be required
- For pulmonary symptoms, a 24-48 hour stay in hospital or a discharge home with detailed information about potential complications is recommended

---

AREAS FOR FURTHER RESEARCH

- The alleged safety of existing riot control agents and of all future innovations in this field
- The delayed toxic effects and potential procarcinogenic risk of repeated exposure
- The effectiveness of decontamination with water (still a matter of debate)
- Development of potential specific treatments and cutaneous therapeutic agents
- Definition of the safety criteria for riot control agents, and discussion of the "rules of engagement" with law enforcement agencies at local and national levels

---

with isotonic sodium chloride (0.9%) and any contact lenses removed.[7] Patients must not touch their face or rub their eyes. Recently, some authors have suggested using air jets to eliminate any remaining particles on the surface of the eye.[7] For persistent symptoms, experts recommend ophthalmological assessment for abrasions.[7]

Most experts propose systematic washing of affected skin surfaces with soap and water.[5 7 25] Nevertheless, this strategy remains controversial. Chlorobenzylidene-malononitrile dissolved in water is said to intensify the irritation, and in one small study, skin vesication was observed with 0.5 mg of chloroacetophenone but only when the skin was moist.[18] [26] In a limited randomised study, baby shampoo provided no

better relief for eye and skin discomfort than water alone.[27] Many decontamination products, such as Diphoterine, are currently being tested for efficacy. However, their cost plus the lack of evidence of effectiveness precludes any proposal for systematic use.[28] Severe skin lesions are treated with the same methods as for an acute irritant dermatitis, by using topical corticoids and antihistamine agents as necessary.[21]

In the event of pulmonary symptoms such as bronchial spasm, short term medical treatment including oxygen therapy, β2-mimetic and ipratropium aerosols may be required.[7] The rare occurrence of delayed pulmonary oedema in patients with pulmonary symptoms has led to some experts recommending a 24-48 hour stay in hospital for observation or a discharge home with detailed information about potential complications and their clinical manifestations.[18] Digestive tract symptoms (table 2) do not pose a big risk and resolve spontaneously, with the exception of rare cases of voluntary or unintentional ingestion, which requires admission to hospital.[29]

What are the ethical considerations?

Medical consequences of the use of riot control agents remain ill defined in terms of morbidity and mortality. In 1998 an editorial in the *Lancet* demanded a moratorium on the use of such agents so that the potential long term consequences of these substances could be studied further, in particular in the area of carcinogenicity.[30]

In Europe the medical research necessary to justify the use of certain crowd control technologies is absent, lacking, or of poor quality. Currently, alternatives to crowd control agents seem to be even more deleterious for demonstrators as well as for law enforcement agencies. Whether tear gases are innocuous will nevertheless continue to be debated.

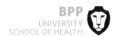

ADDITIONAL EDUCATIONAL RESOURCES

Useful websites

- US Centers for Disease Control and Prevention (www.bt.cdc.gov/agent/riotcontrol)— Information about case definition and about symptoms, signs, and differential diagnosis

Information for the public and patients

- US Centers for Disease Control and Prevention (www.bt.cdc.gov/agent/riotcontrol/pdf/riotcontrol_factsheet.pdf)—Overview of riot control agents, including symptoms, signs, and treatment
- Chemical Weapons Convention (www.opcw.org/chemical-weapons-convention)—Convention on the prohibition of the development, production, stockpiling, and use of chemical weapons and on their destruction

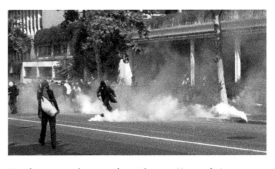

Use of tear gas at demonstration at the 2003 G8 summit, Lausanne, Switzerland

The authors acknowledge Danielle Wyss for proofreading and final translation. The photograph is from the photography archives of the emergency service of the Centre Hospitalier Universitaire Vaudois (CHUV), Lausanne.

Contributors: P-NC did the literature review and wrote the initial draft. BY supervised, reviewed, and contributed to the manuscript. Both authors are guarantors.

Funding: None.

Competing interests: None declared.

Provenance and peer review: Not commissioned; externally peer reviewed.

1. Martin C, Newcombe EA. Emergency care during the 1999 World Trade Organization meeting in Seattle. *J Emerg Nurs* 2001;27:478-80.
2. Weir E. The health impact of crowd-control agents. *Can Med Ass J* 2001;164:1889-90.
3. Wheeler H, MacLehose R, Euripidou E, Murray V. Surveillance into crowd control agents. *Lancet* 1998;352:991-2.
4. Olajos E, Salem H. Riot control agents: pharmacology, toxicology, biochemistry and chemistry. *J Appl Toxicol* 2001;21:355-91.
5. Sanford J. Medical aspects of riot control (harassing) agents. *Annu Rev Med* 1976;27:421-9.
6. OMEGA Foundation. Crowd control technologies (an appraisal of technologies for political control). European Parliament. 2000. (www.europarl.europa.eu/stoa/publications/studies/19991401a_en.pdf)
7. Smith J, Greaves I. The use of chemical incapacitant sprays: a review. *J Trauma* 2002;52:595-600.
8. Recer G, Johnson T, Gleason A. An evaluation of the relative potential public health concern for the self-defense spray active ingredients oleoresin capsicum, o-chlorobenzylidene malononitrile, and 2-chloroacetophenone. *Reg Toxicol Pharma* 2002;36:1-11.
9. McMahon S, Wood J. Increasingly irritable and close to tears: TRPA1 in inflammatory pain. *Cell* 2006;124:1123-5.
10. Kluchinsky T, Savage P, Fitz R, Smith P. Liberation of hydrogen cyanide and hydrogen chloride during high-temperature dispersion of CS riot control agent. *AIHA J* 2002;63:493-6.
11. Euripidou E, MacLehose R, Fletcher A. An investigation into the short term and medium term health impacts of personal incapacitants sprays. A follow up of patients reported to the National Poisons Information Service (London). *Emerg Med J* 2004;21:548-52.
12. Anderson PJ, Lau GS, Taylor WR, Critchley JA. Acute effects of the potent lacrimator o-chlorobenzylidene malononitrile (CS) tear gas. *Hum Exp Toxicol* 1996;15:461-5.
13. Thorburn KM. Injuries after use of lacrymatory agent cloroacetophenone in a confined space. *Arch Environ Health* 1982;37:182-6.
14. Morrone A, Sacerdoti G, Franco R, Corretti R, Fazio M. Tear gas dermatitis. *Clin Exp Dermatol* 2005;230:435-6.
15. Zekri A, King W, Yeung R, Taylor W. Acute mass burns caused by o-chlorobenzylidene malononitrile (CS) tear gas. *Burns* 1995;21:586-9.
16. Watson K, Rycroft R. Unintended cutaneous reactions to CS spray. *Contact Dermatitis* 2005;53:9-13.
17. Vilke G, Chan TC. Less lethal technology: medical issues. *Policing: an International Journal of Police Strategies and Management* 2007;30:341-57.
18. Vaca F, Myers JH, Langdorf M. Delayed pulmonary oedema and bronchospams after accidental lacrimator exposure. *Am J Emerg Med* 1996;14:402-5.
19. Hill AR, Silverberg N, Mayorga D, Baldwin H. Medical hazards of the tear gas CS: a case of persistent, multisystem, hypersensitivity reaction and review of the literature. *Medicine (Baltimore)* 2000;79:234-40.
20. Karagama Y, Newton J, Newbegin C. Short-term and long-term physical effects of exposure to CS spray. *J R Soc Med* 2003;96:172-4.
21. Williams S, Clark R, Dunford J. Contact dermatitis associated with capsaicin: Hunan hand syndrom. *Ann Emerg Med* 1994;25:713-5.
22. Watson W, Stremel K, Westdorp EJ. Oleoresin capsicum (cap-stun) toxicity from aerosol exposure. *Ann Pharmacother* 1996;30:733-5.
23. Horton D, Burgess P, Rossiter S, Kaye W. Secondary contamination of emergency department personnel from o-chlorobenzylidene malononitrile exposure. *Ann Emerg Med* 2005;45:655-8.
24. Horton D, Berkowitz Z, Kaye W. Secondary contamination of ED personnel from hazardous materials events 1995-2001. *Am J Emerg Med* 2003;21:199-204.
25. Kales S, Christiani D. Acute chemical emergencies. *N Engl J Med* 2004;350:800-8.
26. Blaho K, Stark M. Is CS spray dangerous? *BMJ* 2000;321:46.
27. Winslow JE, Hill KD, Bozenman WP. Determination of optimal methods of decontamination after tear gas and pepper spray exposure. *Ann Emerg Med* 2006;48:S51.
28. Viala B, Blomet J, Mathieu L, Hall A. Prevention of CS (tear gas) eye and skin effects and active decontamination with Diphoterine: preliminary studies in five French gendarmes. *J Emerg Med* 2005;29:5-8.
29. Solomon I, Kochba L, Eizenkraft E, Maharshak N. Report of accidental CS ingestion among seven patients in central Israel and review of the current literature. *Arch Toxicol* 2003;77:601-4.
30. "Safety" of chemical batons. *Lancet* 1998;352:159.

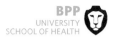

Pain management and sedation for children in the emergency department

Paul Atkinson, consultant in emergency medicine ,
Adam Chesters, specialty registrar in emergency medicine,
Peter Heinz, consultant in paediatric medicine

[1]Emergency Department,
Cambridge University Hospitals
NHS Foundation Trust,
Addenbrooke's Hospital, Cambridge
CB2 0QQ

Correspondence to: P Atkinson Paul.
atkinson@addenbrookes.nhs.uk

Cite this as: *BMJ* 2009;339:b4234

DOI: 10.1136/bmj.b4234

http://www.bmj.com/content/339/
bmj.b4234

Children commonly present for emergency care with painful conditions and injuries. Further painful, distressing, or unpleasant diagnostic and therapeutic procedures may be necessary during the visit. Emergency clinicians are expected to provide safe and effective analgesia and sedation for children, and provision of such analgesia is a primary audit standard of the College of Emergency Medicine.[1] We provide an overview of published evidence to help clinicians assess, manage, and minimise pain in children presenting to hospital.

How is acute pain best assessed in children?

The assessment of pain is a core feature of most international triage systems. National guidelines suggest that children with moderate or severe pain should be triaged as urgent and should wait no longer than 20 minutes for administration of adequate analgesia.[1]

Several methods of assessment have been validated for assessing the severity of pain (table 1).[2] The ability to indicate the presence of pain emerges at around 2 years of age. Children as young as 3 years may be able to quantify pain using simple validated pain scales,[3] such as verbal rating scales, visual analogue scales, and faces scales (figure).[4] [5] A large observational study found little evidence for using abnormal physiology—such as tachycardia, tachypnoea, and hypertension—to screen for severe pain, although the presence of abnormal physiology may indicate its presence. In the acute setting, behaviour is the main way that infants and preverbal children communicate their pain.[6] Specific distress behaviours such as crying, facial grimacing, certain postures, and inability to be consoled have been associated with pain in young children. Such responses have been incorporated into pain assessment tools for preverbal children. The Children's Hospital of Eastern Ontario pain

scale (CHEOPS) is considered the gold standard, although it is complex and may be difficult to use in the acute setting.[7] The faces legs activity cry consolability (FLACC) scale provides an alternative framework for assessment.[8]

A randomised controlled trial found that parents were more likely than doctors to classify their child's pain as severe when present during a painful procedure; this suggests that it may be useful to involve parents in pain assessment.[9] Parental comforting during the procedure did not relieve pain more effectively than when the parents did not comfort or were absent. Parental presence during a painful procedure did, however, relieve parental anxiety.

What is the role of non-pharmacological methods in paediatric pain relief?

A recent Cochrane review found sufficient evidence to support the efficacy of distraction, hypnosis, and cognitive behavioural techniques in reducing needle related pain and distress in children and adolescents.[10]

The national service framework for children recommends play for children in hospital.[w3] Play specialists have a key role in providing age appropriate support. Parents and carers should be encouraged to stay with their child and offer reassurance at all times. Having a designated children's play area—with books, toys, and a television showing children's programmes—can help to provide distraction and comfort in an unfamiliar and frightening environment.

The use of dressings, slings, and splints are other simple measures that can provide effective analgesia.[11] As well as the physical benefit of dressing a wound or splinting a deformed limb, covering an injury that causes the child distress to look at may provide psychological benefit. Application of cold packs is a standard approach for ligamentous sprains, and pain from insect and marine stings can be treated by applying cold or heat to the affected part. Cold spray and ice packs provide immediate relief, whereas warm water immersion provides longer lasting analgesia.[12]

What is the best initial choice of analgesic drug?

Modern emergency practice aims to provide effective analgesia at the first attempt, on the basis of an accurate assessment of the child's pain.[1]

Children with all levels of pain will benefit from administration of paracetamol (acetaminophen). A loading dose of 30 mg/kg should be given initially, followed by the maintenance dose as required (10-15 mg/kg every four to six hours; maximum 90 mg/kg in 24 hours; reduce in infants and neonates).[w4] For severe pain, national guidelines recommend immediate administration of intravenous opiates in combination with oral drugs and the non-pharmacological methods outlined above.[1] The use of inhaled or intranasal analgesics can be valuable before intravenous access has been secured. Well designed randomised controlled trials found that intranasal diamorphine and fentanyl are absorbed rapidly across the nasal mucosa

---

SOURCES AND SELECTION CRITERIA

We searched Medline, PubMed, and the Cochrane database for evidence from systematic reviews and clinical trials. We searched websites of major international royal colleges and colleges of paediatrics and emergency medicine for published guidelines. We also used our personal experience of practice. Search terms used included "pain", "analgesia", "sedation", "children", and "emergency".

SUMMARY POINTS

- Ensure that children do not experience prolonged or additional pain when presenting for emergency medical care; use a composite assessment tool to assess pain at triage

- Aim to provide effective analgesia at the first attempt—use the appropriate drug, dose, and route; if possible choose painless modes of delivery (nasal route, flavoured syrups)

- Reassess pain scores frequently to ensure that analgesia is effective and allow enough time for it to work

- Use pharmacological and non-pharmacological modalities to manage pain

- Avoid the "routine" use of unnecessary painful invasive procedures

- Use topical, local, and regional anaesthesia along with appropriate safe procedural sedation to avoid further pain

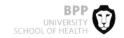

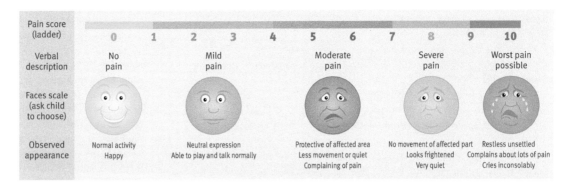

Pain score (ladder)	0	1	2	3	4	5	6	7	8	9	10
Verbal description	No pain		Mild pain			Moderate pain			Severe pain		Worst pain possible
Faces scale (ask child to choose)											
Observed appearance	Normal activity Happy		Neutral expression Able to play and talk normally			Protective of affected area Less movement or quiet Complaining of pain			No movement of affected part Looks frightened Very quiet		Restless unsettled Complains about lots of pain Cries inconsolably

Composite pain assessment tool for children in the emergency department incorporating self reporting; faces and observational scores. Reproduced, with permission, from Elsevier[5]

Table 1 Examples of validated pain assessment tools[2]

Assessment tool	Age range	Assessment
Premature infant pain profile (PPP)[w1]	Term and preterm neonates; may be less reliable in the youngest of preterm neonates	Gestational age, behavioural state, heart rate, oxygen saturation, brow bulge, eye squeeze, nasolabial furrows
Faces, legs, activity, cry and consolability (FLACC)[8]	Non-verbal children other than neonates; can be adapted for use in cognitive impairment	Facial expression, leg position, activity pattern, presence of crying and nature of cry, ability to be consoled
Wong Baker faces[4]	3 years onwards	Five line drawn faces generated from children's drawings
Adolescent pediatric pain tool[w2]	Good for complex pain needs and chronic pain in school age children	Uses a body diagram graphic in conjunction with a word selection tool (includes instructions)
Visual analogue scales	7-8 years to adult	Horizontal or vertical lines on a continuum of increasing pain; may be illustrated by colours when used in paediatrics

and provide initial pain relief comparable to intravenous opiates.[13 14] Oral drugs have a delayed onset of action and their absorption is more variable than parenteral ones, but they can be given painlessly, have a synergistic effect when used with other analgesics, and are usually more acceptable to parents and children. Oral medication alone is reserved for children with mild to moderate pain.[4] Some analgesics are available as a suppository, but administration by this route may prove unacceptable for parents and may add to the child's distress. Intramuscular administration of pain relief has a limited role in the emergency management of pain in children because the injection is often painful, absorption unpredictable, and the onset of effect slow.

How can procedures be carried out without causing further pain?

For a child with a painful condition or injury, further diagnostic or therapeutic procedures may be necessary but can cause additional pain and distress. Simple measures, such as giving a nitrous oxide and oxygen mix (Entonox) to older children or non-nutritive sucking in young infants, can make minor procedures less distressing.[15 16] A randomised double blind placebo controlled clinical trial found single dose oral sucrose to be safe and effective in reducing the behavioural and physiological pain response to a painful stimulus in preterm infants.[w5 w6] For each additional procedure—from needle related to radiological—carefully consider whether the procedure is immediately necessary, and if the available analgesia or psychological techniques (or both) are likely to be sufficient for the child.

For many common minor procedures, less painful alternative techniques are available, which can be combined with the pharmacological and non-pharmacological methods outlined above. For closure of small simple wounds, evidence from randomised controlled trials show that non-invasive alternatives can be as effective as traditional painful procedures. Skin lacerations can be closed with

tissue adhesive rather than sutures with similar medium and long term cosmetic results[17]; similarly, scalp lacerations can be closed using the hair apposition technique, where strands of hair are twisted across the wound and glued together to close the wound.[w7] When necessary, using absorbable sutures prevents the need for future removal.[w8] Comparative clinical studies have shown venous blood gases to be as accurate as the more painful arterial gases for monitoring acid-base status in children with uraemic acidosis and diabetic ketoacidosis.[w9 w10]

Which topical anaesthetics are available for cannulation and venepuncture?

Topical anaesthetic preparations such as EMLA (euteric mixture of local anaesthetics—lidocaine and prilocaine) and Ametop (tetracaine) can be used on intact skin in patients older than one month before minor skin procedures. A recent Cochrane review found that Ametop is superior to EMLA for reducing overall needle insertion pain in children.[18] Ametop takes 45 minutes to anaesthetise the skin, whereas EMLA takes 60 minutes, and this fact has to be incorporated into the emergency department triage assessment for children deemed likely to need blood tests or venous access. Ethyl chloride (coolant) spray is an alternative for minor cutaneous procedures such as venepuncture, especially when urgent, but its efficacy is unclear.[19 20]

What are the topical, local, or regional anaesthesia options for wounds and injuries?

LAT gel (lidocaine, adrenaline, and tetracaine) is useful in providing anaesthesia for the cleaning and repair of open wounds such as skin lacerations. All simple lacerations of the head, neck, limbs, or trunk of less than 5 cm in length can be considered for exploration and repair using LAT gel rather than local anaesthetic infiltration. Several randomised controlled trials have shown that it has a similar efficacy but is less painful to apply.[21]

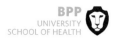

ESSENTIAL RESOURCES AND CONSIDERATIONS FOR PAEDIATRIC PROCEDURAL SEDATION IN THE EMERGENCY DEPARTMENT

- Appropriately trained personnel present:
- Doctor performing sedation (who has received appropriate training and has documented evidence of successful assessment of competency)
- Doctor or practitioner performing procedure
- Children's nurse (who is familiar with sedation procedure, monitoring, and equipment)
- Appropriate indication—painful procedure needed during this attendance at the emergency department
- Would a general anaesthetic be more appropriate (no immediate need for the procedure)?
- Quiet location, monitoring, and equipment available (standards of monitoring set by Royal College of Anaesthetists and the UK Academy of Medical Royal Colleges and Faculties)
- Any contraindications in anaesthetic history or examination?
- ASA (American Society of Anesthesiologists) class 3, 4, or 5
- Recent last meal (<4 hours) or recent fluid intake (<2 hours)—relative contraindication
- Previous adverse reactions to drugs
- Previously known anaesthetic risk (such as difficult airway)
- Explanation and informed consent from parents or legally responsible adult
- Record of drugs used including dosage and timing
- Record of vital signs before, during, and after sedation
- Record of adverse events and interventions
- Record of safe recovery

A PARENT'S PERSPECTIVE

Lucy, my 8 year old daughter, fell off a trampoline and badly injured her right arm. On arrival at the emergency department, she was screaming in agony with any small movement. The triage nurse recognised her severe pain immediately. A sling was applied and she was brought straight into a cubicle in the paediatric area where a paediatric nurse encouraged me to help Lucy use the gas and air (Entonox). She was then given a strong painkiller (diamorphine) intranasally, without the need for needles. Her pain improved quickly. The nurse then placed some gel (Ametop) on the back of her other hand and after a while a doctor was able to put in a needle (an intravenous cannula) while a play specialist distracted Lucy with a puzzle book. The nurse covered up the needle with a bandage with cartoon pictures on it. After her x ray, the consultant explained that Lucy's arm was broken and needed to be manipulated. He offered us the option of having her sedated there and then. Lucy was moved to another room in the children's area and was attached to a monitor. She was given a sedative (ketamine) and she did not feel a thing while they straightened her arm and put it in plaster. Before we went home, the doctor made sure that Lucy had recovered from the sedation and that we had a supply of painkillers to take home.

ADDITIONAL EDUCATIONAL RESOURCES

Resources for healthcare professionals

- American Academy of Pediatrics. The assessment and management of acute pain in infants, children, and adolescents. *Pediatrics* 2001;108:793-7
- American Academy of Pediatrics. Committee on Fetus and Newborn. Committee on Drugs. Section on Anesthesiology. Section on Surgery. Canadian Paediatric Society. Fetus and Newborn Committee. Prevention and management of pain and stress in the neonate. *Pediatrics* 2000;105:454-61
- American College of Emergency Physicians. Clinical policy: critical issues in the sedation of pediatric patients in the emergency department. *Ann Emerg Med* 2008;51:378-99.
- Agency for Health Care Policy and Research. Acute pain management in infants, children, and adolescents: operative and medical procedures. *Clinical practice guideline—quick reference guide for clinicians.* 1992;1B:1-22
- Royal College of Nursing. *The recognition and assessment of acute pain in children.* 2009. www.rcn.org.uk/development/practice/pain
- Royal College of Paediatrics and Child Health. *Recognition and assessment of acute pain in children.* 2001
- Royal College of Paediatrics and Child Health. *Evidence-based guidelines for the safe sedation of children undergoing diagnostic and therapeutic procedures.* 2002

Resources for patients and carers

- Paediatric Pain Profile (www.ppprofile.org.uk/)—Behaviour rating scale for assessing pain in children with severe physical and learning impairments
- Paediatric Pain (http://pediatric-pain.ca/)—Good resource for professionals, children, and parents or carers, with many links to other sites

Commonly used local anaesthetics for infiltration in the emergency department include lidocaine (with or without adrenaline) and bupivacaine. Local nerve blocks (without adrenaline) completely or partially anaesthetise the area supplied by that nerve. Common examples include digital nerve blocks for injuries to the fingers, and the femoral nerve block for femoral shaft fractures. Specific nerve blocks can be performed for minor surgical procedures around the hand, face, and ears. Additional analgesia, procedural sedation, or non-pharmacological techniques can make these procedures more tolerable to the child.

Does procedural sedation have a role in painful emergency procedures in children?

Background and national guidelines

Many procedures performed on children in the emergency department would cause considerable pain and distress without the use of sedation. Common examples include manipulation of a displaced long bone fracture and suturing of complex wounds where the child will not tolerate injection of local anaesthetic or remain still enough for the procedure to be performed effectively and safely. Procedural sedation allows the patient to tolerate unpleasant procedures while independently maintaining airway control, oxygenation, and circulation. Expertise in procedural sedation and analgesia is a core competency for emergency doctors and anaesthetists. In our experience, the key to safe and successful sedation is optimal pain management in the first instance. Sedation is not a replacement for effective pain management. Guidelines and policies approved by the College of Emergency Medicine and the Scottish Intercollegiate Guidelines Network, and a report commissioned by the UK Academy of Medical Royal Colleges and Faculties, support the use of procedural sedation as a safe and appropriate means to facilitate pain and anxiety management during interventional or diagnostic procedures, including emergencies, for all age groups.[22][23][W11]

Drug options

Substantial evidence supports the use of a variety of agents for procedural sedation by trained emergency doctors in the emergency department (table 2).[W12] In particular, ketamine with its combined sedative and analgesic action has been extensively reviewed. A meta-analysis of more than 8000 cases found the use of ketamine as sole sedative agent to be safe in children aged 2-13 years (1-2 mg/kg racemic ketamine intravenously). Short term side effects include "bad dreams," vomiting, and ataxia. Risk factors for airway and respiratory adverse events were high intravenous doses and coadministration of anticholinergics or benzodiazepines.[24] In older children and adults, it is used as an analgesic (0.25-0.5 mg/kg intravenously) to facilitate brief painful interventions and in conjunction with other anaesthetic agents for sedation.[W13] Other drugs commonly used for sedation in children include propofol and combined benzodiazepines and opiates (midazolam and fentanyl).[22] Guidelines recommend fasting for three hours before sedation[23]; however, a prospective observational study has suggested that prolonged pre-sedation fasting is not essential with ketamine.[25]

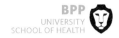

Table 2 Doses and indications for commonly used analgesics and sedatives in children

Drug	Primary use (maximum daily dose)	Dose*	Example indication
Paracetamol	Analgesic (1-3 months: 60 mg/kg; 3 months to 12 years: 90 mg/kg; >12 years: 4 g)	Oral. >32/40 gestational age only: 30 mg/kg loading dose then 10-15 mg/kg every 6-8 h as needed	Used alone in mild pain (for example, a sprained ankle) or as an adjunct in moderate or severe pain
		Rectal. >32/40 gestational age only: 30-40 mg/kg loading dose then 20 mg/kg every 6-8 h as needed	
		Intravenous. <10 kg: 7.5 mg/kg every 6-8 h; 10-50 kg: 15 mg/kg every 6-8 h; >50 kg: 1 g every 6-8 h	
Ibuprofen	Analgesic (30 mg/kg to a maximum of 2.4 g)	Oral. <6 months: 5 mg/kg every 6-8 h, >6 months: 7.5 mg/kg every 6-8 h	Used alone in mild pain (for example, minor head injury) or as an adjunct in moderate or severe pain
Diclofenac sodium	Analgesic (150 mg)	Oral. >1 year: 0.3-1 mg/kg (maximum 50 mg) every 8 h	Used alone in mild pain (for example, small superficial burn or scald) or as an adjunct in moderate or severe pain
		Rectal. >6 years: 0.3-1 mg/kg (maximum 50 mg) every 8 h	
Codeine phosphate	Analgesic (240 mg)	Oral. Neonate to 12 years: 0.5-1 mg/kg every 4-6 h; >12 years: 30-60 mg every 4-6 h	Used in combination with other analgesics in moderate pain (for example, buckle fracture of radius)
Tramadol	Analgesic (400 mg)	Oral (>12 years only): 50-100 mg every 6 h	Used in combination with other analgesics in moderate pain (for example, larger burns and scalds)
Diamorphine	Analgesic (10 mg maximum in a single dose)	Intranasal (>10 kg only): 0.1 mg/kg made up into a 0.2 ml solution	Acute pain in the emergency setting, for short painful procedures (for example, immediate analgesia for deformed fracture to allow splint application and cannulation of a vein)
Morphine	Analgesic	Intravenous. Neonate: 50 μg/kg every 6 hours; 1-6 months: 100 μg/kg every 3 hours; 6 months to 12 years: 100 μg/kg every 4 hours; >12 years: 2.5 mg every 4 hours	Most reliable method to relieve severe pain is by titrated intravenous opiates. Can be used in conjunction with other analgesics (for example, large burns, fractures requiring manipulation)
Midazolam	Sedative	Intravenous. 1 month to 6 years: initially 25-50 μg/kg, increased if necessary in small steps (maximum 6 mg); 6-12 years: initially 25-50 μg/kg, increased if necessary in small steps (maximum 10 mg); 12-18 years: initially 25-50 μg/kg, increased if necessary in small steps (maximum 7.5 mg)	Procedural sedation by appropriately trained staff with necessary equipment and monitoring facilities (for example, suturing of complex wounds that require cooperation and infiltration of local anaesthetic)
		Buccal. 6 months to 10 years: 200-300 μg/kg (maximum 5 mg); 10-18 years: 6-7 mg (maximum 8 mg in those >70 kg)	
Ketamine	Analgesic and sedative	Intravenous. Up to 12 years:1-2 mg/kg produces 5-10 minutes of surgical anaesthesia, adjusted according to response; >12 years: 1-4.5 mg/kg (usually 2 mg/kg) produces 5-10 minutes of surgical anaesthesia, adjusted according to response	Procedural sedation by appropriately trained staff with necessary equipment and monitoring facilities (for example, manipulation of angulated forearm fractures)

*See BNF for Children for preparations, adverse effects, and contraindications.[w12]

QUESTIONS AND AREAS FOR FUTURE RESEARCH

- What are the long term psychological benefits of optimised pain relief for short painful emergency procedures?
- New delivery methods and agents for more immediate analgesia (such as lidocaine iontophoresis, intradermal injection systems)
- How can we implement optimal and age appropriate pain management strategies into daily practice in a busy emergency department?

TIPS FOR NON-SPECIALISTS

Key non-pharmacological interventions
Ensure assessment and treatment in a quiet, calm, child oriented environment; a friendly non-intimidating manner in the approach of staff; and reassurance and explanation to both child and parents
Gentle immobilisation and careful dressings alleviate pressure and movement from the site of pain

Topical anaesthesia
Tetracaine (Ametop) gel can be used from age one month. It acts faster than EMLA. LAT gel (lidocaine, adrenaline, and tetracaine; contains a vasoconstrictor) should be used for open wounds

Intranasal opiates
Some opiate preparations can be given intranasally. This provides rapid bioavailability for faster analgesic effect without requiring a needle or cannula[11 12]
Examples include diamorphine 0.1 mg/kg nasal aerosol (<0.2 ml) and fentanyl 1-2 μg/kg nasal aerosol

Sedation
Do not sedate a child unless you are appropriately trained and certified. Do consider the potential benefits of sedation, however, and seek expert help when needed

Avoiding pain
Consider whether the proposed procedure is necessary; does a less painful option exist? Use steristrips or tissue adhesive rather than sutures, and venous rather than arterial blood gases
Would general anaesthesia be preferable? Some complex or prolonged procedures are better performed on an emergency anaesthetic list rather than in the emergency department or clinic

Training and accreditation in procedural sedation in children
The UK Academy of Medical Royal Colleges and Faculties report on safe sedation practice recommends that instruction in procedural sedation be incorporated into training and revalidation programmes, and that a clinical governance framework should deliver local safe sedation procedures in line with guidelines agreed by the relevant national professional body. The box shows typical components of a local guideline. In particular, multidisciplinary team training is recommended to ensure that all staff involved in procedural sedation understand their roles and that staff who administer the sedative are aware of the possible adverse consequences and have the necessary skills to manage such adverse events.

Conclusions

Safe and effective management of pain and anxiety in children is an essential component of modern emergency practice. Pain can be assessed and treated by a variety of pharmacological and non-pharmacological means (table 3). Children who present in pain can be assessed quickly, treated, and frequently reassessed using an evidence based model of care to ensure that the analgesic strategy is effective (table 1). Several psychological techniques can be used to put the child at ease and lessen the perception of pain. Newer methods of drug delivery will help with the administration of analgesia, and the role of safe procedural sedation in the paediatric emergency department will be consolidated.

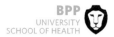

Table 3 Examples of commonly required procedures and options to reduce pain and distress in children

Procedure or injury	Distraction or CBT	Splint or dressing	Topical anaesthesia	Sucking (sucrose or pacifier)	Opioids	Local anaesthesia	Regional anaesthesia	Sedation	General anaesthesia
Venepuncture or cannulation	Yes		Yes	Yes					
Arterial puncture	Yes		Yes	Yes		Yes			
Central venous catheter insertion			Yes	Yes		Yes		Yes	Yes
Suturing	Yes		Yes	Yes		Yes	Yes	Yes	Yes
Dressing change	Yes			Yes	Yes			Yes	
Removal of foreign body	Yes		Yes	Yes		Yes	Yes	Yes	Yes
Joint reduction	Yes	Yes			Yes		Yes	Yes	Yes
Fracture manipulation	Yes	Yes			Yes	Yes	Yes	Yes	Yes
Abdominal pain	Yes				Yes				
Burns	Yes	Yes		Yes	Yes				Yes
Lumbar puncture	Yes		Yes	Yes		Yes		Yes	Yes
Chest drain insertion			Yes		Yes	Yes		Yes	Yes

CBT=cognitive behavioural therapy.

Contributors: PA had the idea for the article, reviewed the literature, co-wrote and revised the article, and is guarantor; AC did the literature search, reviewed the literature, and co-wrote and revised the article; PH reviewed the literature, and co-wrote and revised the article.

Competing interests: None declared.

Provenance and peer review: Commissioned; externally peer reviewed.

Patient consent obtained.

1 College of Emergency Medicine Clinical Effectiveness Committee. *Management of pain in children* . 2004. www.collemergencymed. ac.uk/CEM/Clinical%20Effectiveness%20Committee/Guidelines/ Clinical%20Guidelines/default.asp.

2 Harrop JE. Management of pain in childhood. *Arch Dis Child Educ Pract Ed* 2007;92:ep101-8.

3 Spagrud LJ, Piira T, von Baeyer CL. Children's self report of pain intensity. *Am J Nurs* 2003;103:62-4.

4 Wong D, Baker C. Pain in children: comparison of assessment scales. *Pediatr Nurs* 1988;14:9-17.

5 Atkinson P, Kendall R, Van Rensburg L. *Emergency medicine an illustrated colour text.* 1st ed. Elsevier, 2010:32-3.

6 Büttner W, Finke W. Analysis of behavioral and physiological parameters for the assessment of postoperative analgesic demand in newborns, infants and young children: a comprehensive report on seven consecutive studies. *Paediatr Anaesth* 2000;10:303-18.

7 McGrath PJ, Johnson G, Goodman JT, Schillinger J, Dunn J, Chapman J. CHEOPS: a behavioral scale for rating postoperative pain in children. *Adv Pain Res Ther* 1985;9:395-402.

8 Merkel S, Voepel-Lewis T, Shayevitz J, Malviya S. The FLACC: a behavioral scale for scoring postoperative pain in young children. *Pediatr Nurse* 1997;23:293-7.

9 Bauchner H, Vinci R, Bak S, Pearson C, Corwin MJ. Parents and procedures: a randomized controlled trial. *Pediatrics* 1996;98:861-7.

10 Uman LS, Chambers CT, McGrath PJ, Kisely SR. Psychological interventions for needle-related procedural pain and distress in children and adolescents. *Cochrane Database Syst Rev* 2006;(4):CD005179.

11 O'Donnell JJ, Maurice SC, Beattie TF. Emergency analgesia in the paediatric population. Part III. Non-pharmacological measures of pain relief and anxiolysis. *Emerg Med J* 2002;19:195-7.

12 Atkinson PRT, Boyle A, Hartin D, McAuley D. Is hot water immersion an effective treatment for marine envenomation? *Emerg Med J* 2006;23:503-8.

13 Kendall JM, Reeves BC, Latter VS. Multicentre randomised controlled trial of nasal diamorphine for analgesia in children and teenagers with clinical fractures. *BMJ* 2001;322:261-5.

14 Borland M, Jacobs I, King B, O'Brien D. A randomized controlled trial comparing intranasal fentanyl to intravenous morphine for managing acute pain in children in the emergency department. *Ann Emerg Med* 2007;49:335-40.

15 Ekbom K, Jakobsson J, Marcus C. Nitrous oxide inhalation is a safe and effective way to facilitate procedures in paediatric outpatient departments. *Arch Dis Child* 2005;90:1073-6.

16 Horwitz N. Does oral sucrose reduce the pain of neonatal procedures? *Arch Dis Child* 2002;87:80-1.

17 Quinn J, Wells G, Sutcliffe T, Jarmuske M, Maw J, Stiell I, et al. Tissue adhesive versus suture wound repair at 1 year: randomized clinical trial correlating early, 3-month, and 1-year cosmetic outcome. *Ann Emerg Med* 1998;32:645-9.

18 Lander JA, Weltman BJ, So SS. EMLA and amethocaine for reduction of children's pain associated with needle insertion. *Cochrane Database Syst Rev* 2006;(3):CD004236.

19 Costello M, Ramundo M, Christopher NC, Powell KR. Ethyl vinyl chloride vapocoolant spray fails to decrease pain associated with intravenous cannulation in children. *Clin Pediatr (Phila)* 2006;45:628-32.

20 Farion KJ, Splinter KL, Newhook K, Gaboury I, Splinter WM. The effect of vapocoolant spray on pain due to intravenous cannulation in children: a randomized controlled trial. *CMAJ* 2008;179:31-6.

21 Ferguson C, Loryman B. Topical anaesthetic versus lidocaine infiltration to allow closure of skin wounds in children. *Emerg Med J* 2005;22:507-9.

22 American College of Emergency Physicians. Clinical policy: procedural sedation and analgesia in the emergency department. *Ann Emerg Med* 2005;45:177-96.

23 Scottish Intercollegiate Guidelines Network. *Safe sedation of children undergoing diagnostic and therapeutic procedures* . 2004. www.sign. ac.uk/pdf/sign58.pdf.

24 Green SM, Roback MG, Krauss B, Brown L, McGlone RG, Agrawal D, et al. Predictors of airway and respiratory adverse events with ketamine sedation in the emergency department: an individual-patient data meta-analysis of 8282 children. *Ann Emerg Med* 2009 Online Feb 5.

25 Treston G. Prolonged pre-procedure fasting time is unnecessary when using titrated intravenous ketamine for paediatric procedural sedation. *Emerg Med Aust* 2004;16:145-50.

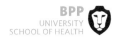
Central venous catheters

Reston N Smith, specialty registrar in anaesthesia and intensive care medicine[1],
Jerry P Nolan, consultant in anaesthesia and intensive care medicine [2]

[1]North Bristol NHS Trust, Bristol, UK

[2]Royal United Hospital NHS Trust, Bath, UK

Correspondence to: J P Nolan jerry.nolan@nhs.net

Cite this as: BMJ 2013;347:f6570

DOI: 10.1136/bmj.f6570

http://www.bmj.com/content/347/bmj.f6570

Central venous catheterisation was first performed in 1929 when Werner Frossman, a German doctor, inserted a ureteric catheter into his antecubital vein. He then walked to the radiography department so that the catheter could be guided into his right ventricle using fluoroscopy. Since then, central venous access has become a mainstay of modern clinical practice. An estimated 200 000 central venous catheters were inserted in the United Kingdom in 1994,[1] and the figure is probably even higher today. Clinicians from most medical disciplines will encounter patients with these catheters. Despite the benefits of central venous lines to patients and clinicians, more than 15% of patients will have a catheter related complication.[2] This review will provide an overview of central venous catheters and insertion techniques, and it will consider the prevention and management of common complications.

What are central venous catheters?

A central venous catheter is a catheter with a tip that lies within the proximal third of the superior vena cava, the right atrium, or the inferior vena cava. Catheters can be inserted through a peripheral vein or a proximal central vein, most commonly the internal jugular, subclavian, or femoral vein.

What are the indications and contraindications to central venous catheterisation?

The indications for central venous catheterisation include access for giving drugs, access for extracorporeal blood circuits, and haemodynamic monitoring and interventions (box 1). Insertion of a catheter solely to measure central venous pressure is becoming less common. A systematic review found a poor correlation between central venous pressure and intravascular volume; neither a single central venous pressure value nor changes in this measurement predicted fluid responsiveness.[3] The need for fluid resuscitation can be evaluated using a test of fluid responsiveness, such as the haemodynamic response to passive leg raising.[4]

Most of the contraindications to central venous catheterisation (box 2) are relative and depend on the indication for insertion.

SOURCES AND SELECTION CRITERIA

We searched the Cochrane Database of Systematic Reviews, Medline, Embase, and Clinical Evidence online. Search terms included central venous catheter, peripherally inserted central catheter, and complication. The reference lists of relevant studies were hand searched to identify other studies of interest. We also consulted relevant reports and national guidelines.

SUMMARY POINTS

- A wide variety of central venous catheters are used
- Complications related to central venous catheters are common and may cause serious morbidity and mortality
- Several strategies can reduce central venous catheter related morbidity; these are implemented at catheter insertion and for the duration of its use
- Peripherally inserted central catheters have the same, or even higher, rate of complications as other central venous catheters

What types of central venous catheter are available and how are they selected?

Four types of central venous catheter are available (table 1): non-tunnelled, tunnelled (fig 1A), peripherally inserted (fig 1C), and totally implantable (fig 2) catheters. Specialist non-tunnelled catheters enable interventions such as intravascular temperature control, continuous monitoring of venous blood oxygen saturation, and the introduction of other intravascular devices (such as pulmonary artery catheters and pacing wires). The catheter type is selected according to the indication for insertion and the predicted duration of use (see table 1).

How are central venous catheters inserted?

Central venous catheters are inserted by practitioners from many different medical specialties and by allied medical practitioners. Someone who is trained and experienced in the technique should be responsible for the line insertion and it should be undertaken in an environment that facilitates asepsis and adequate patient access.

At what anatomical site should I insert the central venous catheter?

The site of insertion depends on several factors: indication for insertion, predicted duration of use, previous line insertion sites (where the veins may be thrombosed or stenosed), and presence of relative contraindications. Ultrasound directed techniques for insertion are now the standard of care in the UK. The site of insertion and indication for the catheter will influence infectious, mechanical, and thrombotic complication rates. A Cochrane systematic review of central venous sites and complications concluded that, in patients with cancer and long term catheters, the risk of catheter related complications was similar for the internal jugular and subclavian routes.[5] For short term central venous catheters, this review concluded that the risk of catheter colonisation (14.2% v 2.2%; relative risk 6.43, 95% confidence interval 1.95 to 21.2) and thrombotic complications (21.6% v 1.9%; 11.53, 2.8 to 47.5) is higher for the femoral route than for the subclavian one.[5]

In contrast, a meta-analysis documented no difference in the risk of infectious complications between the internal jugular, subclavian, and femoral routes.[6] The ease of imaging of the internal jugular vein compared with the subclavian vein has made the first route more popular for short term access. A Cochrane review found that for short term access, for haemodialysis, the femoral and internal jugular sites have similar risks of catheter related complications, although the internal jugular route is associated with a higher rate of mechanical complications.[5] Recent Kidney Disease Improving Global Outcomes (KDIGO) guidelines recommend, in order of preference, the right internal jugular, femoral, left internal jugular, and subclavian veins for insertion of a short term dialysis catheter.[7]

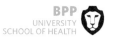
Technique of inserting a cannula into the internal jugular vein

Box 3 describes in detail the technique for inserting a central venous catheter (fig 3).

Skin preparation

The skin is prepared with a solution of 2% chlorhexidine in 70% isopropyl alcohol.[9] A meta-analysis found a reduction in catheter related infections when chlorhexidine is used instead of povidone-iodine.[10] However, a systematic review has highlighted that many of the studies on this topic have compared chlorhexidine in alcohol with aqueous povidone-iodine.[11] The immediate action of alcohol might combine with the more persistent effect of chlorhexidine to produce optimal antisepsis.

Ultrasound guidance

National Institute for Health and Care Excellence (NICE) guidelines recommend using ultrasound guidance for the elective insertion of central venous catheters into the internal jugular vein in adults and children.[12] A meta-analysis indicates that ultrasound guided placement results in lower failure rates, reduced complications, and faster access compared with the landmark technique.[13] Real time imaging of needle passage into the vessel can be performed out of plane (vessel imaged in the transverse plane) or in-plane (vessel imaged in the longitudinal plane). An international expert consensus group concluded that, although no one technique is better than another, a combination of the two may be optimal.[14] The in-plane technique is technically more challenging but enables the position of the tip of the thin walled needle (or cannula) and the wire to be identified precisely (for example, inadvertent penetration of the posterior wall of the vein will be seen clearly). Although ultrasound imaging of the internal jugular and femoral veins is much easier than imaging of the subclavian vein (the view is obscured by the clavicle), ultrasound guided catheterisation of the subclavian vein is possible with the use of a slightly more lateral approach (initially entering the infraclavicular axillary vein).[15][16]

What is the optimal location for the tip of the central venous catheter?

Incorrect placement of the catheter tip increases mechanical and thrombotic complications, but the ideal location of the catheter tip depends on the indications for catheterisation and the site of insertion. No single catheter tip position is ideal for all patients. Patients with cancer are at high risk for developing thrombosis. To reduce rates of thrombosis related to long term catheters in these patients, the catheter tip should lie at the junction of the superior vena cava and right atrium, which is below the pericardial reflection and lower than that recommended for other patients.[17] In other patients, expert opinion suggests that the tip should lie parallel to the wall of a large central vein outside of the pericardial reflection.[8] This reduces the risk of perforation and the risk of cardiac tamponade if perforation occurs. When viewed on a chest radiograph, the catheter tip should be above the level of the carina, which ensures

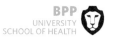

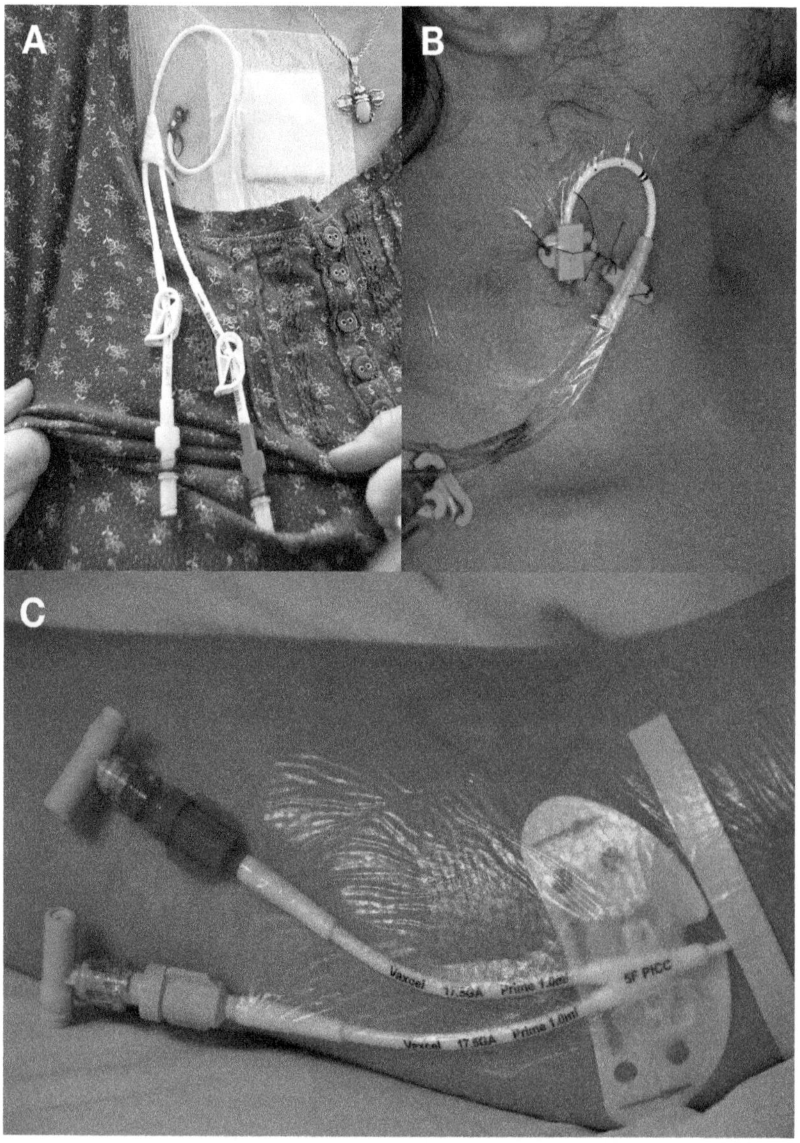

Fig 1 (A) Tunnelled central venous catheter (Hickman line); (B) multi-lumen line in right internal jugular vein secured with sutures and a dressing applied; (C) peripherally inserted central catheter

---

BOX 1 INDICATIONS FOR CENTRAL VENOUS CATHETERISATION

Access for drugs
- Infusion of irritant drugs—for example, chemotherapy
- Total parenteral nutrition
- Poor peripheral access
- Long term administration of drugs, such as antibiotics

Access for extracorporeal blood circuits
- Renal replacement therapy
- Plasma exchange

Monitoring or interventions
- Central venous pressure
- Central venous blood oxygen saturation
- Pulmonary artery pressure
- Temporary transvenous pacing
- Targeted temperature management
- Repeated blood sampling

BOX 2 POTENTIAL CONTRAINDICATIONS TO CENTRAL VENOUS CATHETERISATION
- Coagulopathy
- Thrombocytopenia
- Ipsilateral haemothorax or pneumothorax
- Vessel thrombosis, stenosis, or disruption
- Infection overlying insertion site
- Ipsilateral indwelling central vascular devices

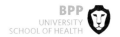

BOX 3 TECHNIQUE OF INSERTING A CENTRAL VENOUS CATHETER INTO THE INTERNAL JUGULAR VEIN

- Explain the procedure to the patient and obtain written informed consent
- Continuously monitor with pulse oximetry (for arterial blood oxygen saturation) and electrocardiography (for early identification of arrhythmias induced by the wire or catheter)
- Using ultrasound, assess the anatomical location and patency of the internal jugular vein (fig 3A and B)
- Place the patient in the Trendelenburg position, with the head slightly rotated to the contralateral side; excess rotation will compress the internal jugular vein, compromising the ability to cannulate the vessel
- Use a strict aseptic technique. After thorough hand washing, put on a sterile gown, gloves, mask, and hat and place a sterile full body drape over the patient. Lay out all equipment on a trolley. Use a sterile ultrasound probe cover and sterile conductive jelly
- Guided by real time ultrasound imaging (ideally, using both in-plane and out of plane views), insert a needle mounted on a syringe into the internal jugular vein (fig 3C)
- Once blood is freely aspirated, set aside the ultrasound probe and remove the syringe from the needle. Blood flow from the needle should be non-pulsatile, but non-pulsatile blood flow does not exclude arterial penetration
- Advance the guide wire through the needle into the vessel, remove the needle, and then confirm the guide wire position with ultrasound imaging (fig 3D). If the guide wire position remains uncertain, insert a short narrow cannula over the wire and into the vessel. Connect the cannula to a transducer system to confirm a venous pressure waveform. Reintroduce the wire through the cannula and then remove the cannula
- If a narrow bore cannula is placed in an artery, remove it and apply pressure. Options for dealing with a large bore catheter introduced into an artery are covered in a recent review.[8] Make a small incision with a scalpel to facilitate the passage of the dilator. Pass the dilator over the wire to a depth a little greater than the predicted vessel depth; this reduces the risk of vessel injury. Maintain control of both the guide wire and dilator at all times
- Remove the dilator. Pass the central venous catheter on to the guide wire and withdraw the guide wire until it protrudes from the end of the catheter
- Advance the catheter into the vessel and remove the guide wire
- Using ultrasound, confirm correct placement of the catheter in the vein
- Secure the catheter and place a dressing over the insertion site
- Obtain a chest radiograph to confirm the location of the catheter tip.

placement above the pericardial sac.[18] High placement of the catheter tip in the superior vena cava increases the risk of thrombosis.[8]

Several techniques can help position the tip correctly during insertion. For short term catheters the insertion depth can be estimated from measurements taken before or during insertion or derived from formulae; alternatively, invasive techniques such as right atrial electrocardiography and transoesophageal echocardiography can be used. Long term catheters are often inserted under radiographic guidance and the catheter tip positioned dynamically.

What are the complications of central venous catheterisation?

Complications are divided into immediate and delayed, then subdivided into mechanical, embolic, and infectious (table 2). Strict attention to insertion technique and correct line-tip positioning reduces the risks of many of the mechanical and embolic complications of catheter insertion. Complications such as air embolism may occur at any point during the lifetime of the line and can be related to poor technique during line insertion, use of the line, or line removal.

Infective complications

The mean central venous catheter bloodstream infection (CVC-BSI) rate documented in a large study of 215 UK intensive care units (ICUs) that submitted data for up to 20 months was 2.0 per 1000 central venous catheter days.[19] In a 2011 UK national point prevalence survey on healthcare associated infections and antimicrobial use, 40% of primary blood stream infections were related to a central venous catheter.[20] An American case-control study of critically ill patients found that nosocomial blood stream infection was associated with increased mortality, length of stay in hospital and intensive care, and economic burden.[21]

What are the clinical signs of line infection?
Clinical signs are unreliable. Fever is the most sensitive clinical finding but is not specific. The presence of inflammation or pus at the catheter exit site is more specific but less sensitive. Consider a diagnosis of CVC-BSI in patients with signs of systemic infection in the absence of another identifiable source or who develop signs of systemic infection after flushing of the line. Box 4 details the laboratory diagnosis of this infection. Maintain a high index of suspicion when blood cultures are positive for organisms associated with central venous catheter infection: *Staphylococcus aureus*, coagulase negative staphylococci, or candida with no other obvious source for bacteraemia.[22]

What are the common causes of central venous catheter infection or colonisation?
Colonisation occurs on the endoluminal or extraluminal surface of the line. Extraluminal colonisation occurs early after line insertion—micro-organisms from the skin colonise the line during insertion or migrate along the catheter tract. Less often, extraluminal colonisation occurs by haematogenous seeding of infection from a distant site. Endoluminal contamination occurs late and is caused by manipulation of the catheter hubs during interventions or more rarely from contamination of infusate. The organisms causing catheter colonisation and infection are most commonly coagulase negative staphylococci (particularly *S epidermidis*), enterococci, *S aureus*, and *Candida* spp.

Table 1 Types of central venous catheter

Type of line	Sites of insertion	Expected duration	Comments	Examples of use
Non-tunnelled	Internal jugular vein, subclavian vein, axillary vein, femoral vein	Short term (several days to 3 weeks)	Line and ports protrude directly from entry site; multi-lumen line	Difficult intravenous access; infusion of irritant drugs, vasopressors, inotropes; short term total parenteral nutrition
Peripherally inserted	Basilic vein, cephalic vein, brachial vein	Medium term (weeks to months)	Line and ports protrude directly from entry site; uncuffed; single, dual, or triple lumen; requires adequate peripheral venous access	Difficult intravenous access; blood sampling; medium term drug administration (for example, antibiotics); administration of irritant drugs (such as chemotherapy); total parenteral nutrition
Tunnelled (for example, Hickmann, Groshong)	Internal jugular vein, subclavian vein	Long term (months to years)	Subcutaneous tunnel from vessel entry site; line access ports sit externally; cuff to reduce line colonisation along tract; the 3 way valve in a Groshong line restricts blood backflow and air embolism	Long term administration of irritant drugs (such as chemotherapy)
Totally implantable (such as implanted port)	Internal jugular vein, subclavian vein	Long term (months to years)	Entire line and port lie subcutaneously; port accessed by non-coring needle; lower rates of CVC-BSIs compared with other central venous catheters	Long term intermittent access (for example, regular hospital admissions with poor intravenous access); administration of irritant drugs (such as chemotherapy)

CVC-BSIs=central venous catheter bloodstream infections.

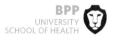

Table 2 Complications of central venous catheterisation

| Immediate complications | | Delayed complications | | |
Mechanical	Thromboembolic	Mechanical	Infectious	Thromboembolic
Arterial puncture	Air embolism	Cardiac tamponade	Catheter colonisation	Catheter related thrombus
Intra-arterial placement of catheter	Wire embolism	Erosion or perforation of vessel	Catheter related bloodstream infection	Pulmonary embolism
Haemorrhage		Venous stenosis		Air embolism
Pneumothorax		Line fracture and embolism		
Haemothorax				
Arrhythmia				
Thoracic duct injury				
Cardiac tamponade				

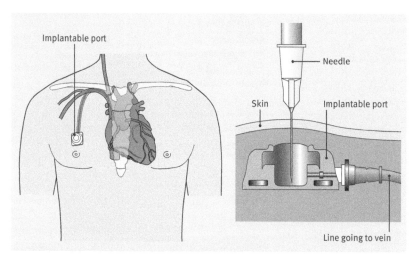

Fig 2 Illustration of a totally implantable central venous catheter

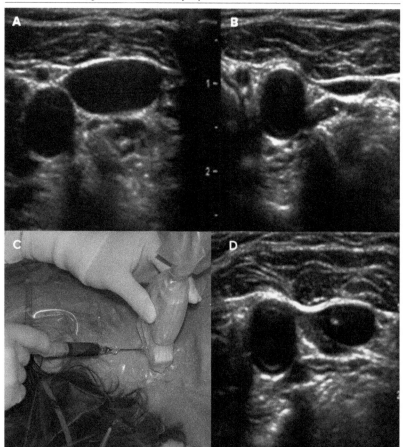

Fig 3 (A) Ultrasound image of the right internal jugular vein (no compression). (B) Ultrasound image of the right internal jugular vein compressed by the probe. (C) Insertion of needle under real time ultrasound guidance (out of plane). (D) Ultrasound image (out of plane) of needle in right internal jugular vein (echogenic (white) spot in centre of vein)

It is not always possible to prove that the central line is the source of infection. For the purposes of research and epidemiological surveillance, two terms are used to describe CVC-BSI (box 4): catheter related bloodstream infection and central line associated bloodstream infection.

Establishing the criteria for catheter related bloodstream infection requires specialist microbiological testing or line removal (box 4). It is often not possible to remove the catheter or gain access to quantitative blood cultures. Unlike catheter related bloodstream infection, central line associated bloodstream infection does not require direct microbiological evidence of line contamination to identify the catheter as the cause, so this diagnosis often overestimates the rate of catheter infection.

Do antimicrobial or antiseptic impregnated catheters reduce the rate of CVC-BSI?
Impregnating the surface of the catheter with antiseptic or antimicrobial substances (such as chlorhexidine and silver sulfadiazine) reduces CVC-BSI. A Cochrane review of the effectiveness of this approach for reducing CVC-BSI in adults included 56 studies and 16 512 catheters with 11 different types of impregnation, bonding, or coating.[23] Catheter impregnation reduced the risk of catheter related bloodstream infections and catheter colonisation. The rate of sepsis or all cause mortality was not reduced, and the benefit of impregnation varied with the clinical setting, being most beneficial in the ICU. The draft epic 3 guidelines recommend that impregnated lines should be used only in patients who are expected to have a catheter in place for more than five days and in units where the CVC-BSI rate remains high despite implementation of a package to reduce it.[24]

Do multi-lumen central venous catheters increase the risk of infection?
A meta-analysis of all the available evidence concluded that multi-lumen catheters may be associated with a slightly higher risk of infection than single lumen ones. However, when only high quality studies (which controlled for patient differences) were considered, there was no increase in infection risk.[25] Therefore, insert a catheter with the minimum number of lumens considered essential for patient care.[24]

Does antibiotic prophylaxis reduce infection rates?
A Cochrane review concluded that prophylactic vancomycin or teicoplanin given before insertion of a tunnelled catheter in patients with cancer did not significantly reduce the number of early Gram positive line infections.[26] A review of 16 randomised controlled trials found insufficient evidence to recommend the routine use of antibiotic lock solutions for preventing CVC-BSI.[27]

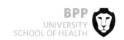
Do not use prophylactic antibiotics before line insertion, antibiotic lock solutions, or antibiotic ointments applied to the insertion site. These strategies do not reduce rates of CVC-BSI and, theoretically, routine use could alter patterns of antimicrobial resistance.

What interventions will reduce infective complications?

There is no evidence that the type of dressing placed over the insertion site influences the rate of catheter related infection. A Cochrane review of two small studies found no difference between gauze and tape versus transparent polyurethane dressings.[28] The draft epic 3 national evidence based guidelines for preventing healthcare associated infections recommend use of a transparent semipermeable polyurethane dressing.[24] If there is bleeding or excessive moisture, a sterile gauze dressing can be used initially and replaced with a transparent dressing when possible. The dressing is not changed unless it is dislodged or there is pooling of fluid or blood under the dressing.

Intraluminal contamination of the catheter occurs through its access sites, so more frequent access through the catheter hub increases the likelihood of microbial contamination. Decontaminate the catheter hub or access port with 2% chlorhexidine in 70% alcohol before and after access.

The catheter can be exchanged over a guide wire or inserted at a different site. Evidence does not support the routine exchange of central venous catheters. A systematic review of exchange techniques showed that guide wire exchange was associated with a reduction in mechanical complications but also an increase in the frequency of catheter colonisation and CVC-BSI; however, none of these associations were significant.[29] Four trials comparing prophylactic catheter exchange at three days versus exchange at seven days, or as needed, found no differences in rates of catheter colonisation or CVC-BSI. Do not guide wire exchange a new catheter through a line that is known to be infected; however, if the risk of mechanical complications related to line insertion is high, and the current catheter is not infected, guide wire replacement is reasonable.

A meta-analysis has shown that daily bathing of ICU patients with chlorhexidine gluconate reduces healthcare related infection and central line associated bloodstream infection,[30] but in our experience this is not common practice in the UK.

The duration that a line should remain in situ before elective exchange or removal is not known. Review the ongoing requirement for a central line daily. Consider removal if it is no longer essential, the catheter is non-functioning, or there is associated infection or thrombosis. The decision to remove the line is made in the context of its clinical indication, the difficulty of establishing further central venous access, and the risk of it remaining in situ.

System based strategies to reduce rates of CVC-BSI

In a collaborative cohort study, implementation of a bundle of evidence based interventions significantly reduced CVC-BSI in 103 ICUs in Michigan, US; the benefit persisted for 18 months.[31] The interventions comprised:

- Hand washing
- Using full barrier precautions during insertion
- Cleaning the skin with chlorhexidine
- Avoiding the femoral site if possible
- Removing unnecessary catheters.

The ICU staff also implemented a daily goals sheet to improve communication between clinicians, an intervention to reduce the incidence of ventilator associated pneumonia, and a comprehensive safety programme to improve the safety culture. The reduction in CVC-BSI was maintained 36 months after implementation of the interventions.[32] Using a similar approach, in the UK, a two year stepped intervention programme (Matching Michigan) was associated with a marked reduction in rates of CVC-BSI in 196 adult ICUs (mean 3.7 CVC-BSIs/1000 catheter patient days in the first cluster to mean 1.48 CVC-BSIs/1000 catheter patient days for all clusters combined; P<0.0001).[19]

What are the risks and complications of central venous catheter related thrombosis?

The presence of a central venous catheter is an independent risk factor for venous thromboembolism,[33] but many of the indications for placement of a catheter are also risk factors for the development of thromboembolism (box 5).

Catheter related thrombosis can be symptomatic or asymptomatic. The thrombus is present on the catheter itself or on the vessel wall. Symptomatic thrombosis is diagnosed with duplex ultrasonography or contrast venography. It is associated with symptoms and signs such as swelling of the affected limb, discomfort, erythema, low grade fever, and dilation of collateral veins. Asymptomatic thrombosis is diagnosed on screening or coincidental imaging in the absence of associated signs or symptoms. Asymptomatic thrombosis may present with line occlusion. Reported rates of catheter related thrombosis vary widely—from 2% to 67%; the incidence of symptomatic catheter related thrombosis is 0-28%.[34]

BOX 4 CRITERIA FOR THE DIAGNOSIS OF CENTRAL VENOUS CATHETER RELATED INFECTIONS (CENTERS FOR DISEASE CONTROL AND PREVENTION (CDC) DEFINITIONS)

Catheter related bloodstream infection*

- Presence of an intravascular device
- Evidence of systemic infection—pyrexia, tachycardia, or hypotension in the absence of another source of infection
- Laboratory evidence that the catheter is the source:
- If the catheter has been removed: quantitative or semiquantitative culture of the catheter
- If the catheter remains in situ: quantitative paired blood cultures (peripheral cultures and cultures drawn from central catheter) or differential time to positivity of paired blood cultures

Central line associated bloodstream infection*

- Evidence of systemic infection
- Central line has been in situ during the 48 hours before blood being cultured
- Laboratory confirmed bloodstream infection on peripheral blood culture
- No evidence of infection from another site

All criteria needed for a diagnosis.

BOX 5 RISK FACTORS FOR CENTRAL VENOUS CATHETER RELATED THROMBOSIS

Patient related factors

- Hypercoagulable state (acute or chronic)
- Cancer
- Cancer treatment
- Age
- Previous deep vein thrombosis

Device related factors

- Line material
- Number of lumens (catheter diameter)
- Position of catheter tip
- Presence of line infection
- Line insertion site

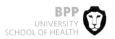

Potential complications of catheter related thrombosis are thromboembolism, interruption of venous flow, line infection, and catheter occlusion. The thrombus may embolise to the right heart or pulmonary circulation. The reported incidence of symptomatic pulmonary embolism is 0-17% in patients with catheter related thrombosis.[34] The thrombus may act as a site for bacterial growth.

The post-thrombotic syndrome is well described in deep vein thrombosis unrelated to central venous catheterisation and is characterised by venous hypertension, swelling, and pain. There is little evidence to establish the risk of the post-thrombotic syndrome and recurrent thrombosis after catheter related thrombosis.

How can catheter related thrombosis be prevented?

The use of prophylactic anticoagulants to prevent catheter related thrombosis has been studied extensively. A Cochrane review of anticoagulation in patients with cancer and a central venous catheter found no significant effect of low dose vitamin K antagonists or low dose unfractionated heparin on mortality, infection, bleeding, or thrombocytopenia.[35]

A meta-analysis of 15 studies (10 of patients with cancer and five of patients receiving long term parenteral nutrition) found that anticoagulant prophylaxis reduced the risk of all catheter related thromboses (symptomatic and asymptomatic) but not the rate of pulmonary embolism or mortality.[36]

On the basis of these data, use of anticoagulant prophylaxis to prevent catheter related thrombosis is not recommended.[17]

How should I treat catheter related thrombosis?

Treatment of catheter related thrombosis includes prevention of complications and management of the central venous catheter. Therapeutic anticoagulation reduces the risk of embolic complications and of the post-thrombotic syndrome, and it prevents recurrent thrombosis. Consider anticoagulation in any patient with a demonstrable deep vein thrombosis on imaging. International evidence based guidelines recommend that patients with cancer and symptomatic catheter related thrombosis are given anticoagulants for three months—low molecular weight heparin or vitamin K antagonists.[17] Thrombolytic treatment has the potential to restore venous patency and catheter patency. Although a Cochrane review found inadequate evidence to support or refute the use of thrombolysis to restore catheter patency, this strategy is commonly used.[37] If the catheter is positioned correctly, functioning, and not infected, it may be left in situ. Remove the catheter if distal limb swelling is not resolving.

Peripherally inserted central catheters

Peripherally inserted central catheters (fig 1C) provide intravenous access for long term antibiotics—particularly for patients with difficult intravenous access and for those receiving intravenous antibiotics in the community—and for parenteral nutrition, chemotherapy, blood products, and blood sampling. They can be left in situ for several months. Their recent popularity probably reflects improved access to this technique delivered at the bedside by dedicated vascular access teams, as well as a belief that these lines combine the advantages of central access with a reduction in the risks associated with traditional central venous catheters. Although these lines are associated with fewer mechanical complications at insertion,[38] a recent systematic review and meta-analysis of 64 studies found that the rates of upper extremity deep vein thrombosis are higher with peripherally inserted central catheters than with central venous catheters.[39] This increase in risk is greatest in critically ill patients and those with cancer.

Two further reviews comparing complication rates with these two types of catheter have challenged the established belief that peripheral lines are safer.[40] [41] The authors of one review concluded that malpositioning of the catheter tip, thrombophlebitis, and catheter dysfunction were more common with these lines than with central venous catheters,[40] and the authors of both reviews conclude that there is no difference in rates of infection associated with either line in hospital inpatients.

Although often considered a safe and convenient solution to difficult intravenous access in the long term, the risks and benefits of peripherally inserted lines must be considered carefully before insertion.

Caring for central venous catheters

Responsibility for the daily care of long term central lines is often delegated to patients and their relatives or carers. Meticulous attention to detail in care will reduce the likelihood of a line related complication. The sterile, transparent, semipermeable dressing is removed weekly, or sooner if it is soiled or not intact. Before replacing the dressing, clean the insertion site with 2% chlorhexidine in 70% alcohol[24]. If the line is not used regularly, aspirate and flush all lumens weekly. To reduce the risk of line infection, patients are advised to shower and not bathe (if bathing, do not submerge the line in water). Swimming is not recommended because the line will be completely submerged. Vigorous physical activity involving the upper body may cause the line to be displaced and should be avoided. Patients with long term central venous catheters with implanted ports are free from all of these restrictions.

ADDITIONAL EDUCATIONAL RESOURCES

Resources for healthcare professionals

- Ortega R, Song M, Hansen CJ, Barash P. Ultrasound-guided internal jugular vein cannulation. *N Engl J Med* 2010;362:e57. Video showing insertion of an internal jugular central venous catheter
- University of West London. Epic 3 national evidence based guidelines for preventing healthcare associated infections. 2013. www.uwl.ac.uk/sites/default/files/Academic-schools/ College-of-Nursing-Midwifery-and-Healthcare/Web/Epic3/ epic3_Consultation_Draft.pdf

Resources for patients

- New South Wales Government, Australia (http:// intensivecare.hsnet.nsw.gov.au/central-venous-lines)— Patient information on central venous lines
- Macmillan (www.macmillan.org.uk/Cancerinformation/ Cancertreatment/Treatmenttypes/Chemotherapy/Linesports/ Centrallines.aspx)—Patient information on tunnelled central lines
- Christie NHS Foundation Trust (www.christie.nhs.uk/ booklets/10.pdf)—A guide for patients and their carers on the care of central venous catheters

---

QUESTIONS FOR FUTURE RESEARCH

- Do peripherally inserted central catheters have a higher rate of complications than traditional central venous catheters?
- Should routine screening be used to detect asymptomatic catheter related thrombosis?
- What is the optimal way to manage asymptomatic catheter related thrombosis?
- What is the optimal technique for ultrasound directed subclavian vein catheterisation?

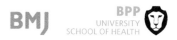

Contributors: All authors helped plan and write this review. JPN is guarantor.

Competing interests: We have read and understood the BMJ Group policy on declaration of interests and declare the following interests: None.

Provenance and peer review: Commissioned; externally peer reviewed.

1 Waghorn DJ. Intravascular device-associated systemic infections: a 2 year analysis of cases in a district general hospital. *J Hosp Infect* 1994;28:91-101.

2 McGee DC, Gould MK. Preventing complications of central venous catheterization. *N Engl J Med* 2003;348:1123-33.

3 Marik PE, Baram M, Vahid B. Does central venous pressure predict fluid responsiveness? A systematic review of the literature and the tale of seven mares. *Chest* 2008;134:172-8.

4 Monet X, Teboul J-L. Passive leg raising. *Intensive Care Med* 2008;34:659-63.

5 Ge X, Cavallazzi R, Li C, Pan SM, Wang YW, Wang FL. Central venous access sites for the prevention of venous thrombosis, stenosis and infection. *Cochrane Database Syst Rev* 2012;3:CD004084.

6 Marik PE, Flemmer M, Harrison W. The risk of catheter-related bloodstream infection with femoral venous catheters as compared to subclavian and internal jugular venous catheters: a systematic review of the literature and meta-analysis. *Crit Care Med* 2012;40:2479-85.

7 Kellum JA. KDIGO clinical practice guideline for acute kidney injury. *Kidney Int Suppl* 2012;2(1).

8 Gibson F, Bodenham A. Misplaced central venous catheters: applied anatomy and practical management. *Br J Anaesth* 2013;110:333-46.

9 Pratt RJ, Pellowe CM, Wilson JA, Loveday HP, Harper PJ, Jones SR, et al. epic2: National evidence-based guidelines for preventing healthcare-associated infections in NHS hospitals in England. *J Hosp Infect* 2007;65(suppl 1):S1-64.

10 Chaiyakunapruk N, Veenstra DL, Lipsky BA, Saint S. Chlorhexidine compared with povidone-iodine solution for vascular catheter-site care: a meta-analysis. *Ann Intern Med* 2002;136:792-801.

11 Maiwald M, Chan ES. The forgotten role of alcohol: a systematic review and meta-analysis of the clinical efficacy and perceived role of chlorhexidine in skin antisepsis. *PloS One* 2012;7:e44277.

12 National Institute for Health and Care Excellence. Guidance on the use of ultrasound locating devices for placing central venous catheters. TA49. 2002. http://guidance.nice.org.uk/TA49.

13 Hind D, Calvert N, McWilliams R, Davidson A, Paisley S, Beverley C, et al. Ultrasonic locating devices for central venous cannulation: meta-analysis. *BMJ* 2003;327:361.

14 Lamperti M, Bodenham AR, Pittiruti M, et al. International evidence-based recommendations on ultrasound-guided vascular access. *Intensive Care Med* 2012;38:1105-17.

15 Sharma A, Bodenham AR, Mallick A. Ultrasound-guided infraclavicular axillary vein cannulation for central venous access. *Br J Anaesth* 2004;93:188-92.

16 Fragou M, Gravvanis A, Dimitriou V, Papalois A, Kouraklis G, Karabibis A, et al. Real-time ultrasound-guided subclavian vein cannulation versus the landmark method in critical care patients: a prospective randomized study. *Crit Care Med* 2011;39:1607-12.

17 Debourdeau P, Farge D, Beckers M, Baglin C, Bauersachs RM, Brenner B, et al. International clinical practice guidelines for the treatment and prophylaxis of thrombosis associated with central venous catheters in patients with cancer. *J Thromb Haemost* 2013;11:71-80.

18 Albrecht K, Nave H, Breitmeier D, Panning B, Troger HD. Applied anatomy of the superior vena cava—the carina as a landmark to guide central venous catheter placement. *Br J Anaesth* 2004;92:75-7.

19 Bion J, Richardson A, Hibbert P, Beer J, Abrusci T, McCutcheon M, et al. "Matching Michigan": a 2-year stepped interventional programme to minimise central venous catheter-blood stream infections in intensive care units in England. *BMJ Qual Safe* 2013;22:110-23.

20 Hopkins S, Shaw K, Simpson L. English national point prevalence survey on healthcare associated infections and antimicrobial use, 2011: preliminary data. Health Protection Agency, 2012. www.hpa.org.uk/webc/hpawebfile/hpaweb_c/1317134304594.

21 Pittet D, Tarara D, Wenzel RP. Nosocomial bloodstream infection in critically ill patients. Excess length of stay, extra costs, and attributable mortality. *JAMA* 1994;271:1598-601.

22 Mermel LA, Allon M, Bouza E, Craven DE, Flynn P, O'Grady NP, et al. Clinical practice guidelines for the diagnosis and management of intravascular catheter-related infection: 2009 update by the Infectious Diseases Society of America. *Clin Infect Dis* 2009;49:1-45.

23 Lai NM, Chaiyakunapruk N, Lai NA, O'Riordan E, Pau WSC, Saint S. Catheter impregnation, coating or bonding for reducing central venous catheter-related infections in adults. *Cochrane Database Syst Rev* 2013;6:CD007878.

24 Loveday HP, Wilson JA, Pratt RJ, Golsorkhi M, Tingle A, Bak A, et al. epic3 National evidence-based guidelines for preventing healthcare-associated infections in NHS hospitals in England. 2013. www.uwl.ac.uk/sites/default/files/Academic-schools/College-of-Nursing-Midwifery-and-Healthcare/Web/Epic3/epic3_Consultation_Draft.pdf.

25 Dezfulian C, Lavelle J, Nallamothu BK, Kaufman SR, Saint S. Rates of infection for single-lumen versus multilumen central venous catheters: a meta-analysis. *Crit Care Med* 2003;31:2385-90.

26 Van de Wetering MD, van Woensel JB. Prophylactic antibiotics for preventing early central venous catheter Gram positive infections in oncology patients. *Cochrane Database Syst Rev* 2007;1:CD003295.

27 Snaterse M, Ruger W, Scholte Op Reimer WJ, Lucas C. Antibiotic-based catheter lock solutions for prevention of catheter-related bloodstream infection: a systematic review of randomised controlled trials. *J Hosp Infect* 2010;75:1-11.

28 Webster J, Gillies D, O'Riordan E, Sherriff KL, Rickard CM. Gauze and tape and transparent polyurethane dressings for central venous catheters. *Cochrane Database Syst Rev* 2011;11:CD003827.

29 Cook D, Randolph A, Kernerman P, Cupido C, King D, Soukup C, et al. Central venous catheter replacement strategies: a systematic review of the literature. *Crit Care Med* 1997;25:1417-24.

30 O'Horo JC, Silva GL, Munoz-Price LS, Safdar N. The efficacy of daily bathing with chlorhexidine for reducing healthcare-associated bloodstream infections: a meta-analysis. *Infect Control Hosp Epidemiol* 2012;33:257-67.

31 Pronovost P, Needham D, Berenholtz S, Sinopoli D, Chu H, Cosgrove S, et al. An intervention to decrease catheter-related bloodstream infections in the ICU. *N Engl J Med* 2006;355:2725-32.

32 Pronovost PJ, Goeschel CA, Colantuoni E, Watson S, Lubomski LH, Berenholtz SM, et al. Sustaining reductions in catheter related bloodstream infections in Michigan intensive care units: observational study. *BMJ* 2010;340:c309.

33 Shivakumar SP, Anderson DR, Couban S. Catheter-associated thrombosis in patients with malignancy. *J Clin Oncol* 2009;27:4858-64.

34 Rooden CJ, Tesselaar ME, Osanto S, Rosendaal FR, Huisman MV. Deep vein thrombosis associated with central venous catheters—a review. *J Thromb Haemostas* 2005;3:2409-19.

35 Akl EA, Vasireddi SR, Gunukula S, Yosuico VED, Barba M, Sperati F, et al. Anticoagulation for patients with cancer and central venous catheters. *Cochrane Database Syst Rev* 2011;4:CD006468.

36 Kirkpatrick A, Rathbun S, Whitsett T, Raskob G. Prevention of central venous catheter-associated thrombosis: a meta-analysis. *Am J Med* 2007;120:901e1-13.

37 Van Miert C, Hill R, Jones L. Interventions for restoring patency of occluded central venous catheter lumens. *Cochrane Database Syst Rev* 2012;4:CD007119.

38 Gallieni M, Pittiruti M, Biffi R. Vascular access in oncology patients. *CA Cancer J Clin* 2008;58:323-46.

39 Chopra V, Anand S, Hickner A, Buist M, Rogers MAM, Saint S, et al. Risk of venous thromboembolism associated with peripherally inserted central catheters: a systematic review and meta-analysis. *Lancet* 2013;382:311-25.

40 Pikwer A, Akeson J, Lindgren S. Complications associated with peripheral or central routes for central venous cannulation. *Anaesthesia* 2012;67:65-71.

41 Chopra V, Anand S, Krein SL, Chenoweth C, Saint S. Bloodstream infection, venous thrombosis, and peripherally inserted central catheters: reappraising the evidence. *Am J Med* 2012;125:733-41.

Related links

bmj.com/archive
Previous articles in this series
- The diagnosis and management of gastric cancer (BMJ 2013;347:f6367)
- Management of nocturnal enuresis (BMJ 2013;347:f6259)
- An introduction to advance care planning in practice (BMJ 2013;347:f6064)
- Post-mastectomy breast reconstruction (BMJ 2013;347:f5903)
- Identifying brain tumours in children and young adults (BMJ 2013;347:f5844)

bmj.com
- Get Cleveland Clinic CME credits for this article

BMJ

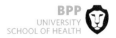

Management of paracetamol poisoning

Robin E Ferner, honorary professor of clinical pharmacology[12],
James W Dear, consultant clinical pharmacologist[34],
D Nicholas Bateman, professor of clinical toxicology[3]

[1]West Midlands Centre for Adverse Drug Reactions, City Hospital, Birmingham, UK

[2]School of Clinical and Experimental Medicine, College of Medical and Dental Sciences, University of Birmingham, Birmingham, UK

[3]National Poisons Information Service, Royal Infirmary of Edinburgh, Edinburgh EH16 4SA, UK

[4]University/BHF Centre for Cardiovascular Science, Edinburgh University, Queen's Medical Research Institute, Edinburgh, UK

Correspondence to: D N Bateman
nick.bateman@luht.scot.nhs.uk

Cite this as: BMJ 2011;342:d2218

DOI: 10.1136/bmj.d2218

http://www.bmj.com/content/342/bmj.d2218

Paracetamol (acetaminophen) is an effective oral analgesic, with few adverse effects when used at the recommended dose. Nevertheless, paracetamol poisoning is common and potentially fatal.[1] It is a leading cause of acute liver failure in the United Kingdom[2] and the United States.[3] Potential liver damage, predicted from blood paracetamol concentration and time from ingestion, can be prevented by prompt treatment with antidote. However, young and otherwise healthy patients still risk serious liver injury, especially if they present more than a few hours after overdose or take staggered overdoses over hours or days.[4]

How does paracetamol cause damage and who is at risk?

The recommended therapeutic dosage of paracetamol depends on age (table 1). Therapeutic doses of paracetamol are mainly metabolised by conjugation to inactive metabolites. Paracetamol predominantly damages the liver.[6] The reactive metabolite, N-acetyl-p-benzoquinoneimine (NAPQI), formed when paracetamol is oxidised by the cytochrome P450 enzyme family, is the key to hepatic injury. NAPQI binds covalently to sulphydryl groups, which can be provided by glutathione; but when glutathione stores are depleted NAPQI binds to cellular proteins (fig 1). Toxicity is therefore affected by the rate of enzyme catalysed formation of NAPQI, which can be induced by several drugs and chronic alcoholism, and by the availability of glutathione, which depends crucially on nutritional status. Thus, some patients are more susceptible than others to liver injury from paracetamol ingestion—box 1 lists the risk factors. After covalent binding of NAPQI to cellular proteins, cell injury is mediated by free radicals. An inflammatory response follows cell death and may determine the outcome once liver injury is established.[7]

Serious liver damage after a single 75 mg/kg body weight dose of paracetamol is rare, even in patients at increased risk. In patients without risk factors, a dose less than 150 mg/kg body weight is unlikely to cause serious liver damage.[5]

Severe paracetamol induced liver injury can be associated with renal failure.[8] Isolated renal dysfunction occurs only rarely, and mostly in patients with glutathione depletion, or those who have taken nephrotoxic compounds as well, become dehydrated, or have pre-existing renal insufficiency.[4]

How do patients with paracetamol overdose present?

Many patients who present do so within a few hours of taking an overdose, when symptoms and signs are absent or confined to nausea and vomiting. Lactic acidosis and coma can, exceptionally, occur soon after ingestion of massive amounts of paracetamol.[9] Their presence usually implies mixed overdose. Right upper quadrant tenderness is common in patients presenting with established liver damage. Patients who present after 24 hours may already have signs of liver failure—hepatic tenderness, jaundice, impaired consciousness, asterixis, foetor hepaticus, and haemorrhage. Overt liver failure can, however, be delayed for two or three days. It is important not to overlook paracetamol in those who have signs suggesting overdose with another agent.

How should the patient with suspected paracetamol poisoning be investigated?

The history is crucial in patients who do not yet have liver failure because it determines the risk of serious liver damage, and hence treatment strategy. Ascertain the dose and timing of ingestion, and whether a patient may be more susceptible than average to the toxic effects of paracetamol (box 1).

Dose of paracetamol

After a single overdose, the patient may be able to say how many tablets have been taken. Difficulties arise if the tablets have been taken over a period, or if the patient is unable or unwilling to give the relevant information.

Time of ingestion

Knowing the time of tablet ingestion is crucial for calculating whether treatment with antidote is needed. Because it takes some time to swallow a substantial number of tablets, take the start of ingestion as the relevant time if all tablets were taken during a period shorter than one hour, otherwise treat as a staggered overdose. In cases of staggered overdose, more than one supratherapeutic dose, or if the patient has been poisoned with an intravenous or modified release formulation,[10] decisions regarding treatment are more difficult.

Physical examination

As well as eliciting signs of liver damage from paracetamol, the examination may indicate that the patient is more susceptible to developing such damage (see box 1)—for example, because the patient is malnourished.[11] It may also identify an antecedent liver disorder.

SOURCES AND SELECTION CRITERIA

We based our review on a PubMed search for articles on paracetamol (or acetaminophen) and acetylcysteine or (N-acetylcysteine) published between 1 January 1990 and 31 December 2010, without language limits. The search was limited to human clinical trials, meta-analyses, randomised controlled trials, reviews, and case reports. We also searched a newspaper database for reports published after 1988 of coroners' inquests and procurators' fiscal inquiries into fatal cases of paracetamol poisoning. In addition, we used a bibliography and our own collections of relevant references.[5]

SUMMARY POINTS

- Patients still die from paracetamol poisoning because they are not recognised to be at risk of harm or present too late for effective treatment
- Patients who are malnourished, have been fasting, take enzyme inducing drugs, or regularly drink alcohol to excess are at higher risk of liver damage
- Treat patients who have ingested too much paracetamol within eight hours of ingestion whenever possible
- If the time of ingestion is known, treatment can be based on blood tests taken after four hours
- If the timing is uncertain or unknown, treatment should be started immediately in all patients who are at potential risk
- Treat patients as high risk unless factors that increase risk of harm are known to be absent

Investigation

The crucial investigations are the timed serum paracetamol concentration, to determine risk of liver damage, and tests of liver function (including prothrombin time or international normalised ratio) and kidney function. These tests are needed to assess risk and monitor progress. Prognosis is worse if they are abnormal at presentation.[4][12] Paracetamol concentration in venous blood should be measured between four and 16 hours after ingestion of a single dose to allow the patient's risk to be determined from the standard nomograms (discussed below). Values obtained earlier than four hours cannot be interpreted because absorption is not yet complete. Values taken after 16 hours may be high because of acute liver injury that delays paracetamol metabolism,[13] or falsely reassuring, even though irreversible liver damage has already occurred. In untreated patients with negative tests for paracetamol and normal hepatic and renal function 24 hours after exposure, serious harm is unlikely.

Ketones on urinalysis and low blood urea concentration can indicate starvation or poor nutrition, which increases the risk of liver damage. Raised γ-glutamyl transpeptidase activity is a potentially useful indicator of hepatic enzyme induction.

What is the initial approach to treatment?

Out of hospital treatment

Treatment depends on adequate assessment, first aid measures, and transfer of at risk patients for antidotal treatment. Activated charcoal taken soon after overdose should reduce absorption of paracetamol.[14] It is unlikely to help more than an hour after overdose.[15]

Acetylcysteine

The mainstay of treatment for patients who have taken a potentially toxic dose of paracetamol is the antidote acetylcysteine, which is a sulphydryl donor.[16] It is given intravenously in three sequential infusions, each containing a different dose of antidote, and is based on the patient's body weight (up to a maximum dose equivalent to a weight of 110 kg) (table 2).

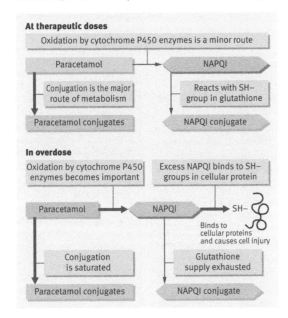

Fig 1 At therapeutic doses, paracetamol is mainly metabolised by conjugation to inactive metabolites. A reactive metabolite, N-acetyl-p-benzoquinoneimine (NAPQI), is formed by oxidation. When a large dose of paracetamol is taken, more NAPQI is formed, sulphation conjugation pathways are saturated, and NAPQI binds covalently to sulphydryl (SH-) groups. These can be provided by glutathione, but when hepatic glutathione stores are depleted, NAPQI binds to cellular proteins and causes cell injury

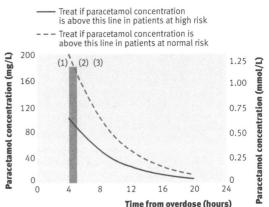

Fig 2 The graph shows how a relatively small inaccuracy in timing could result in the wrong course of action. Paracetamol concentration is shown on the y axes (as both mg/L (left hand axis) and mmol/L (right hand axis)) and time from overdose on the x axis for patients at high risk (lower line) and normal risk (upper line). In this example, the sample is thought to have been taken at four hours (1) after overdose, in which case no treatment would be needed (in a patient at normal risk). If, however, the wrong time had been given and the sample had actually been taken at five hours (2) after overdose—and more clearly if had been taken at eight hours (3)—it would require treatment

Table 1 Recommended maximum doses of paracetamol

Patients	Maximum single dose	Minimum dosing interval (hours)	Maximum dose in 24 hours
Adults	1 g	4	4 g
Children 6-12 years	500 mg	4	2 g
Children 1-5 years	240 mg	4	960 mg
Infants 3-12 months	120 mg	4	480 mg

Table 2 Recommended doses of acetylcysteine as antidote to paracetamol poisoning in adults. Adapted from the summary of product characteristics for Parvolex[17]

Recommended sequential doses*	Dose according to patient's weight		
	70 kg	110 kg	140 kg†
150 mg/kg in 200 mL over first 0.25 hours	10.5 g	16.5 g	16.5 g
50 mg/kg over next 4 hours in 500 mL	3.5 g	5.5 g	5.5 g
100 mg/kg over next 16 hours in 1000 mL	7 g	11 g	11 g
Total dose (300 mg/kg in 20 hours)	21 g	33 g	33 g

*Acetylcysteine in glucose 5% solution.
†A ceiling weight of 110 kg is recommended when calculating the dosage for obese patients.

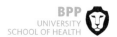

Acetylcysteine replenishes glutathione stores, which at least partly explains its antidotal efficacy. A large multicentre study of efficacy published in 1988 found that the antidote is uniformly effective if given within eight hours of a single overdose, but subsequently its efficacy falls.[18] A controlled trial provided evidence that acetylcysteine can improve outcome even in patients with encephalopathy,[19] so those who present more than eight hours after overdose are still treated with the antidote if they are deemed at risk of liver damage or if liver function is already abnormal.

A retrospective cohort study of more than 4000 patients showed that intravenous treatment is at least as effective as oral treatment but takes less time to administer.[20] Intravenous treatment can be administered reliably even if the patient is vomiting.

Findings from animal studies suggest that the alternative sulphydryl donor methionine is less effective than acetylcysteine.[21]

The treatment nomogram

Decisions to treat paracetamol overdose with acetylcysteine are based on an assessment of the risk of serious liver damage. The treatment nomogram, originally derived from a study of just 32 patients, separates those who will develop serious hepatotoxicity (transaminase activity >1000 U/L) from those who will not on the basis of a graph of paracetamol concentration against time from ingestion as it falls from 200 mg/L at four hours (the "200" line) (fig 2).[13] Healthcare professionals can consult their poisons information service (in the UK and Ireland: www.toxbase.org/) for treatment recommendations.

In the US, Australia, and New Zealand a similar semi-logarithmic plot at paracetamol concentrations 25% lower (the "150" line) is used to permit a wider margin of error.[22][23] Some patients reportedly come to harm even if the paracetamol concentration falls below the 200 or 150 lines.[24] An appreciation of the factors that increased the risk of liver damage led to the introduction in the UK of a second (high risk) line, running from 100 mg/L at four hours after ingestion (fig 2). We strongly advise that all patients be treated according to the high risk line unless factors that increase the risk of harm (box 1) are known to be absent.

BOX 1 FACTORS THAT INCREASE THE RISK OF LIVER INJURY AFTER AN OVERDOSE OF PARACETAMOL

- High chance of glutathione depletion:
- Malnourished (for example, not eating because of dental pain or fasting for more than a day)
- Eating disorders (anorexia or bulimia)
- Failure to thrive or cystic fibrosis in children
- AIDS
- Cachexia
- Alcoholism
- Clinical clues: history, low body mass index, urinalysis positive for ketones, low serum urea concentration
- Hepatic enzyme induction:
- Long term treatment with enzyme inducing drugs, such as carbamazepine, phenobarbital, phenytoin, primidone, rifampicin, rifabutin, efavirenz, nevirapine, and St John's wort
- Regular consumption of ethanol in excess of recommended amounts
- Clinical clues: history, abnormal liver function tests, increased international normalised ratio, increased γ-glutamyl transpeptidase
- Abnormal renal or hepatic function at presentation

BOX 2 CRITERIA FOR POSSIBLE LIVER TRANSPLANTATION*[30]

- Arterial pH less than 7.3
- Hepatic encephalopathy grade III or IV and serum creatinine concentration >300 µmol/L and prothrombin time >100 seconds
- Arterial lactate concentration >3.5 mmol/L on admission or >3.0 mol/L 24 hours after paracetamol ingestion or after fluid resuscitation

It is best to discuss transplantation with a liver transplant unit as soon as the possible need is identified

---

BOX 3 CASE SCENARIO 1

A 19 year old woman with a rare syndrome, which meant she weighed just five and a half stone (35 kg) and was only four feet tall, was admitted to a neurology ward. She was prescribed intravenous paracetamol 1 g, when the correct (weight adjusted) dose was 525 mg. She received a total of 20 doses. When she developed fatal liver failure as a result, this was initially ascribed to Reye's syndrome. (*Evening Times (Glasgow)* 2010 September 17; http://news.stv.tv/scotland/west-central/186253-doctor-tells-court-of-battle-to-save-danielle-welsh/)

BOX 4 CASE SCENARIOS 2 AND 3

A 72 year old woman died after taking capsules of Lemsip Max cold relief as well as her prescribed paracetamol. She was taking the daily dose of paracetamol for pain and had been mixing it with the Lemsip Max for about a week—almost doubling her normal dose. After the court hearing, her husband urged people to read the labels carefully and called for large warnings about the dangers of paracetamol overdose to be printed on the front of packets. "[My wife] knew too much paracetamol was dangerous but she did not realise there was paracetamol in Lemsip. If you go into a chemist and ask for something the first thing they ask is if you are taking any medication. But if you go into a supermarket there is no proper dispensary counter and the people at the check-out don't know anything about it." (This is Bradford 2004 July 21.) A 43 year old woman with a history of polymyositis was prescribed a paracetamol based painkiller known as Kapake by her general practitioner for a dental abscess, but she was also taking standard paracetamol tablets. She was admitted to hospital with a suspected recurrence of the polymyositis, but tests showed she had serious liver damage, from which she later died. (This is Lancashire 2004 November 23.)

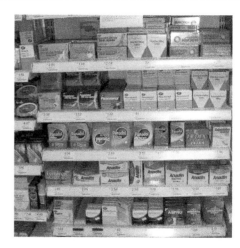

Fig 3 A wide range of branded products on open sale, many of which contain paracetamol. Mistakes can be made when estimating the risk of hepatic damage after paracetamol overdose. Whenever risk assessment is difficult or uncertain, we recommend that the patient is taken to be at high risk

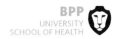

The risk assessment nomogram requires the time from ingestion to be known with reasonable accuracy (fig 2). The efficacy of the antidote declines from about eight hours after overdose, so it is important not to delay treatment of potentially poisoned patients beyond eight hours even if the paracetamol concentration is not known. The nomogram is misleading or unhelpful if the overdose was repeated or staggered, if the exact timing is unclear, or if the patient received an intravenous preparation, because the pharmacokinetics of such preparations are different. In these circumstances, the initial treatment decision has to be based on the total dose, taking any risk factors into account; subsequently, abnormalities in renal and hepatic function tests will guide treatment.

Treating adverse events related to acetylcysteine

Acetylcysteine is sulphurous and commonly causes vomiting when given by mouth or nausea when given intravenously. It can also provoke an anaphylactoid reaction, which is mediated by histamine and depends on blood acetylcysteine concentrations. Such reactions may be more common in patients with asthma, those with a family history of drug allergy, and women.[25] Almost all reactions can be treated effectively by interrupting the acetylcysteine infusion and providing symptomatic relief with an antihistamine such as chlorphenamine and nebulised salbutamol if needed. In severe reactions where the patient becomes haemodynamically unstable resuscitation may be needed. Once the reaction has subsided, however, ensure that the entire dose of acetylcysteine is given in due course, possibly at a slower rate of infusion (for example, at a rate of 50 mg/kg/h).

Acetylcysteine has, very rarely, been associated with fatal adverse reactions; some reported cases have been caused by miscalculation of the dose, which has led to overdose with the antidote.[26]

The risk of an anaphylactoid reaction is higher in patients with lower plasma concentrations of paracetamol[27]; this suggests that treating patients who are unlikely to benefit from the antidote may increase the frequency of adverse reactions. Neither cost-benefit analysis,[28] nor experience in Denmark,[29] supports a policy of universal treatment with acetylcysteine.

What supportive treatment should be given?

Fluid replacement and symptomatic treatment for nausea and vomiting are often needed. When acute liver failure has already occurred, or seems likely, intensive supportive treatment and—in the appropriate circumstances—liver transplantation will be needed. A transplant is most likely to be successful if the need for one is identified early, so swift referral is important (box 2).

How to manage the patient after administering the antidote

Liver damage can be detected by measuring international normalised ratio, serum creatinine concentration, and liver function at the end of acetylcysteine treatment; some units also measure paracetamol concentration because appreciable concentrations can indicate a risk of continuing damage. UK guidelines, which have extrapolated from the study of acetylcysteine in encephalopathy,[16] suggest that if the international normalised ratio exceeds 1.3, or transaminases have increased to more than double baseline values, then the antidote should continue to be infused at a dose of 100 mg/kg over 16 hours until results are acceptable. Patients with renal dysfunction after paracetamol poisoning require ongoing monitoring and may need renal support.

Why do patients still die from paracetamol poisoning?

Most deaths in the UK occur because patients present to hospital too late for the antidote to be effective. The diagnosis of paracetamol poisoning may be missed in patients who take a dose only slightly higher than therapeutic but have one or several factors that increase the risk of hepatotoxicity (box 3), when drug errors occur,[9] and in patients who have inadvertently taken more than the recommended dose of paracetamol in two or more different preparations containing paracetamol (box 4; fig 3). Paracetamol poisoning may also be missed in patients who have taken a mixed overdose and are unconscious, because unconsciousness is rare in paracetamol poisoning.

Mistakes can be made when estimating the risk of hepatic damage after paracetamol overdose.[31] Whenever risk assessment is difficult or uncertain, we recommend that the patient is assumed to be at high risk.

Treatment errors can occur when paracetamol concentrations are misunderstood. The cardinal measurement in ascertaining risk is the timed plasma paracetamol concentration. Patients have died when doctors have thought that results quoted in mmol/L are actually in mg/L (151 mg=1 mmol) and have therefore withheld acetylcysteine.[32] The acetylcysteine regimen is complex, and errors are common.[33] Errors also arise when absorption of paracetamol is delayed because co-ingestion of a drug such as codeine or an anticholinergic antihistamine has slowed gastric emptying and thus delayed absorption of paracetamol, or a modified release formulation has been taken. In such circumstances, toxic paracetamol concentrations may be reached much longer than four hours after overdose.[34]

Patients also come to harm when non-immunological adverse reactions to acetylcysteine are interpreted as anaphylaxis and the antidote is withheld.

Areas of uncertainty

The optimal dosage of acetylcysteine and the appropriate dose adjustment for body weight remain unclear and are difficult to study in patients. Because the initial rapid infusion seems to cause most adverse effects, some people advocate giving the loading dose over one hour, although this is of no confirmed benefit.[35]

Better indicators of prognosis both at presentation and as a warning of impending liver failure, and more secure criteria for liver transplantation, are needed.[30]

Drugs that prevent mitochondrial injury[36] and drugs that target key inflammatory mediators[7] have been shown to prevent injury from paracetamol in experimental models and represent potential new therapeutic targets.

ADDITIONAL EDUCATIONAL RESOURCES

Resources for healthcare professionals

- TOXBASE e-learning site (www.toxbase.co.uk/)—An e-learning resource for NHS and public health staff on Toxbase and the clinical management of poisoned patients
- BMJ Learning (http://learning.bmj.com/learning/channel-home.html)—Includes an update of the management of paracetamol overdose
- WiKi Tox (http://curriculum.toxicology.wikispaces.net/)—Provides a set of resources that can be used as tools to learn or teach clinical toxicology
- National Institute for Health and Clinical Excellence (www.nice.org.uk/Guidance/CG16)—National UK guideline on self harm

Resources for patients

- X-PIL. (http://xpil.medicines.org.uk/)—Product information leaflets: give advice on quantities of paracetamol in over the counter preparations
- Samaritans (www.samaritans.org/) and MIND (www.mind.org.uk/)—Both organisations provide information to patients and relatives on self harm

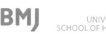

Contributors: The article was originally conceived by REF and DNB. All authors helped search the literature, structure the article, and draft the article. All have seen and approved the final manuscript. REF and DNB are guarantors.

Competing interests: All authors have completed the Unified Competing Interest form at www.icmje.org/coi_disclosure.pdf (available on request from the corresponding author) and declare: no support from any organisation for the submitted work; no financial relationships with any organisations that might have an interest in the submitted work in the previous three years; REF and DNB are members of the Pharmacovigilance Expert Advisory Group of the Commission for Human Medicines, and JWD and DNB are consultants to the National Poisons Information Service.

Provenance and peer review: Not commissioned; externally peer reviewed.

1   Bronstein AC, Spyker DA, Cantilena LR Jr, Green JL, Rumack BH, Giffin SL. 2009 Annual Report of the American Association of Poison Control Centers' national poison data system (NPDS): 27th annual report. *Clin Toxicol (Phila)* 2010;48:979-1178.
2   Khan LR, Oniscu GC, Powell JJ. Long-term outcome following liver transplantation for paracetamol overdose. *Transpl Int* 2010;23:524-9.
3   Larson AM, Polson J, Fontana RJ, Davern TJ, Lalani E, Hynan LS, et al. Acetaminophen-induced acute liver failure: results of a United States multicenter, prospective study. *Hepatology* 2005;42:1364-72.
4   Pakravan N, Simpson K, Waring WS, Bates CM, Bateman DN. Renal injury at first presentation as a predictor for poor outcome in severe paracetamol poisoning referred to a liver transplant unit. *Eur J Clin Pharmacol* 2009;65:163-8.
5   Prescott LF. Paracetamol (acetaminophen): a critical bibliographic review. 2nd ed. Taylor & Francis. 2001:587-88.
6   Hinson JA, Roberts DW, James LP. Mechanisms of acetaminophen-induced liver necrosis. *Handb Exp Pharmacol* 2010;196:369-405.
7   Imaeda AB, Watanabe A, Sohail MA, Mahmood S, Mohamadnejad M, Sutterwala FS, et al. Acetaminophen-induced hepatotoxicity in mice is dependent on Tlr9 and the Nalp3 inflammasome. *J Clin Invest* 2009;119:305-14.
8   Jones AF, Vale JA. Paracetamol poisoning and the kidney. *J Clin Pharm Ther* 1993;18:5-8.
9   Shah AD, Wood DM, Dargan PI. Understanding lactic acidosis in paracetamol (acetaminophen) poisoning. *Br J Clin Pharmacol* 2010;71:20-8.
10 Beringer RM, Thompson JP, Parry S, Stoddart PA. Intravenous paracetamol overdose: two case reports and a change to national treatment guidelines. *Arch Dis Child* 2011;96:307-8.
11 Fernando WK, Ariyananda PL. Paracetamol poisoning below toxic level causing liver damage in a fasting adult. *Ceylon Med J* 2009;54:16-7.
12 Green TJ, Sivilotti ML, Langmann C, Yarema M, Juurlink D, Burns MJ, et al. When do the aminotransferases rise after acute acetaminophen overdose? *Clin Toxicol (Phila)* 2010;48:787-92.
13 Prescott LF, Roscoe P, Wright N, Brown S. Plasma paracetamol half-life and hepatic necrosis in patients with paracetamol overdosage. *Lancet* 1971;1:519-22.
14 Teece S, Hogg K. Best evidence topic reports. Gastric lavage in paracetamol poisoning. *Emerg Med J* 2004;21:75-6.
15 Chyka PA, Seger D, Krenzelok EP, Vale JA. Position paper: single-dose activated charcoal. *Clin Toxicol (Phila)* 2005;43:61-87.
16 Prescott LF, Illingworth RN, Critchley JA, Stewart MJ, Adam RD, Proudfoot AT. Intravenous N-acetylcystine: the treatment of choice for paracetamol poisoning. *BMJ* 1979;2:1097-100.
17 eMC. Summary of product characteristics. Parvolex 200 mg/ml concentrate for solution for infusion. 2011. www.medicines.org.uk/EMC/medicine/1127/SPC/Parvolex+200+mg+ml+Concentrate+for+Solution+for+Infusion/.
18 Smilkstein MJ, Knapp GL, Kulig KW, Rumack BH. Efficacy of oral N-acetylcysteine in the treatment of acetaminophen overdose. Analysis of the national multicenter study (1976 to 1985). *N Engl J Med* 1988;319:1557-62.
19 Keays R, Harrison PM, Wendon JA, Forbes A, Gove C, Alexander GJ, et al. Intravenous acetylcysteine in paracetamol induced fulminant hepatic failure: a prospective controlled trial. *BMJ* 1991;303:1026-9.
20 Yarema MC, Johnson DW, Berlin RJ, Sivilotti ML, Nettel-Aguirre A, Brant RF, et al. Comparison of the 20-hour intravenous and 72-hour oral acetylcysteine protocols for the treatment of acute acetaminophen poisoning. *Ann Emerg Med* 2009;54:606-14.
21 Boobis AR, Tee LB, Hampden CE, Davies DS. Freshly isolated hepatocytes as a model for studying the toxicity of paracetamol. *Food Chem Toxicol* 1986;24:731-6.
22 Rumack BH, Matthew H. Acetaminophen poisoning and toxicity. *Pediatrics* 1975;55:871-6.
23 Daly FF, Fountain JS, Murray L, Graudins A, Buckley NA. Guidelines for the management of paracetamol poisoning in Australia and New Zealand—explanation and elaboration. A consensus statement from clinical toxicologists consulting to the Australasian poisons information centres. *Med J Aust* 2008;188:296-301.
24 Bridger S, Henderson K, Glucksman E, Ellis AJ, Henry JA, Williams R. Deaths from low dose paracetamol poisoning. *BMJ* 1998;316:1724-5.
25 Sandilands EA, Bateman DN. Adverse reactions associated with acetylcysteine. *Clin Toxicol (Phila)* 2009;47:81-8.
26 Mant T, Tempowski J, Volans G, Talbot J. Adverse reactions to acetylcysteine and effects of overdose. *BMJ* 1984;289:217-9.
27 Waring WS, Stephen AF, Robinson OD, Dow MA, Pettie JM. Lower incidence of anaphylactoid reactions to N-acetylcysteine in patients with high acetaminophen concentrations after overdose. *Clin Toxicol (Phila)* 2008;46:496-500.
28 Beer C, Pakravan N, Hudson M, Smith LT, Simpson K, Bateman DN, et al. Liver unit admission following paracetamol overdose with concentrations below current UK treatment thresholds. *QJM* 2007;100:93-6.
29 Dalhoff K, Gesser K, Rasmussen M. Should you treat every paracetamol-poisoned patient? *Clin Toxicol (Phila)* 2009;47:440.
30 Craig DG, Ford AC, Hayes PC, Simpson KJ. Systematic review: prognostic tests of paracetamol-induced acute liver failure. *Aliment Pharmacol Ther* 2010;31:1064-76.
31 Pearce B, Grant IS. Acute liver failure following therapeutic paracetamol administration in patients with muscular dystrophies. *Anaesthesia* 2008;63:89-91.
32 Flanagan RJ, de Wolff FA, Mills IM. Principles, practice and paracetamol: when units matter. *Ann Clin Biochem* 2000;37:16-9.
33 Ferner RE, Langford NJ, Anton C, Hutchings A, Bateman DN, Routledge PA. Random and systematic medication errors in routine clinical practice: a multicentre study of infusions, using acetylcysteine as an example. *Br J Clin Pharmacol* 2001;52:573-7.
34 Tighe TV, Walter FG. Delayed toxic acetaminophen level after initial four hour nontoxic level. *J Toxicol Clin Toxicol* 1994;32:431-4.
35 Kerr F, Dawson A, Whyte IM, Buckley N, Murray L, Graudins A, et al. The Australasian Clinical Toxicology Investigators Collaboration randomized trial of different loading infusion rates of N-acetylcysteine. *Ann Emerg Med* 2005;45:402-8.
36 Reid AB, Kurten RC, McCullough SS, Brock RW, Hinson JA. Mechanisms of acetaminophen-induced hepatotoxicity: role of oxidative stress and mitochondrial permeability transition in freshly isolated mouse hepatocytes. *J Pharmacol Exp Ther* 2005;312:509-16.

Related links

bmj.com/archive
- The challenge of managing coexistent type 2 diabetes and obesity (2011;342:d1996)
- Post-acute care and secondary prevention after ischaemic stroke (2011;342:d2083)
- Diagnosis and management of transient ischaemic attack and ischaemic stroke in the acute phase (2011;342:d1938)
- Investigation and management of unintentional weight loss in older adults (2011;342:d1732)

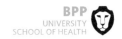

Hyperkalaemia

Moffat J Nyirenda, MRC clinician scientist/honorary consultant physician[1],
Justin I Tang, research fellow[1],
Paul L Padfield, professor of hypertension[2],
Jonathan R Seckl, professor of molecular medicine[1]

[1]Endocrinology Unit, Centre for Cardiovascular Science, Queen's Medical Research Institute, University of Edinburgh, Edinburgh EH16 4TJ

[2]Metabolic Unit, Western General Hospital, Lothian University Hospitals NHS Trust, Edinburgh

Correspondence to: M Nyirenda
m.nyirenda@ed.ac.uk

Cite this as: BMJ 2009;339:b4114

DOI: 10.1136/bmj.b4114

http://www.bmj.com/content/339/bmj.b4114

Hyperkalaemia is defined as serum potassium concentration greater than 5.5 mmol/l. Its prevalence in the general population is unknown, but it is thought to occur in 1-10% of patients admitted to hospital.[1] The rate of morbidity and mortality associated with hyperkalaemia has risen greatly with the use of drugs that target the renin-angiotensin system, and since publication 10 years ago of a randomised trial that showed that adding an aldosterone receptor antagonist to usual treatment for congestive failure improved outcomes.[2] [3] [4] [5]

Potassium is the most abundant cation in the human body and has key roles in the excitatory properties needed for conduction of nerve impulses and muscle contraction. Ninety eight per cent of the body's potassium is in the intracellular fluid (concentration about 140 mmol/l), with only 2% in extracellular fluid (3.8-5.0 mmol/l). A complex interplay of regulatory mechanisms is needed to maintain normal potassium balance, which involves the transfer of potassium between the extracellular and intracellular compartments (fig 1). In the long term potassium homoeostasis is mainly governed by regulation of renal potassium excretion, notably by the actions of aldosterone (fig 2). These mechanisms ensure that although total daily potassium intake could range from 40 mmol to 200 mmol per day, potassium levels in serum remain within the relatively narrow normal range. Derangements in potassium regulation, and resultant changes in serum potassium concentration, may alter membrane excitability. Disorders of plasma potassium can therefore have profound effects on nerve, muscle, and cardiac function.

What are the common causes of hyperkalaemia?

Multiple factors are often involved in the pathogenesis of hyperkalaemia, which commonly results from decreased potassium excretion or increased release of potassium from cells.[6] Hyperkalaemia can be spurious, and this possibility should be excluded first, except in severe cases when immediate treatment is needed.

Spurious hyperkalaemia

Spurious hyperkalaemia (also called pseudohyperkalaemia) occurs when the reported laboratory potassium values do not reflect actual in vivo concentrations—usually because platelets, leucocytes, or erythrocytes have released intracellular potassium in vitro. It can be excluded by

SOURCES AND SELECTION CRITERIA

We searched PubMed for articles whose titles included the terms "hyperkalaemia" or "potassium homoeostasis" and restricted the search to articles published in English in the past 15 years. We also searched contemporary textbooks.

sending a new sample for analysis or by simultaneously measuring potassium in plasma and serum; serum potassium concentration is usually 0.2-0.4 mmol/l higher than that in plasma, owing to release during normal clotting. Box 1 lists common causes of spurious hyperkalaemia.

Hyperkalaemia due to increased potassium intake

Excessive dietary intake of potassium is an uncommon cause of hyperkalaemia, unless concurrent decreased excretion is a factor. High potassium intake should be avoided in patients with compromised renal function. Box 2 lists foods rich in potassium. Hyperkalaemia can also occur with blood transfusion (due to release of potassium from haemolysis), when intravenous potassium is administered too rapidly in treatment of hypokalaemia, or when total parenteral nutrition contains high concentrations of potassium.

Hyperkalaemia caused by shift of potassium out of cells

Several endogenous and exogenous factors can affect transfer of potassium between the extracellular and intracellular fluid to raise the concentration in serum. However, this mechanism is rarely the sole cause of severe hyperkalaemia, except when excessive release of intracellular potassium occurs with tissue injury or necrosis—for example, in rhabdomyolysis, tumour lysis, and severe burns. Box 3 shows causes of hyperkalaemia due to potassium redistribution.

Hyperkalaemia caused by reduced excretion of potassium

The kidneys are the main route of potassium elimination, and renal failure is the major cause of hyperkalaemia, accounting for up to 75% of cases of severe hyperkalaemia.[1] In patients with chronic kidney disease, the capacity to excrete potassium is reasonably well maintained until renal failure is advanced (glomerular filtration rate <15-20 ml/min); until then hyperkalaemia is not usually seen unless intake of potassium is high or the patient is taking a drug that promotes hyperkalaemia.

Damage to the juxtaglomerular apparatus with resulting deficit in renin production can cause hyporeninaemic hypoaldosteronism, which can also cause hyperkalaemia in the absence of severe renal failure. Hyporeninaemic hypoaldosteronism is also known as type 4 renal tubular acidosis because it is often, but not always, associated with mild to moderate metabolic acidosis with a normal anion gap. Diabetic nephropathy is the most common underlying cause. Hypoaldosteronism can also be caused by primary disorders of the adrenal gland (such as Addison's disease or congenital steroidogenic enzyme defects, most commonly 21 hydroxylase deficiency) or by reduced mineralocorticoid activity due to

---

SUMMARY POINTS

- Hyperkalaemia is usually caused by a combination of factors, but renal failure and drugs are often implicated
- Increased use of drugs that interact with the renin-angiotensin-aldosterone system has caused the prevalence of hyperkalaemia to rise
- Hyperkalaemia can cause life threatening cardiac arrhythmias and should be urgently managed
- ECG changes correlate poorly with the degree of potassium disturbance

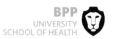

resistance to the action of aldosterone action in the kidney. The latter problem is often seen in sickle cell anaemia, systemic lupus erythematosus, amyloidosis, and obstructive nephropathy or with use of potassium sparing diuretics. In rare cases, it is caused by mutations of the gene encoding the mineralocorticoid receptor or its major downstream targets, including the epithelial sodium channel ENaC.

In general, an abnormality in mineralocorticoid level by itself does not produce hyperkaelemia if sufficient amount of sodium is delivered to the distal nephron. Thus, patients with Addison's disease do not usually exhibit hyperkalaemia if they have adequate salt intake; it is only when sodium intake is restricted or they otherwise become volume depleted that hyperkalaemia develops. Disturbances of urinary flow rate or delivery of sodium to the distal

nephron are therefore also important in the pathogenesis of hyperkalaemia. These defects can be intrinsic or (more commonly) caused by drugs (box 3, box 4).

Which drugs cause hyperkalaemia?

Drugs can interfere with potassium homoeostasis by promoting transcellular potassium shift or by impairing renal potassium excretion (for example, through effects on aldosterone action, sodium delivery to the distal nephron, or function of collecting tubules).[1][3][6] In a prospective study of 242 consecutive patients admitted with hyperkalaemia, 63% were taking drugs that interfere with potassium balance.[1] The risk of hyperkalaemia is particularly great when such drugs are given to patients with underlying renal insufficiency. The elderly and patients with diabetes are especially susceptible. Doctors should therefore prescribe such drugs with caution in these populations; it is best to start with low doses and to recheck serum potassium within a week of starting the drug, and with each increase in dose. There are no consensus guidelines as to what constitutes timely follow-up, but the frequency with which serum potassium is monitored will depend on the level of renal impairment, the presence of diabetes, and concurrent use of other hyperkalaemia inducing medications. Particular caution should be exercised in patients with underlying cardiac conduction defects, in whom even minor increases in serum potassium can precipitate severe arrhythmias. A comprehensive list of drugs associated with hyperkalaemia is given in box 4. We will briefly discuss some of the most commonly prescribed ones.

Angiotensin converting enzyme (ACE) inhibitors and angiotensin II receptor blockers (ARBs) are increasingly used for renoprotection and to reduce cardiovascular mortality in patients at high risk, particularly those with diabetes. They also are standard treatment in the management of patients with chronic heart failure. ACE inhibitors and ARBs predispose to hyperkalaemia because they impair aldosterone secretion and reduce renal perfusion (and thus glomerular filtration rate), both of which decrease excretion

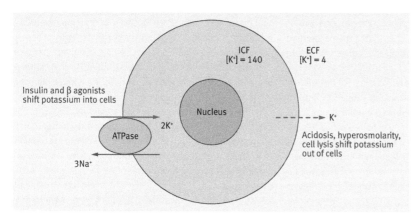

Fig 1 Schematic representation of regulation of transcellular potassium movement. Cellular potassium concentration is controlled by an active uptake mechanism regulated by Na-K-ATPase and a passive leak mechanism driven by the electrochemical gradient favouring potassium exit from the cell. The rate of leak is dependent on the permeability of the potassium channels in the cell membrane. Insulin and β_2 adrenergic agonists (acting via cyclic AMP) promote potassium uptake into cells by stimulating the Na-K-ATPase pump. Insulin deficiency and β blockers increase potassium movement out of cells leading to hyperkalaemia. Acidosis, hyperosmolarity, or cell lysis also cause potassium to leave cells and can cause hyperkalaemia. ECF=extracelluar fluid; ICF=intracellular fluid.

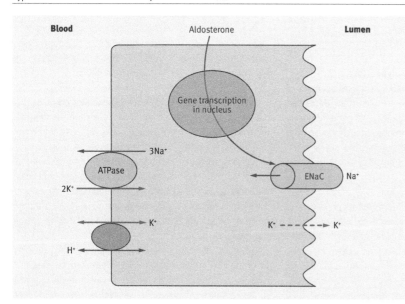

Fig 2 Schematic representation of mineralocorticoid action in target cell in renal cortical collecting duct. On entering the cell, aldosterone binds to the mineralocorticoid receptors (MR). The ligand-receptor complex translocates to the nucleus and binds to hormone response elements, increasing transcription of specific genes, which in turn signal to increase activities of apical sodium channels (ENaC) and the basolateral Na-K-ATPase. This leads to increased intracellular potassium concentration and a greater diffusion gradient for potassium to diffuse into the lumen. Increased uptake of sodium leads to more negative lumen charge, facilitating the diffusion of potassium into the lumen. Disorders of aldosterone action are common causes of hyperkalaemia. Renal potassium excretion is also affected by urine flow rate and delivery of sodium to the distal nephron.

BOX 1 CAUSES OF SPURIOUS HYPERKALAEMIA

- Laboratory error
- Delayed analysis
- Blood collected from vein into which potassium is infused
- Excessive tourniquet or repeated fist clenching
- Haemolysis via small needle or traumatic venepuncture
- Prolonged storage of blood
- Severe leucocytosis or thrombocytosis
- Uncommon genetic disorders (familial pseudohyperkalaemia)

BOX 2 FOODS WITH HIGH POTASSIUM CONTENT

- Salt substitutes
- Figs
- Molasses
- Seaweed
- Chocolates
- Bran cereal, wheat germ
- Vegetables (such as spinach, tomatoes, mushrooms, carrots, potatoes, broccoli, lima beans, cauliflower)
- Dried fruit, nuts, and seeds
- Fruits (such as banana, kiwi fruit, orange, mango, cantaloupe)

Adapted from the National Kidney Foundation website (www.kidney.org/ news/newsroom/fs_new/potassiumCKD.cfm)

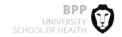

of potassium by the kidneys. However, in general, they do not cause hyperkalaemia in patients with normal renal function; indeed, the degree of aldosterone suppression is usually not sufficient to substantially impair potassium excretion unless pre-existing hypoaldosteronism from other causes (disease state or from other drugs) is present. Unfortunately, most patients targeted for renovascular benefits of these drugs (such as those with diabetes, renal failure, or heart failure) are at high risk of developing hyperkalaemia. About 10% of outpatients develop hyperkalaemia within a year of starting treatment with ACE inhibitors or ARBs.[1][3][7][8] Moreover, these drugs contribute to hyperkalaemia in 10-38% of patients admitted to hospital with the condition, with the risk increasing substantially when higher doses are used or when they are used in combination or with other hyperkalaemia inducing drugs.[5]

Aldosterone (mineralocorticoid) receptor antagonists are also commonly prescribed to treat patients with congestive cardiac failure since the Randomized Aldactone Evaluation Study showed that the addition of spironolactone to standard treatment is associated with significant reduction in morbidity and mortality.[2] Serious hyperkalaemia occurred in only 2% of patients in the study, where the average serum creatinine concentration was 106 μmol/l and the dose of spironolactone did not exceed 25 mg daily. By contrast, population based time-series analyses have demonstrated significant increases in rates of hospitalisation and mortality from hyperkalaemia.[4][9][10] This is probably because these studies included patients with more severe renal dysfunction who were given higher doses of spironolactone. These patients were also more likely than those in the clinical trial to be taking potassium supplements or other drugs that impair potassium excretion. The risk was highest in patients who took spironolactone in combination with ACE inhibitors or ARBs, particularly in elderly patients with renal failure.[11][12]

Non-steroidal anti-inflammatory drugs (NSAIDs) inhibit renin secretion (leading to hypoaldosteronism and reduced potassium excretion) and can impair renal function. These agents should be prescribed judiciously in patients with diabetes or renal insufficiency, particularly if they are concurrently receiving ACE inhibitors or ARBs.[13]

How is hyperkalaemia diagnosed?

Hyperkalaemia is often asymptomatic and discovered on routine laboratory tests. When symptoms are present, they are non-specific and predominantly related to muscular function (paresthesiae, muscle weakness, fatigue) or cardiac function (palpitations). Hyperkalaemia may produce progressive abnormalities on the electrocardiogram (ECG), including peaked T waves, flattening or absence of P waves, widening of QRS complexes, and sine waves (fig 3).[14] However, electrocardiography is not a sensitive method for detecting hyperkalaemia. In a study by Acer and colleagues nearly half the patients with serum potassium concentration greater than 6.5 mmol/l did not have ECG changes.[1] Moreover, whereas some patients show gradual progression in changes, others progress from benign to potentially fatal ventricular arrhythmias without warning.

Assessment of a patient with hyperkalaemia should include a thorough review of the medical history to identify potential contributing factors such as renal failure, diabetes, adrenal insufficiency, and use of drugs that cause hyperkalaemia. Laboratory blood tests should be directed towards causes suggested by the history and physical examination, and should include urea, creatinine, electrolytes, and serum osmolarity (acute increase in osmolarity can cause potassium to exit from cells). Analysis of urine potassium concentrations could help to ascertain whether renal potassium elimination is appropriate. In selected patients, additional specialised tests such as measurement of the fractional excretion of potassium or transtubular potassium gradient may be useful in distinguishing between renal and non-renal causes of hyperkalaemia.[15]

BOX 3 CAUSES OF HYPERKALAEMIA

Potassium redistribution (intracellular to extracellular fluid)
- Exercise
- Tissue necrosis or lysis (rhabdomyolysis, tumour lysis syndrome, severe burns)
- Insulin deficiency
- Metabolic acidosis (especially with mineral acids)
- Hyperosmolarity (hyperglycaemia, mannitol infusion)
- Drugs (for example, succinylcholine, β blockers, digoxin toxicity)
- Hyperkalaemic periodic paralysis

Decreased excretion of potassium
- Renal failure (glomerular filtration rate <20 ml/min)
- Decreased mineralocorticoid activity
- Hyporeninaemic hypoaldosteronism (chronic renal failure, diabetic nephropathy, NSAIDs)
- Adrenal insufficiency (Addison's disease, congenital enzyme defects)
- Aldosterone blocking drugs (see box 4)
- End organ unresponsiveness to aldosterone (sickle cell anaemia, systemic lupus erythematosus, amyloidosis, and obstructive nephropathy)

Decreased urine flow rate or sodium delivery to distal nephron
- Severe volume contraction
- Rare genetic disorders, such as Gordon's syndrome

BOX 4 DRUG INDUCED HYPERKALAEMIA

Drugs that alter transmembrane potassium movement
- β blockers
- Digoxin
- Hyperosmolar solutions (mannitol, glucose)
- Suxamethonium
- Intravenous cationic amino acids

Potassium containing agents
- Potassium supplements
- Salt substitutes
- Herbal medicines (such as alfalfa, dandelion, horsetail, milkweed, and nettle)
- Stored red blood cells (haemolysis releases potassium)

Drugs that reduce aldosterone secretion
- ACE inhibitors
- Angiotensin II receptor blockers
- NSAIDs
- Heparins
- Antifungals (ketoconazole, fluconazole, itraconazole)
- Ciclosporin
- Tacrolimus

Drugs that block aldosterone binding to mineralocorticoid receptor
- Spironolactone
- Eplerenone
- Drospirenone

Drugs that inhibit activity of epithelial sodium channel
- Potassium sparing diuretics (amiloride, triamterene)
- Trimethoprim
- Pentamidine

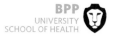

How is severe hyperkalaemia managed?

Guidelines for treatment of hyperkalaemia are based on consensus or expert opinion because of a lack of controlled clinical trials.[16] Treatment should be aimed at restoring normal potassium balance, preventing serious complications, and treating the underlying causes. Figure 4 shows a general approach in management of patients with hyperkalaemia.

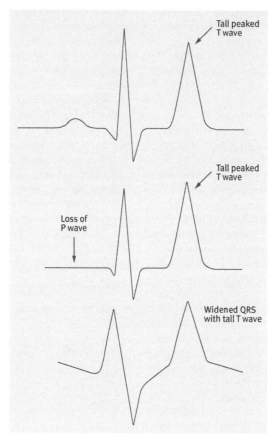

Fig 3 ECG changes in patients with hyperkalaemia[14]

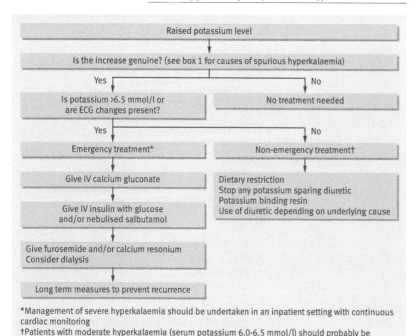

*Management of severe hyperkalaemia should be undertaken in an inpatient setting with continuous cardiac monitoring

†Patients with moderate hyperkalaemia (serum potassium 6.0-6.5 mmol/l) should probably be admitted to hospital for supervised lowering of serum potassium

Fig 4 Algorithm for diagnosis of hyperkaelemia. IV=intravenous.

Mild to moderate hyperkalaemia can be treated with a loop diuretic to increase urinary potassium excretion. Dietary potassium is restricted and hyperkalaemic drugs should be minimised or withdrawn. If a patient has renal failure a diuretic may not be effective and other measures, including dialysis, may be needed.

Severe hyperkalaemia is a life threatening state because it can cause catastrophic cardiac and neuromuscular effects, such as cardiac arrest and paralysis of the respiratory muscles. Therefore prompt and aggressive treatment is necessary. Most authorities consider that serum potassium concentration of greater than 6.0 mmol/l with ECG changes, or greater than 6.5 mmol/l regardless of the ECG, represents severe hyperkalaemia that warrants urgent treatment.[17] [18] If the patient's ECG suggests hyperkalaemia, or in a clinical scenario such as cardiac arrest in a patient having chronic dialysis, for example, therapy is frequently started without waiting for laboratory confirmation. Other factors that might necessitate pre-emptive treatment of hyperkalaemia include a rapid rise of serum potassium, the presence of significant acidosis, and rapid deterioration in renal function.

Most guidelines and experts advise that severe hyperkalaemia should be treated in an inpatient setting to allow continuous cardiac monitoring, because even patients without symptoms or ECG changes can swiftly develop life threatening arrhythmias. Although urgent dialysis to remove potassium from the body would be the definitive treatment, delays in starting this treatment are inevitable. A 2005 Cochrane systematic review of emergency interventions for hyperkalaemia recommended that immediate temporising treatment incorporates three key measures.[19]

The first step is to stabilise the myocardium to reduce its susceptibility to ventricular arrhythmias. Intravenous calcium is used to directly antagonise the membrane effects of hyperkalaemia, stabilising cardiac conduction. Calcium gluconate in a volume of 10 ml of 10% solution is infused over 3–5 minutes with cardiac monitoring. Calcium infusion does not affect serum potassium level, but beneficial ECG changes can be seen after 1-3 minutes of administration and the effect can last for 30-60 minutes. The infusion can be repeated if no effect is seen within 5-10 minutes. Caution should be exercised when replacing calcium in patients taking digoxin because calcium potentiates myocardial toxicity to digoxin.[20]

The second step is to shift potassium from the extracellular to the intracellular fluid compartment so as to rapidly decrease serum potassium. This shift is achieved by administration of insulin or β2 agonist, both of which stimulate the Na+/K+ pump. Insulin is given as an intravenous bolus along with sufficient glucose to prevent development of hypoglycaemia (usually 10 units of insulin with 50 ml of 50% dextrose given over 5 minutes). The hypokalaemic effect of this treatment can be seen within 20 minutes, peaking between 30 and 60 minutes, and it may last for 6 hours. Salbutamol is the most commonly used selective β2 agonist. It is usually given through a nebuliser (10-20 mg in 4 ml of saline). An effect may be seen in 30 minutes, with maximum effect at 90–120 minutes. Salbutamol can be used alone or to augment the effect of insulin. Patients with acidosis may also be treated with intravenous sodium bicarbonate (500 ml of a 1.26% solution [75 mmol] over 60 minutes) although the benefit is uncertain and routine bicarbonate treatment for hyperkalaemia remains controversial.[18] [21]

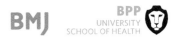

Thirdly, further interventions are undertaken to remove potassium from the body. Potent loop diuretics (for example, 40-80 mg of intravenous furosemide) enhance renal potassium excretion by increasing urine flow and sodium delivery to the distal nephron. However, diuretics only work if the patient has adequate renal function, and many patients with hyperkalaemia have acute or chronic renal failure. Cation exchange resins, which remove potassium from extracellular fluid via the gut in exchange for sodium, are also commonly used, although their effectiveness is debatable.[22] They act more quickly when given as enemas (for example, calcium resonium 30 g) than when given orally (15 g four time a day); it may take 6 hours to achieve a full effect. Dialysis is the definitive treatment for patients with severe hyperkalaemia and advanced chronic kidney disease.

Long term management of hyperkalaemia

After acute treatment, measures should be established to prevent recurrence of hyperkalaemia. The first step is to carefully review the patient's medication and to avoid or minimise drugs that increase potassium retention. Because ACE inhibitors and ARBs slow the progression of chronic renal disease, use of other measures to control the hyperkalaemia or dose reduction are preferable to discontinuing these drugs. Dietary advice to restrict potassium intake to 40-60 mmol a day is prudent. Diuretics may be effective in promoting renal potassium loss to prevent recurrence of hyperkalaemia. Thiazide diuretics may be used in patients with preserved renal function, but are usually ineffective when the glomerular filtration rate is less than 40 ml/min, when a loop diuretic such as furosemide is preferable. Fludrocortisone may be used in patients with hyporeninaemic hypoaldosteronism. However, this drug can cause fluid retention and hypertension, and should be used with caution—particularly in patients with type 2 diabetes, who often have co-existing hypertension.

Contributors: MJN wrote the first draft. All authors took part in researching and writing the paper. MJN edited the final manuscript and is guarantor.

Competing interests: None declared.

Provenance and peer review: Commissioned, externally peer reviewed.

---

1 Acker CG, Johnson JP, Palevsky PM, Greenberg A. Hyperkalemia in hospitalized patients: causes, adequacy of treatment, and results of an attempt to improve physician compliance with published therapy guidelines. *Arch Intern Med* 1998;158:917-24.
2 Pitt B, Zannad F, Remme WJ, Cody R, Castaigne A, Perez A, et al. The effect of spironolactone on morbidity and mortality in patients with severe heart failure. *N Engl J Med* 1999;341:709-17.
3 Perazella MA. Drug-induced hyperkalemia: old culprits and new offenders. *Am J Med* 2000;109:307-14.
4 Juurlink DN, Mamdani MM, Lee DS, Kopp A, Austin PC, Laupacis A, et al. Rates of hyperkalemia after publication of the randomized aldactone evaluation study. *N Engl J Med* 2004;351:543-51.
5 Yusuf S, Teo KK, Pogue J, Dyal L, Copland I, Schumacher H, et al. Telmisartan, ramipril, or both in patients at high risk for vascular events. *N Engl J Med* 2008;358:1547-59.
6 Hollander-Rodriguez JC, Calvert JF Jr. Hyperkalemia. *Am Fam Physician* 2006;73:283-90.
7 Ahuja T, Freeman D Jr, Mahnken JD, Agraharkar M, Siddiqui M, Memon A. Predictors of the development of hyperkalemia in patients using angiotensin-converting enzyme inhibitors. *Am J Nephrol* 2000;20:268-72.
8 Reardon LC, Macpherson DS. Hyperkalemia in outpatients using angiotensin-converting enzyme inhibitors. *Arch Intern Med* 1998;158:26-32.
9 Cruz CS, Cruz AA, Marcilio de Souza CA. Hyperkalemia in congestive heart failure patients using ACE inhibitors and spironolactone. *Nephrol Dial Transplant* 2003;18:1814-9.
10 Bozkurt B, Agoston I, Knowlton AA. Complications of inappropriate use of spironolactone in heart failure: when an old medicine spirals out of new guidelines. *J Am Coll Cardiol* 2003;41:211-4.
11 Svensson M, Gustafsson F, Galatius S, Hildebrandt PR, Atar D. How prevalent is hyperkalemia and renal dysfunction during treatment with spironolactone in patients with congestive heart failure? *J Card Fail* 2004;10:297-303.
12 Navaneethan SD, Nigwekar SU, Sehgal AR, Strippoli GF. Aldosterone antagonists for preventing the progression of chronic kidney disease. *Cochrane Database Syst Rev* 2009;(3):CD007004.
13 Perazella MA, Tray K. Selective cyclooxygenase-2 inhibitors: a pattern of nephrotoxicity similar to traditional nonsteroidal anti-inflammatory drugs. *Am J Med* 2001;111:64-7.
14 Slovis C, Jenkins R. ABC of clinical electrocardiography: conditions not primarily affecting the heart. *BMJ* 2002;324:1320-3.
15 Ethier JH, Kamel KS, Magner PO, Lemann J, Halperin ML. The transtubular potassium concentration in patients with hypokalemia and hyperkalemia. *Am J Kid Dis* 1990;4:309-15.
16 Kim H-J, Han S-W. Therapeutic approach to hyperkalaemia *Nephron* 2002;92(suppl 1):33-40.
17 Charytan D, Goldfarb DS. Indications for hospitalization of patients with hyperkalemia. *Arch Intern Med* 2000;160:1605-11.
18 Greenberg A. Hyperkalaemia: treatment options. *Semin Nephrol* 1998;18:46-57.
19 Mahoney BA, Smith WA, Lo DS, Tsoi K, Tonelli M, Clase CM. Emergency interventions for hyperkalaemia. *Cochrane Database Syst Rev* 2005;(2):CD003235.
20 Davey M. Calcium for hyperkalemia in digoxin toxicity. *Emerg Med J* 2002;19:183.
21 Allon M, Shanklin N. Effect of bicarbonate administration on plasma potassium in dialysis patients: interactions with insulin and albuterol. *Am J Kidney Dis* 1996;28:508-14.
22 Kamel KS, Wei C. Controversial issues in the treatment of hyperkalaemia. *Nephrol Dial Transplant* 2003;18:2215-8.

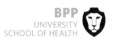

Managing anaemia in critically ill adults

Timothy S Walsh, professor of critical care[1], Duncan LA Wyncoll, consultant in critical care[2],
Simon J Stanworth, consultant haematologist[3]

[1]Royal Infirmary of Edinburgh, Edinburgh EH16 2SA

[2]Guy's and St Thomas' NHS Foundation Trust, London SE1 7EH

[3]NHS Blood and Transplant, Oxford Radcliffe Hospitals Trust, Oxford OX3 9BQ

Correspondence to: T S Walsh twalsh@staffmail.ed.ac.uk

Cite this as: BMJ 2010;341:c4408

DOI: 10.1136/bmj.c4408

http://www.bmj.com/content/341/bmj.c4408

Anaemia (haemoglobin <120 g/l for women, and <130 g/l for men) is common in acutely unwell patients. Maintaining sufficient oxygen transport to the tissues is fundamental to survival and recovery from acute illness, and in the United Kingdom 8-10% of the blood supply is used to treat patients in intensive care.[1] Red blood cells transport more than 97% of the oxygen content of blood—about 200 ml/l—and anaemia greatly reduces oxygen delivery, especially if patients also have cardiovascular and respiratory compromise.[2]

Transfusion of donor (allogeneic) red blood cells is the standard method for rapidly correcting anaemia in acutely unwell patients, but the risk-benefit balance of this intervention is a subject of continuing debate, controversy, and concern.[3] We highlight uncertainties in the management of anaemia in critically ill patients, especially in relation to the use of red cells, and summarise current evidence from observational studies and randomised trials. We focus on the management of anaemia in critically ill patients without active bleeding, such as those who are in adult medical and surgical intensive care units, high dependency units, and other acute units. We do not discuss the management of patients with major haemorrhage, for which recent evidence is available elsewhere.[w1-w3]

How common is anaemia in patients with critical illness?

Observational studies have shown that anaemia affects 60-80% of patients cared for in intensive care units, and 50-70% develop moderate to severe anaemia (haemoglobin concentration <90 g/l) during their stay.[4][5] Most patients have a normochromic, normocytic anaemia with high ferritin concentrations and low serum iron, transferrin, and transferrin saturation.[5][6] Only 10-15% of patients have a history of chronic anaemia before admission to intensive care, which highlights the importance of acute factors in its development.[7][8]

SOURCES AND SELECTION CRITERIA

We searched randomised controlled trials and systematic reviews identified by the Systematic Reviews Initiative, NHS Blood and Transplant, Oxford (updated December 2009), which includes the Cochrane Library, Medline, Embase, and the SRI Systematic Review Handsearch Database. We supplemented this with searches of Medline and Embase using the terms "intensive care" or "critical care" and "blood transfusion" or "anaemia". We also reviewed recently published clinical guidelines and searched for current transfusion related trials on clinicaltrials.gov and the ISRCTN register.

SUMMARY POINTS

- Acute anaemia is common in critically ill patients
- Several factors, including blood sampling and reduced red cell production associated with systemic inflammation, can contribute to anaemia
- The risk-benefit profile for red cell transfusions to treat anaemia in non-bleeding critically ill adults is uncertain, but they may contribute to adverse patient outcomes in some situations
- Best evidence suggests that using single unit red cell transfusions when haemoglobin is close to 70 g/l and aiming for a haemoglobin of 70-90 g/l is not harmful in most patients
- Aiming for a haemoglobin nearer to 90-100 g/l might be better for patients with acute cardiac disease and the early stages of severe sepsis

Why do critically ill patients become anaemic?

Unless modified by blood transfusions, haemoglobin values typically decrease by about 5 g/l/day during critical illness,[9] and 20-50% of critically ill patients receive transfusions.[4][5] Box 1 lists the factors that contribute to anaemia during critical illness. In individual patients several factors usually contribute in varying degrees. When intravenous fluids are given plasma volume expands and the haemoglobin concentration decreases without a major change in red cell mass. This is important to consider when resuscitating a patient (fig 1). Blood sampling typically results in the loss of 30-60 ml of blood each day,[7] and loss from artificial circuits, such as haemofiltration circuits, or occult loss may increase daily losses.[10] Several high quality observational studies have shown impaired erythropoiesis during critical illness. The healthy response to acute blood loss, the reticulocyte response, is usually absent,[11] probably because of the failure of the kidneys to increase erythropoietin production and a hyporeactive bone marrow.[10][w4][w5] These biochemical characteristics are almost identical to the anaemia of chronic disease, which suggests that they result from systemic inflammation.[5][11][12] Absolute iron deficiency is rare, but many patients have a functional iron deficiency from redistribution of iron into macrophages and reticuloendothelial cells, which may limit availability of iron for red cell production. Inflammation makes iron studies difficult to interpret. Reduced red cell survival is likely in critically ill patients, especially those with sepsis, because red cells become less deformable as a result of oxidative damage and cell membrane changes.[13]

Are there risks associated with blood transfusions?

Observational studies have found it difficult to measure clinical benefit from red cell transfusion in patients with acute severe illness and have often found higher complication rates in transfused patients than in otherwise similar patients who received fewer or no transfusions.[2][4] These studies found associations between receiving red cells and a range of adverse outcomes including higher rates of hospital acquired infections, organ dysfunction, longer stays in the intensive care unit and hospital, and increased mortality.[14] However, observational studies are open to confounding bias because patients who are more severely ill are more likely to die and also more likely to be transfused, so the association between transfusion and mortality may not be causal.[6]

Several small randomised trials have explored the relation between red cell transfusion and complications, but most were inconclusive. The largest randomised trial to compare different haemoglobin transfusion "triggers" (the Transfusion Requirements In Critical Care, TRICC trial, described below) found that using red cells more restrictively was at least as effective as a more liberal approach.[15] It found a trend towards lower mortality in patients managed with a restrictive approach, especially if they were younger or less severely unwell, and patients in the liberally transfused group had higher rates of organ dysfunction and cardiac complications.

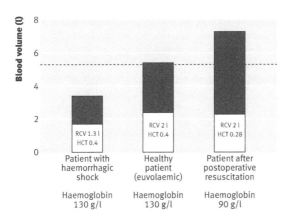

Fig 1 The relation between red cell volume (RCV), plasma volume (PV), haemoglobin concentration, and haematocrit (HCT) during haemorrhage, healthy euvolaemia, and fluid resuscitation with clear fluids indicating the important effect of changes to plasma volume on the haemoglobin concentration

---

BOX 1 FACTORS CONTRIBUTING TO ANAEMIA DURING CRITICAL ILLNESS

Pre-existing chronic anaemia (about 10-15% of patients)
- Renal impairment, liver disease
- Pre-existing medical conditions
- Recent surgery
- Myelodysplasia

Acquired anaemia
- Haemodilution
- Blood loss
- Blood sampling
- Haemorrhage
- Loss from extracorporeal circuits, such as haemofiltration circuits
- Reduced red cell survival
- Haemolysis
- Damage by inflammatory processes
- Reduced red cell production
- Abnormal iron metabolism
- Nutritional deficiencies
- Inappropriately low erythropoietin production
- Bone marrow hyporeactivity

BOX 2 MEASURES TO REDUCE ANAEMIA
- Minimise iatrogenic blood loss from extracorporeal circuits
- Avoid unnecessary blood tests and sampling
- Use blood conservation devices to return the "deadspace" sample to the patient when sampling from indwelling arterial or venous catheters[19]
- Use paediatric blood sampling tubes

Table 1 lists known risks associated with red cell transfusion.[2] [3] The contribution of blood transfusions to complications such as hospital acquired infections and organ failure is difficult to quantify, partly because these complications are common in critically ill patients, and because red cell products vary across different studies and blood services.[16] Red cells can be stored in different types of solution, subjected to different processing steps (for example, the timing and process of removing white blood cells), and stored for varying durations before transfusion. All these factors could alter the risk-benefit profile, but at present the mechanisms and relative clinical importance are poorly understood.[2] [17]

Maintaining adequate supplies of donor blood is increasingly challenging and expensive for blood transfusion services as more potential donors are excluded and greater testing and processing are undertaken.[16] Demand for blood is likely to increase as the population ages.[18] [w6] Using blood transfusion safely and appropriately is therefore a priority for health systems for economic reasons and to maximise benefit to the patient. Quality improvement reports have shown that some interventions can decrease iatrogenic blood loss in patients and reduce the incidence and severity of anaemia in critically ill patients (box 2).[19]

When should a patient receive a blood transfusion?

Physiological reserve

Oxygen delivery to tissues is typically 1000 ml per minute in healthy people, but only 250 ml per minute is used, so there is a large "safety margin." In controlled experimental conditions, young healthy adults can compensate for haemoglobin concentrations of 40-50 g/l if the circulating blood volume is maintained with fluids.[20] [w7] [w8] Older acutely unwell people are less likely to tolerate this level of anaemia, especially if they have coexisting disease.

Many studies, varying widely in quality, have examined the effect of red cell administration on various physiological measures of oxygen supply in critically ill patients.[4] Typically the haemoglobin concentration was increased from 70-90 g/l to more than 100 g/l, and most studies failed to show clinically important changes to the selected end points. This probably means that transfusion is not needed for most patients at these haemoglobin concentrations, but it could also be an indication of the insensitivity of available measures of oxygenation. Table 2 shows physiological and biochemical measures that can help guide blood transfusion decisions, although they lack specificity as diagnostic tests and transfusion triggers. A high or rising lactate concentration and a low or falling central venous haemoglobin oxygen saturation (measured from a central

---

Table 1 Risks associated with blood transfusions

Risk	Mechanism and prevalence[2] [3]
Transfusion process errors resulting in the wrong blood being transfused	Errors in the process and administration of transfusion are still the most common cases reported to the UK national haemovigilance scheme (www.shotuk.org)
Transfusion reactions	Acute transfusion reactions may occur because of haemolytic reactions or anaphylaxis
Transfusion transmitted infections (eg, hepatitis B, hepatitis C, HIV, variant Creutzfeldt-Jakob disease (vCJD)	Transfusion transmitted bacterial infections are more common than viral risks, which are now very low in developed countries. The exact risk of vCJD transmission is unclear
Transfusion associated circulatory overload	Standardised reporting has been inconsistent and the true prevalence is unknown
Transfusion associated lung injury	Acute lung injury related to transfusion still occurs, although many transfusion services have taken measures to reduce this risk, such as use of male only plasma (antileucocyte antibodies, found mostly in parous women, are thought to be responsible for most cases of transfusion associated lung injury)
Transfusion associated immunomodulation	Studies have suggested that such risks exist (for example, increased overall rates of infection), but the size of this effect is unclear
Increased incidence of hospital acquired infections	This may occur as a consequence of several of the mechanisms described above

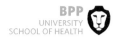

venous catheter) are clinically useful triggers that signal the need to increase oxygen delivery. When faced with evidence of poor oxygenation, clinicians must decide whether to increase the cardiac output (with fluids or inotropic drugs, or both) or improve the oxygen carrying capacity of blood (with red cells). The lack of reliable clinical or laboratory tests to indicate when transfusion is needed means that clinicians rely heavily on the haemoglobin concentration as the primary trigger for transfusion. The problem is that the correct trigger haemoglobin is usually unknown for an individual patient and might vary depending on their clinical condition.

Table 2 Useful clinical symptoms, signs, and tests when deciding if red cell transfusion is needed

Clinical symptom, sign, or test	Considerations
Most useful	
Lactic acidosis	This is a useful indicator of inadequate oxygen delivery, especially early in critical illness (during the "resuscitation phase"). It commonly results from hypoxia or inadequate cardiac output rather than anaemia, so careful cardiorespiratory assessment is needed. Lactic acidosis can also result from poisoning and other conditions causing critical illness
Low central venous oxygen saturations (from a central venous catheter)	These measures are invasive, but low saturations (less than 70%) imply that the body is extracting more oxygen from arterial blood than normal. This may mean oxygen delivery is insufficient to meet demand. As for lactic acidosis, correct hypoxia and ensure that cardiac output is optimised before blood transfusion unless haemoglobin concentrations are ‹70-80 g/l or the patient is bleeding
Haemoglobin value	This is the most commonly used transfusion "trigger." The best evidence to guide the appropriate value comes from the "TRICC" trial (see box 2)
Less useful	
Fatigue and breathlessness	Although common in patients with chronic anaemia, these symptoms can be caused by the disease causing critical illness. Patients may also be unable to provide a history
Pallor	Pallor does not reliably predict the haemoglobin concentration and can also result from hypovolaemia and excessive adrenergic activity (eg, anxiety)
High heart rate	Many other factors, such as pain, anxiety, dehydration, hypovolaemia, and adrenergic drugs, can increase heart rate in critically ill patients

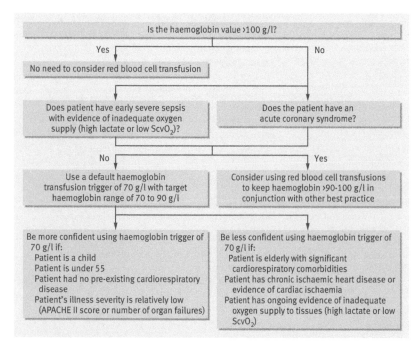

Fig 2 Suggested approach to making transfusion decisions in critically ill patients with no evidence that haemorrhage is causing cardiovascular instability. ScvO2=oxygen saturation of less than 70% in central venous blood

What haemoglobin concentration should trigger blood transfusion in critically ill patients?

The best evidence on what haemoglobin concentration should trigger transfusions in critically ill patients comes from a well performed non-blinded multicentre Canadian trial published in 1999 (the TRICC trial; summarised in box 3),[15] which is widely considered the most important trial in transfusion medicine. Patients with a haemoglobin 90 g/l or less were randomised to either a relatively high haemoglobin transfusion trigger of less than 100 g/l with a target of 100-120 g/l (the "liberal" group) or a lower haemoglobin transfusion trigger of less than 70 g/l with a target of 70-90 g/l ("restrictive" group). The findings strongly support using red cells only to maintain a haemoglobin concentration of 70-90 g/l, especially in younger or less severely ill patients. The generalisability of these findings are unclear, however, and this might explain why clinical practice still varies. This trial has never been replicated in adult critical care, and a recent Cochrane systematic review noted the need for further trials.[21]

We recommend using a haemoglobin transfusion trigger close to 70 g/l as the default position but to modify this using clinical judgment in individual patients. We consider a single unit transfusion followed by reassessment of the haemoglobin value before further transfusion to be best practice unless the patient is actively bleeding or has a haemoglobin concentration substantially lower than 70 g/l.

Some evidence exists to support using a higher transfusion trigger than 70 g/l in the following clinical scenarios.

Patients with chronic ischaemic heart disease

Coronary blood flow occurs mainly during diastole. The heart muscle has a high metabolic rate and normally extracts 60-70% of available oxygen to meet its needs. If coronary stenoses limit blood flow it is logical to suppose that anaemia will increase the risk of myocardial ischaemia, especially if tachycardia and shock limit perfusion further. Several large cohort studies found that in patients with chronic ischaemic heart disease haemoglobin concentrations less than 90 g/l were associated with higher mortality during surgery and critical illness.[22] [W9] [W10] No high quality randomised trials have confirmed this association. A subgroup analysis of patients in the TRICC trial who had pre-existing ischaemic heart disease found a non-significant trend towards lower mortality for the liberally transfused group.[23] However, in the entire study cohort the rates of new cardiac complications were lower in the restrictive group.[15] A lack of high quality evidence means that clinicians have to make decisions on the basis of the severity of coronary artery disease in the individual patient, on whether electrocardiography shows evidence of ischaemia, and on whether coronary blood flow is likely to be adequate.

Patients with acute coronary syndrome

Several cohort studies have found associations between anaemia and higher mortality after acute coronary syndrome,[22] [W11-W13] but no evidence is available from randomised controlled trials to suggest what haemoglobin value should be targeted. The most recent highest quality cohort studies do not show benefit from transfusion when the haemoglobin concentration is more than 80 g/l, but the overall quality of evidence is low and controlled trials are needed, especially because bleeding and anaemia are both common in patients who are treated for acute coronary syndrome.[24]

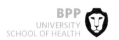

We agree with current recommendations to keep the haemoglobin concentration no lower than 80-90 g/l in patients with an acute coronary syndrome, although the supporting evidence is weak and based largely on physiological reasoning.[4][22]

BOX 3 SUMMARY OF KEY FINDINGS OF THE TRICC TRIAL

PICO details

Population
- Non-bleeding critically ill patients whose haemoglobin value was 90 g/l or less during the first three days in the intensive care unit

Intervention and comparator
- The trial compared a restrictive strategy (haemoglobin transfusion trigger <70 g/l; target value 70-90 g/l) with a liberal strategy (haemoglobin trigger 100 g/l; target value 100-120 g/l) for managing anaemia with blood transfusions during the intensive care unit stay

Outcomes
- The restrictive group received 54% fewer units of blood and 33% received no blood transfusions in the intensive care unit, whereas all of the liberal group were transfused
- The restrictive group showed a non-significant trend towards lower mortality (18.7% v 23.3%; P=0.11)
- The restrictive group had lower rates of cardiac complications (13.2% v 21.0%) and new organ failures (difference in multiple organ dysfunction score of 1 between the groups)
- The liberal group showed a trend towards higher rates of acute respiratory distress syndrome (11.4% v 7.7%)

Predefined subgroup analyses
- Younger patients (<55 years) and patients with lower illness severity during the first 24 hours in the intensive care unit (APACHE II score <20) had significantly better outcomes when they were in the restrictive group (these patients were more anaemic and received fewer blood transfusions)

Subgroup analyses that were not predefined (post hoc analyses)
- There was a trend for patients with known ischaemic heart disease to have better outcomes in the liberal group
- No differences in outcomes were seen in the subgroup of patients who were mechanically ventilated[w17]

Uncertainties about the generalisability of the findings
- The blood used was not leucodepleted. Transfused leucocytes may have adverse effects in critically ill patients and most countries now routinely leucodeplete blood before storage[w18]
- The storage age of the blood was unknown. Longer storage times might affect patient outcomes, especially if the blood was not leucodepleted[17]
- The study could not prove that the restrictive approach was safe for all patient subgroups, especially those with heart disease and sicker older patients
- Improvements in critical care and blood processing over the past decade might mean the findings would be different if the trial were repeated now

---

ADDITIONAL EDUCATIONAL RESOURCES

Resources for healthcare professionals
- NHS Scotland (www.learnbloodtransfusion.org.uk/)—An interactive eLearning resource relating to safe transfusion practice, which is ideal for training of healthcare staff who prescribe or administer blood products
- Scottish Intercollegiate Guidelines Network. Perioperative blood transfusion for elective surgery. Guideline no 54. 2001. www.sign.ac.uk/guidelines/fulltext/54/index.html

Resource for patients
- NHS Choices (www.nhs.uk/Conditions/Blood-transfusion/Pages/Introduction.aspx)—UK based website providing information in lay terms on blood transfusions, when they are needed, and what questions to ask healthcare professionals when they recommend a blood transfusion
- National Heart Lung and Blood Institute. (www.nhlbi.nih.gov/health/dci/Diseases/bt/bt_whatis. html)—US based website providing a wide range of information about blood transfusions using lay terminology

---

Patients with early sepsis

Patients with sepsis are at risk of inadequate oxygen delivery to the tissues, particularly during the first six to 12 hours after onset. After this time, abnormalities in the utilisation of cellular oxygen probably become more important than oxygen supply. One single centre, non-blinded, randomised controlled trial used oxygen saturation of less than 70% in central venous blood (measured via a central venous catheter) as a trigger for a resuscitation protocol that included giving red cells to keep the haemoglobin concentration more than 90-100 g/l.[25] Fifty per cent more patients in the intervention group received blood during the first six hours of care compared with controls, but patients also received more fluids and inotropic drugs. The intervention improved hospital survival from 30.5% to 46.5%, but the relative importance of blood transfusion was uncertain. Until additional evidence emerges it is reasonable to consider transfusing patients with early sepsis to haemoglobin values of 90-100 g/l in addition to resuscitation with fluids and adrenergic drugs, but only if there is clear evidence that oxygen supply may be inadequate (oxygen saturation of <70% in central venous blood, or severe or worsening lactic acidosis). Once patients are haemodynamically stable, a haemoglobin of 70-90 g/l is probably adequate.

Acute neurological disease

The quality of evidence to guide transfusion in patients with intracerebral haemorrhage, thrombotic stroke, subarachnoid haemorrhage, and traumatic brain injury is low and no randomised trials exist.[4][26] Anaemia and the need for blood transfusion are associated with greater disability and mortality in these patients, but clinicians must judge on a case by case basis whether blood transfusion is necessary. Using direct measures of brain oxygenation may help.[w14]

Figure 2 presents an approach to making decisions about transfusion in critically ill adults.

What alternatives to blood transfusions are available to treat anaemia?

Several large well conducted randomised trials have evaluated the effect of using recombinant human erythropoietin, which is not currently licensed for use in this setting, to treat anaemia in people with critical illness.[27] [w15] [w16] The dose and frequency of treatment, the use of supplemental iron, and the haemoglobin transfusion triggers used differed between trials. This treatment resulted only in a modest reduction in the use of red cells in early smaller trials, and in the largest most recent trial transfusion was not significantly reduced.[27] Although thrombotic events increased, which is a concern, overall mortality decreased, especially in patients with trauma, so this treatment may have other beneficial effects.[27]

TIPS FOR NON-SPECIALISTS

- Before giving a blood transfusion consider the potential risks and benefits for the individual patient
- Most critically ill patients can safely tolerate a haemoglobin concentration of 70-90 g/l
- If the patient is not bleeding a haemoglobin value of 70-80 g/l is a safe transfusion trigger, with a target value of 70-90 g/l
- In patients who are not bleeding transfuse a single unit of red cells and re-measure the haemoglobin concentration before considering more

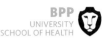

23 Hebert PC, Yetisir E, Martin C, Blajchman MA, Wells G, Marshall J, et al. Is a low transfusion threshold safe in critically ill patients with cardiovascular diseases? *Crit Care Med* 2001;29:227-34.
24 Bassand JP. Bleeding and transfusion in acute coronary syndromes: a shift in the paradigm. *Heart* 2008;94:661-6.
25 Rivers E, Nguyen B, Havstad S, Ressler J, Muzzin A, Knoblich B, et al. Early goal-directed therapy in the treatment of severe sepsis and septic shock. *N Engl J Med* 2001;345:1368-77.
26 Leal-Noval SR, Munoz-Gomez M, Murillo-Cabezas F. Optimal hemoglobin concentration in patients with subarachnoid hemorrhage, acute ischemic stroke and traumatic brain injury. *Curr Opin Crit Care* 2008;14:156-62.
27 Corwin HL Gettinger A, Fabian TC, et al. Efficacy and safety of epoetin alfa in critically ill patients. *N Engl J Med* 2007;357:965-76.

ONGOING RESEARCH

- A large multicentre trial in critically ill patients is comparing the effect of fresh red cells (stored for fewer than eight days) with red cells of standard age (typically 18-21 days' storage) on mortality and other outcomes (ABLE study; ISRCTN44878718)
- A multicentre trial in patients who have undergone cardiac surgery is comparing the effect of transfusing red cells stored for up to 10 days with red cells stored for 21 days or more on mortality and other important clinical outcomes (RECESS study; NCT00991341)
- Trials in the US (ProCESS trial), Australia (ARISE), and the UK (ProMISe) are all evaluating goal directed early "bundles" of care for severe sepsis with current standard care
- Several research trials and programmes are re-evaluating the effect of different transfusion triggers on patient outcomes—for example, in cardiac surgery (TiTRE2 trial; ISRCTN70923932), hip fracture surgery (FOCUS trial; NCT00071032), and intensive care (RELIEVE trial; NCT 00944112)

Contributors: TSW wrote the first draft of the manuscript and finalised all revisions. DW and SJS made revisions and suggestions to the drafts. All authors searched the literature. TSW is guarantor.

Competing interests: None declared.

Provenance and peer review: Commissioned; externally peer reviewed.

1 Walsh TS, Garrioch M, Maciver C, Lee RJ, MacKirdy F, McClelland DB, et al. Red cell requirements for intensive care units adhering to evidence-based transfusion guidelines. *Transfusion* 2004;44:1405-11.
2 Madjdpour C, Spahn DR. Allogeneic red blood cell transfusions: efficacy, risks, alternatives and indications. *Br J Anaesth* 2005;95:33-42.
3 Klein HG, Spahn DR, Carson JL. Red blood cell transfusion in clinical practice. *Lancet* 2007;370:415-26.
4 Napolitano LM, Kurek S, Luchette FA, Corwin HL, Barie PS, Tisherman SA, et al. Clinical practice guideline: red blood cell transfusion in adult trauma and critical care. *Crit Care Med* 2009;37:3124-57.
5 Walsh TS, Saleh EE. Anaemia during critical illness. *Br J Anaesth* 2006;97:278-91.
6 Carson JL, Reynolds RC, Klein HG. Bad bad blood? *Crit Care Med* 2008;36:2707-8.
7 Vincent JL, Baron JF, Reinhart K, Gattinoni L, Thijs L, Webb A, et al. Anemia and blood transfusion in critically ill patients. *JAMA* 2002;288:1499-507.
8 Corwin HL, Gettinger A, Pearl RG, Fink MP, Levy MM, Abraham E, et al. The CRIT study: anemia and blood transfusion in the critically ill—current clinical practice in the United States. *Crit Care Med* 2004;32:39-52.
9 Nguyen BV, Bota DP, Melot C, Vincent JL. Time course of hemoglobin concentrations in nonbleeding intensive care unit patients. *Crit Care Med* 2003;31:406-10.
10 Von Ahsen N, Muller C, Serke S, Frei U, Eckardt KU. Important role of nondiagnostic blood loss and blunted erythropoietic response in the anemia of medical intensive care patients. *Crit Care Med* 1999;27:2630-9.
11 Scharte M, Fink MP. Red blood cell physiology in critical illness. *Crit Care Med* 2003;31:S651-7.
12 Weiss G, Goodnough LT. Anemia of chronic disease. *N Engl J Med* 2005;352:1011-23.
13 Piagnerelli M, Boudjeltia KZ, Vanhaeverbeek M, Vincent JL. Red blood cell rheology in sepsis. *Intensive Care Med* 2003;29:1052-61.
14 Marik PE, Corwin HL. Efficacy of red blood cell transfusion in the critically ill: a systematic review of the literature. *Crit Care Med* 2008;36:2667-74.
15 Hebert PC, Wells G, Blajchman MA, Marshall J, Martin C, Pagliarello G, et al. A multicenter, randomized, controlled clinical trial of transfusion requirements in critical care. Transfusion Requirements in Critical Care Investigators, Canadian Critical Care Trials Group. *N Engl J Med* 1999;340:409-17.
16 Cardigan R, Williamson LM. Production and storage of blood components. In: *Practical transfusion medicine*. 3rd ed. Blackwell publishing, 2009:209-24.
17 Zimrin AB, Hess JR. Current issues relating to the transfusion of stored red blood cells. *Vox Sanguinis* 2009;96:93-103.
18 Wells AW, Mounter PJ, Chapman CE, Stainsby D, Wallis JP. Where does blood go? Prospective observational study of red cell transfusion in north England. *BMJ* 2002;325:803-4.
19 Mukhopadhyay A, Yip HS, Prabhuswamy D, Chan YH, Phua J, Lim TK, et al. The use of a blood conservation device to reduce red blood cell transfusion requirements: before and after study. *Crit Care* 2010;14:R7.
20 Weiskopf RB, Viele MK, Feiner J, Kelley S, Lieberman J, Noorani M, et al. Human cardiovascular and metabolic response to acute, severe isovolemic anemia. *JAMA* 1998;279:217-21.
21 Hill SR, Carless PA, Henry DA, Carson JL, Hebert PC, Henderson KM, et al. Transfusion thresholds and other strategies for guiding allogeneic red blood cell transfusion. *Cochrane Database Syst Rev* 2002;2:CD002042.
22 Gerber DR. Transfusion of packed red blood cells in patients with ischemic heart disease. *Crit Care Med* 2008;36:1068-74.

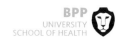
Laryngitis

John M Wood, ENT registrar[1], Theodore Athanasiadis, laryngologist[2], Jacqui Allen, laryngologist[3]

[1]Otolaryngology Head Neck Surgery, Princess Margaret Hospital, Subiaco, WA, Australia

[2]Adelaide Voice Specialists, Adelaide, SA 5000, Australia

[3]North Shore Hospital, Auckland, New Zealand

Correspondence to: T Athanasiadis
theoathans@gmail.com

Cite this as: *BMJ* 2014;349:g5827

DOI: 10.1136/bmj.g5827

http://www.bmj.com/content/349/bmj.g5827

Laryngitis describes inflammation of the larynx, and a variety of causes result in the presentation of common symptoms. Laryngitis may be acute or chronic, infective or inflammatory, an isolated disorder, or part of systemic disease, and often includes symptoms such as hoarseness. Commonly, laryngitis is related to an upper respiratory tract infection and can have a major impact on physical health, quality of life, and even psychological wellbeing and occupation if symptoms persist.[1] Overall, laryngitis incorporates a cluster of non-specific laryngeal signs and symptoms that can also be caused by other diseases. Consequently diagnosis can be difficult and requires correlation of history, examination, and, if necessary, specialised assessment, including visualisation of the larynx and stroboscopy. Acute laryngitis is typically diagnosed and managed at the primary care level. In at risk populations, or those with persisting symptoms, referral to a specialist otolaryngologist should be considered. The aim of this review is to assist non-specialists in assessing and managing people with laryngitis and to identify the cohort that requires specialist input.

What is laryngitis?

The larynx is a complex organ that is important for airway protection and maintaining safe swallowing and positive pressure in the pulmonary system. It is integral to cough, straining, and swallowing, and has immunological[2] and even hormonal[3] functions. Disease related changes in the larynx can impair some or all of these functions. The term laryngitis is descriptive and refers to inflammation of the larynx. It is typically used to describe acute infective laryngitis, one of the most common diseases of the larynx.[4] However, a multitude of other causes of laryngeal inflammation present with similar signs and symptoms. Typically, laryngitis includes dysphonia, air wasting (excessive loss of air through the incompletely closed glottis resulting in a breathy voice), and pain or discomfort in the anterior neck, and it may include other symptoms such as cough, throat clearing, globus pharyngeus (feeling of a lump in the throat), fever, myalgia, and dysphagia.

SOURCES AND SELECTION CRITERIA

We searched Medline, PubMed, and the Cochrane Database of Systematic Reviews, using the search terms "laryngitis", "laryngeal inflammation", and "dysphonia". In addition we searched for specific conditions: "laryngopharyngeal reflux", "sarcoidosis", "pemphigoid", and "tuberculosis". Studies were limited to adult populations and where possible included systematic reviews and randomised controlled trials; we also included case reports to emphasise important problems.

SUMMARY POINTS

- The cause of laryngitis is varied and determines appropriate treatment
- Acute laryngitis is common and generally self limiting
- Clinicians should re-visit the diagnosis and ensure endoscopic examination has been performed if symptoms persist or red flag symptoms develop
- Initial assessment must consider airway patency and rule out malignancy
- Patients with compromised immunity may be at increased risk of infectious causes
- The impact of laryngopharyngeal reflux is becoming widely recognised, with research focused on improving diagnosis and treatment

How common is it?

The prevalence of laryngitis is difficult to estimate. A review conducted by the Royal College of General Practitioners in the United Kingdom in 2010 reported an average incidence of 6.6 cases of laryngitis and tracheitis per 100 000 patients (all ages) per week.[5]

How is it assessed?

Laryngeal symptoms may have many causes. They are usually driven by four broad disease processes: inflammation, neoplastic and structural abnormalities, imbalance in muscle tension, and neuromuscular dysfunction.[6] Laryngeal symptoms arise from one or a combination of these processes. A careful history and examination is crucial in determining the primary factor and helping to identify other factors leading to persisting symptoms.

The first consideration in the initial assessment of patients with laryngeal symptoms should be airway patency. Patients with stridor or respiratory distress need urgent assessment in a setting where airway support can be provided quickly if needed.

Having assessed the airway, the history should cover the nature and chronology of voice symptoms, any exacerbating and relieving factors, and the patient's voice use and requirements. In addition to the description of vocal problems, it is important to ask about associated symptoms of dysphagia, odynophagia, otalgia, reflux, globus pharyngeus, weight loss, pulmonary health, and choking. Box 1 outlines the red flag symptoms that should prompt an urgent referral to exclude malignancy. Contributing medical conditions or the effects of treatment should be considered, as should lifestyle factors, including smoking, diet, and hydration. The impact on quality of life and psychosocial wellbeing should also be addressed.

Investigations include a general head and neck examination covering the oral cavity, oropharynx, and neck, and an assessment of the patient's voice. This can be done by way of a simple scale: grade 1 (subjectively normal voice), grade 2 (mild dysphonia), grade 3 (moderate dysphonia), grade 4 (severe dysphonia), and grade 5 (aphonic), with additional qualifiers used as necessary—for example, breathy, strained. Alternatively, a widely used grading system is the GRBAS (grade, roughness, breathiness, asthenia, strain) scale. It is a simple and reproducible method to assess voice change and quality. This tool grades hoarseness, roughness, breathiness, aesthenia (weakness), and strain on a scale of 0-3, with 0 representing normal, 1 mild degree, 2 moderate degree, and 3 high degree.[8] Either scale may be used by practitioners to track changes in voice over time and also allows other practitioners to understand the degree of voice dysfunction from notation.

What are the causes of acute laryngitis?

Acute laryngitis is commonly caused by infection (viral, bacterial, or fungal) or trauma.[9] Inflammation and oedema of the larynx impairs vibration of the vocal folds, with

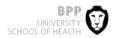

resulting symptoms.[9] Inflammation may involve any area within the larynx, including the supraglottis (epiglottis, arytenoids, and false vocal folds), the glottis (true vocal folds), and subglottic regions. The larynx may be affected directly by inhaled material or by haematogenous spread, infective secretions, or as a consequence of irritation from contact trauma—for example, coughing. Symptoms may persist but are usually self limiting, with a duration of less than two weeks. In general practice, treatment is generally supportive, with voice rest, adequate hydration, and mucolytics.

Viral laryngitis

Viruses are the most common cause of acute laryngitis, most often rhinovirus, adenovirus, influenza, and parainfluenza. Other viruses should be considered, particularly in patients who are immunocompromised (for example, due to herpes species, human immunodeficiency virus, coxsackievirus). Rarely, severe infections such as herpes simplex can result in laryngeal erosion and necrosis.[10]

Bacterial laryngitis

Bacteria are also an important cause of acute laryngitis, and distinction between viral and bacterial infections can be difficult. The two may coexist, with viral illness allowing opportunistic bacterial superinfection to occur. Commonly identified bacteria include *Haemophilus influenzae B (HiB)*, *Streptococcus pneumoniae*, *Staphylococcus aureus*, β haemolytic streptococci, *Moraxella catarrhalis*, and *Klebsiella pneumoniae*.[4] [11] Production of pseudomembrane or serous casts, purulence, marked erythema, and co-involved distant sites (for example, lung, tonsils) are often suggestive of bacterial disease. Historically, diphtheria was associated with a pathognomonic grey membranous cast that could actually cause airway obstruction. With vaccination this is rarely seen nowadays. Viral illness may manifest blisters, particularly herpes zoster, and can be associated with nerve paresis involving the lower cranial nerves. Equally, erythema and pain disproportionate to the mucosal appearances can be representative of viral disease. Fever may be present in both, as can systemic symptoms. Reaction to antibiotics can indicate viral disease in retrospect—for example, production of rash when amoxicillin is given in the presence of Epstein Barr virus infection.

Unusual causes of bacterial laryngitis in developed nations include mycobacterial and syphilitic disease, although these are still seen in developing countries or areas with large immigrant populations.[12] Diagnosis can be difficult, as lesions may appear ulcerative, mimic neoplasia or candidiasis, or have a non-specific inflammatory appearance. Ultimately tissue diagnosis is essential to assess for tumour, which is considerably common, or to identify acid-fast bacilli on microscopy. Suspicion should be high in patients from developing countries with high rates of tuberculosis and those who are immunocompromised.[13]

Supraglottitis and epiglottitis—Owing to the rapid progression of airway compromise, especially in children, much of the literature on acute bacterial laryngitis concerns supraglottitis and epiglottitis, particularly in the context of *H influenzae*.[14] Patients present with rapidly progressing odynophagia, dysphagia, hoarseness, drooling, and stridor. This constellation of symptoms indicates a high risk of impending airway compromise and requires emergency

---

> **BOX 1 RED FLAG SYMPTOMS FOR EARLY REFERRAL (ADAPTED FROM SCHWARTZ ET AL[7])**
>
> - Stridor—emergency referral
> - Recent surgery involving the neck or recurrent laryngeal nerve
> - Recent endotracheal intubation
> - Radiotherapy to the neck
> - History of smoking
> - Professional voice user (for example, singer, actor, teacher)
> - Weight loss
> - Dysphagia or odynophagia
> - Otalgia
> - Serious underlying concern by clinician

---

assessment and airway management. Treatment for less severe cases includes humidification through nebulised normal saline, or constant humidified oxygen, corticosteroids, intravenous antibiotics, and nebulised adrenaline. HiB vaccination has altered the epidemiology and incidence of supraglottitis and epiglottitis, most notably in the paediatric population, with a substantial decrease in presentations.[14]

Fungal laryngitis

Laryngeal candidiasis is a common yet under-diagnosed disease, presenting in both immunocompromised and immunocompetent patients and accounting for up to 10% of presentations.[15] Risk factors include recent use of antibiotics and use of inhaled corticosteroids.[16] Laryngeal examination usually demonstrates whitish speckling of the supraglottis or glottis. At times, diffuse laryngeal erythema and oedema may be seen without these plaques. Candidiasis may mimic other disorders, particularly hyperkeratosis, leucoplakia, and malignancy, and these must be ruled out by biopsy or imaging. Although such infections most often occur in immunocompromised patients, they can occur in patients with normal immunity when there are alterations to the mucosal barrier,[16] such as after chemoradiotherapy, prolonged use of inhalers, or laryngopharyngeal reflux. Biopsy can be difficult to obtain and culture may take several weeks, although fungal elements may be detected more rapidly on Gram stains. Consequently some experts have recommended the diagnosis is implied from a combination of strong clinical suspicion with adequate treatment response to oral antifungal tablets and antifungal solution.

Phonotrauma

Laryngeal inflammation can arise from collision forces of the vocal folds. Such injury can occur with excessive voice use or misuse during phonation.[17] Yelling, screaming, forceful singing, and strained voicing may result in diffuse inflammation and erythema within the larynx.[18] Consequently those in professions with high vocal demands, such as professional singers, actors, and teachers are at much greater risk of developing voice disorders.[18] [19] Although injury is most often limited to the superficial layers of the vocal fold, and endoscopic findings may be minimal, wound healing after repeated episodes can lead to long term changes and persistent symptoms. The larynx may be traumatised in other ways, including blunt or penetrating trauma, chronic coughing, or habitual throat clearing.[18] These may be acute or may persist, with development of chronic laryngitis.

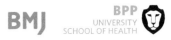

How is acute laryngitis treated?

Management of laryngitis varies depending on the severity. Patients with acute airway compromise or presumed epiglottitis should be referred for urgent management. Most cases of acute laryngitis are self limiting and typically resolve within two weeks. Management options include vocal hygiene and antibiotics.

Vocal hygiene refers to measures such as voice rest, hydration, humidification, and limiting caffeine intake. These measures are invaluable in the symptomatic treatment of laryngeal inflammation. Care of the voice should be recommended to all presenting with vocal difficulties as this provides symptomatic relief and is good practice to carry forward, even as laryngitis resolves. Periods of voice rest may be as short as 48 hours or as long as a week, and a simple rule of thumb can be to recommend voice rest until patients find it comfortable to hum. Then modest speech can be resumed. Hydration is vital, particularly in those who snore or mouth-breathe at night. Hydration may be achieved just by chewing sugar-free gum, or increasing total fluid intake during waking hours (250 mL per waking hour). Caffeine is dehydrating and increases reflux and therefore exacerbates both snoring and pharyngolaryngeal irritation. Fewer than two standard espressos a day is recommended. Many sodas and "smart drinks" also contain high levels of caffeine.

BOX 2 COMMON CAUSES OF CHRONIC LARYNGITIS

Inflammatory

Allergic
- Unclear whether symptoms related to allergic rhinitis or asthma, or primarily from larynx[24][25]
- Diagnosis can be difficult: non-specific findings, hard to differentiate from laryngopharyngeal reflux

Laryngopharyngeal reflux
- Non-specific cluster of laryngeal manifestations
- Evidence of different pathophysiology to gastro-oesophageal reflux disease

Autoimmune

Autoimmune disorders
- Chronic laryngitis may be a manifestation of systemic disease such as rheumatoid arthritis, pemphigoid, systemic lupus erythematosus, and amyloidosis
- High degree of suspicion is needed in the setting of other systemic symptoms, such as arthritis, cutaneous changes, and mucous membrane lesions

Rheumatoid arthritis
- The prevalence of laryngeal symptoms in people with rheumatoid arthritis is reported to be between 30% and 75%[26]
- Includes cricoarytenoid joint fixation, recurrent laryngeal nerve neuropathy, myositis, and laryngeal nodules

Mucous membrane pemphigoid
- Rare chronic autoimmune vesiculobullous disease
- Manifests as blisters or bullae of the ocular and oral mucous membranes, with involvement of aerodigestive tract
- Laryngeal involvement is a rare but life threatening complication, affecting 12% of patients[27]
- Managed with cyclophosphamide and prednisolone; role of surgery unclear

Granulomatous

Sarcoidosis
- Laryngeal sarcoidosis is present in 0.5-5% of patients with sarcoidosis[28]
- Commonly presents with non-specific laryngeal symptoms[29]
- Dysphonia may be present due to recurrent laryngeal nerve palsy from mediastinal lymphadenopathy
- Examination may reveal oedematous laryngeal mucosa, with supraglottis being the most commonly involved site. The vocal folds are rarely involved
- Biopsy is required to confirm the diagnosis
- Treated with systemic corticosteroids; or more rarely intralesional injections or laser resection[28]

Vocal difficulties can result from hyperfunctional vocal behaviours, which in professional voice users can limit or even end their career. High risk groups include singers, performers, and teachers. Holistic voice hygiene programmes encompass a multifactorial approach. Most programmes focus on four main tenets: dealing with the amount and type of voice use, reducing phonotraumatic behaviours, improving hydration, and enhancing lifestyle to improve vocal health, such as reducing caffeine and alcohol intake, smoking cessation, and managing medical conditions. The role of local lubrication, systemic hydration, control of laryngopharyngeal reflux, and allergies are often addressed.[20] A study of teachers found such programmes demonstrated a reduction in vocal misuse and resulting voice symptoms.[21] However, reviews conducted on the benefit of vocal hygiene found limited data for either therapeutic or preventive techniques.[20]

Antibiotics

Treatment of acute laryngitis with antibiotics is widely debated, with frequent reports of inappropriate prescribing of antibiotics for upper respiratory tract infections.[22] A Cochrane systematic review of two trials involving a total of 206 adults found no benefit in treating acute laryngitis with antibiotics, as measured by differences in objective voice scores at one and two weeks' follow-up.[4] The first included study compared a five day course of penicillin V with placebo and reported no difference in patient reported symptoms at 2-6 months' follow-up. The second study compared erythromycin with placebo and found a subjective reduction in voice disturbance at one week and a reduction in cough at two weeks in the erythromycin group. Signs and symptoms such as persistent fever (>48 hours), purulent sputum, membrane formation, or associated distant disease should prompt consideration of antibiotic treatment.

When should people with laryngitis be referred?

Patients with acute airway compromise or suspected epiglottitis or supraglottitis should be assessed in hospital as an emergency. Acute laryngitis is often self limiting and typically resolves within two weeks. The persistence of laryngeal symptoms beyond three weeks is defined as chronic laryngitis. It can indicate additional laryngeal disease and warrants examination. Acute laryngitis may become chronic, with a shift in the underlying pathophysiology. It may be a direct consequence of the initial acute laryngitis episode or have a completely different or concomitant or superimposed cause. A recent retrospective study found that three quarters of patients referred to an otolaryngologist with an initial diagnosis of acute laryngitis had a different final laryngeal diagnosis.[23] Importantly, nearly half the patients with laryngeal cancer had an initial diagnosis by their primary care doctor of either acute laryngitis or non-specific dysphonia. This highlights the need for adequate laryngeal examination by an otolaryngologist in all patients with persisting symptoms, or in those who generate a high degree of suspicion, such as heavy smokers.

There is debate as to how long dysphonia may be present before warranting laryngoscopy. Many otolaryngologists would recommend laryngoscopy if dysphonia is present for more than three weeks without an obvious cause, such as acute illness or intubation. Interestingly, guidelines from the American Academy currently state that direct laryngeal

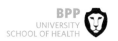

examination is warranted for dysphonia that is present for up to three months, or sooner if there are concerns.[7] This recommendation is based on a cohort study, which found that a delay in diagnosis of laryngeal cancer greater than three months led to poorer survival outcomes.[7] The statement is also qualified by highlighting certain groups that require more urgent review, particularly if the cause may be life threatening or reduce professional viability or voice related quality of life[7]; these groups include people with red flag symptoms and those who rely on their voice for their occupation (box 1). If symptoms persist for longer than three weeks, we recommend that patients should be referred to an otolaryngologist to exclude malignancy.

What are the causes of chronic laryngitis?

Chronic laryngitis is defined as laryngitis that persists beyond three weeks. It can be due to a range of different disease processes, ranging from inflammatory processes, such as allergic laryngitis and laryngopharyngeal reflux, to autoimmune disorders such as rheumatoid arthritis, and granulomatous disease such as sarcoidosis. Chronic laryngitis is less prevalent in primary practice but is the primary indication for referral. By definition, chronic laryngitis implies persistent laryngeal problems, and the glottis should be directly visualised in this situation. While a detailed description of each cause of chronic laryngitis is outside the scope of this review, box 2 summarises the features of the common causes of chronic laryngitis.

Laryngopharyngeal reflux/extraoesophageal reflux

Over the past 30 years it has been increasingly recognised that extraoesophageal manifestations of gastro-oesophageal reflux disease (GORD) may include laryngitis. Large population based studies have reported that patients with GORD are at increased risk for associated laryngeal or pulmonary complications.[30] Symptoms of laryngopharyngeal reflux include non-specific laryngeal manifestations, such as hoarseness, dysphagia, odynophagia, globus pharyngeus, chronic cough, and throat clearing. Furthermore, laryngopharyngeal reflux has been associated with other conditions, such as vocal cord nodules, both premalignant and malignant changes in the larynx, and even sinusitis and otitis media.[31] There is increasing evidence that the pathophysiology of laryngopharyngeal reflux differs from that of GORD, with patients affected by laryngopharyngeal reflux experiencing more daytime (upright) reflux without oesophagitis.[31]

The prevalence of laryngopharyngeal reflux is difficult to determine, particularly as typical heartburn is absent in 57-94% of patients.[32] However, it has been estimated to be present in 10% of patients presenting to an otolaryngologist[33] and over half the patients referred with voice disorders.[34] The diagnosis of laryngopharyngeal reflux is controversial as no ideal test is available. The results of dual probe pH monitoring have varied,[32] with some studies showing, particularly in chronic cough, that the pH of refluxate is not important.[35] Recent studies have considered the utility of pH-metry with intraluminal impedance testing and symptom association probability scores. Impedance allows consideration of non-acid and mixed reflux episodes in relation to symptom generation. This improves temporal association of symptoms with reflux episodes of any pH, which may be relevant in atypical symptoms of reflux such as cough or globus pharyngeus. New diagnostic tools including the lateral flow pepsin

assay or Peptest (RDBiomed, Hull, United Kingdom), and the Restech pharyngeal probe (Respiratory Technology Core, San Diego, CA) are currently in validation studies and may prove to be of clinical use in future.[36] Several studies have identified pepsin as one of the injurious agents in laryngopharyngeal reflux, with injury compounded in the presence of an acidic environment.[37] Pepsin can be endocytosed by hypopharyngeal cells and may be reactivated later. Furthermore, it is not inactivated until the pH is greater than 8 and retains around 20% activity at a pH of 6.8, the average pH of the laryngopharynx.

Despite acknowledgment that reflux laryngitis is not merely an acid phenomenon, management still centres on high dose use of proton pump inhibitors (PPIs), both as a therapeutic and as a diagnostic technique. A significant percentage of patients with laryngopharyngeal symptoms fail to improve with use of PPIs and may require physical reflux barriers such as Gaviscon liquid (Reckitt Benckiser, Hull, United Kingdom). In addition, the duration of treatment with PPIs is uncertain. A recent systematic review, including eight randomised controlled trials, found only two studies where PPIs were significantly more effective than placebo. The studies concluded that the current body of literature is insufficient to make reliable conclusions about the benefits of PPIs in laryngopharyngeal reflux. Antisecretory drugs also present an important side effect profile, including bloating, epigastric discomfort, inhibition of calcium and magnesium absorption, atrophic gastritis, and drug induced acid hypersecretion. PPIs should only be prescribed for a defined period and then symptoms reviewed. Where symptoms remain, further investigation should be considered, including pH-metry, impedance, laryngoscopy, gastroscopy, manometry, and videofluoroscopic swallowing study, depending on the cluster of symptoms. Hyperacidity, association of symptoms with or after meals should prompt pH study with impedance. Where there is associated solid food dysphagia, gagging, or choking a videofluoroscopic assessment of swallowing is recommended. If symptoms are dyspeptic in nature (bloating, belching, food triggered) then gastroscopy may help.

Overall, the treatment of extraoesophageal reflux should include dietary and behaviour modification, with judicious use of antisecretory drugs. Liquid alginate preparations and H2 receptor antagonists have been used in combination with PPIs in recalcitrant cases.[36] The role of laparoscopic fundoplication is well established in patients with GORD and typical symptoms. Some investigators recommend antireflux surgery for patients with laryngeal symptoms.[38] However, a review of 893 consecutive patients who underwent a laparoscopic fundoplication identified 93 with throat symptoms. Those who experienced typical GORD symptoms in addition to "throat" symptoms improved similarly to those with only typical GORD symptoms of heartburn or regurgitation. Patients with objective evidence of GORD, dual channel pH monitoring and laryngeal examination suggesting laryngopharyngeal reflux, and only experiencing throat symptoms were less likely to benefit from surgery. Less than half in this group benefited from surgery, and patients should be counselled appropriately if this option is being considered.[20][33] Failure to respond to optimal combined antireflux treatment should prompt consideration of alternative causes of laryngeal symptoms.

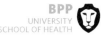

18 Dworkin JP. Laryngitis: types, causes, and treatments. *Otolaryngol Clin N Am* 2008;41:419-36.
19 Williams NR. Occupational groups at risk of voice disorders: a review of the literature. *Occup Med* 2003;53:456-60.
20 Behlau M, Oliveira G. Vocal hygiene for the voice professional. *Curr Opin Otolaryngol Head Neck Surg* 2009;17:149-54.
21 Pasa G, Oates J, Dacakis G. The relative effectiveness of vocal hygiene training and vocal function exercises in preventing voice disorders in primary school teachers. *Logoped Phoniatr Vocol* 2007;32:128-40.
22 Xu KT, Roberts D, Sulapas I, Martinez O, Berk J, Baldwin J. Over-prescribing of antibiotics and imaging in the management of uncomplicated URIs in emergency departments. *BMC Emerg Med* 2013; published online 17 Apr.
23 Cohen SM, Dinan MA, Roy N, Kim J, Courey M. Diagnosis change in voice-disordered patients evaluated by primary care and/or otolaryngology: a longitudinal study. *Otolaryngol Head Neck Surg* 2014;150:95-102.
24 Barker E, Haverson K, Stokes CR, Birchall M, Bailey M. The larynx as an immunological organ: immunological architecture in the pig as a large animal model. *Clin Exp Immunol* 2006;143:6-14.
25 Roth D, Ferguson BJ. Vocal allergy: recent advances in understanding the role of allergy in dysphonia. *Curr Opin Otolaryngol Head Neck Surg* 2010;18:176-81.
26 Hamdan AL, Sarieddine D. Laryngeal manifestations of rheumatoid arthritis. *Autoimmune Dis* 2013; published online 25 Jun.
27 Higgins TS, Cohen JC, Sinacori JT. Laryngeal mucous membrane pemphigoid: a systematic review and pooled-data analysis. *Laryngoscope* 2010;120:529-36.
28 Van den Broek EMJM, Heijnen BJ, Verbist BM, Sjögren EV. Laryngeal sarcoidosis: a case report presenting transglottis involvement. *J Voice* 2013;27:647-9.
29 Mrówka-Kata K, Kata D, Lange D, Namyslowski G, Czecuir E, Banert K. Sarcoidosis and its otolaryngological implications. *Eur Arch Otorhinolaryngol* 2010;267:1507-14.
30 Vakil N, van Zanten SV, Kharilas P, Dent J, Jones R, Global Consensus Group. The Montreal definition and classification of gastroesophageal reflux disease: a global evidence-based consensus. *Am J Gastroenterol* 2006;101:1900-20.
31 Wood JM, Hussey DJ, Woods CM, Watson DI, Carney AS. Biomarkers and laryngopharyngeal reflux. *J Laryngol Otol* 2011;125:1218-24.
32 Hom C, Vaezi MF. Extra-esophageal manifestations of gastroesophageal reflux disease: diagnosis and treatment. *Drugs* 2013;73:1281-95.
33 Ratnasingam D, Irvine T, Thompson SK, Watson DI. Laparoscopic antireflux surgery in patients with throat symptoms: a word of caution. *World J Surg* 2011;35:342-8.
34 Powell J, Cocks HC. Mucosal changes in laryngopharyngeal reflux—prevalence, sensitivity, specificity and assessment. *Laryngoscope* 2013;123:985-91.
35 Athanasiadis T, Allen JE. Chronic cough: an otorhinolaryngology perspective. *Curr Opin Otolaryngol Head Neck Surg* 2013;21:517-22.
36 Watson MG. Review article: laryngopharyngeal reflux—the ear, nose and throat patient. *Aliment Pharmacol Ther* 2011;33(Suppl 1):53-7.
37 Johnston N, Wells CW, Samuels TL, Blumin JH . Rationale for targeting pepsin in the treatment of reflux disease. *Ann Otol Rhinol Laryngol* 2010;119:547-58.
38 Salminen P, Karvonen J, Ovaska J. Long-term outcomes after laparoscopic Nissen fundoplication for reflux laryngitis. *Dig Surg* 2010;27:509-14.

Related links

bmj.com/archive
Previous articles in this series
- Managing the care of adults with Down's syndrome (BMJ 2014;349:g5596)
- Managing common symptoms of cerebral palsy in children (BMJ 2014;349:g5474)
- Bariatric surgery for obesity and metabolic conditions in adults (BMJ 2014;349:g3961)
- Diagnosis and management of prolactinomas and non-functioning pituitary adenomas (BMJ 2014;349:g5390)
- Vitamin B12 deficiency (BMJ 2014;349:g5226)

TIPS FOR NON-SPECIALISTS
- Dysphonia of duration more than three weeks requires direct laryngoscopy
- Dysphonia associated with otalgia, stridor, neck mass, or dysphagia should be considered related to malignancy until proved otherwise
- Failure to respond to proton pump inhibitor treatment does not exclude a diagnosis of reflux laryngitis
- Behavioural modification and hydration or humidification are invaluable in symptomatic treatment of inflammatory laryngitis

ADDITIONAL EDUCATIONAL RESOURCES

Resources for healthcare professionals
- Reveiz L, Cardona AF. Antibiotics for acute laryngitis in adults. *Cochrane Database Syst Rev* 2013;3:CD004783—highest level evidence suggests that antibiotics are not useful for acute laryngitis

Resources for patients
- Egton Medical Information Systems. Laryngitis (www.patient.co.uk/health/laryngitis-leaflet)—well written leaflet for patients, summarising laryngitis
- American Accreditation HealthCare Commission. Laryngitis (www.ncbi.nlm.nih.gov/pubmedhealth/PMH0002361/)—bullet points on laryngitis, which provide useful patient information

Contributors: JMW drafted and revised the manuscript. TA designed the article outline and critically revised and edited the manuscript. He is guarantor. JA drafted and reviewed the manuscript.

Competing interests: We have read and understood the BMJ policy on declaration of interests and declare the following: none.

Provenance and peer review: Commissioned; externally peer reviewed.

1   Cheung TK, Lam PKY, Wei WI, Wong WM, Ng ML, Gu Q, et al. Quality of life in patients with laryngopharyngeal reflux. *Digestion* 2009;79:52-7.
2   Birchall MA, Bailey M, Gutowska-Owsiak D, Johnston N, Inman CF, Stokes CR, et al. Immunologic response of the laryngeal mucosa to extraesophageal reflux. *Ann Otol Rhinol Laryngol* 2008;117:891-5.
3   Kadakia S, Carlson D, Sataloff RT. The effect of hormones on the voice. *J Sing* 2013;69:571-4.
4   Reveiz L, Cardona AF. Antibiotics for acute laryngitis in adults. *Cochrane Database Syst Rev* 2013;3:CD004783.
5   Royal College of General Practitioners. *Communicable and respiratory disease report for England and Wales* . RCGP, 2001-10.
6   McGlashan JA. Clinical assessment of voice disorders. In: Bhattacharyya AK, Nerurkar NK, eds. *Laryngology: otorhinolaryngology—head and neck surgery series* . Thieme, 2014.
7   Schwartz SR, Cohen SM, Dailey SH, Rosenfeld RM, Deutsch ES, Gillespie MB, et al. Clinical practice guideline: hoarseness (dysphonia). *Otolaryngol Head Neck Surg* 2009;141:S1-31.
8   Omori K. Diagnosis of voice disorders. *Jpn Med Assoc J* 2011;54:248-53.
9   Myerson D, DeFatta R, Sataloff RT. Acute laryngitis superimposed on chronic laryngitis. *Ear Nose Throat J* 2013;92:60-2.
10 Sims JR, Massoll NA, Suen JY. Herpes simplex infection of the larynx requiring laryngectomy. *Am J Otolaryngol Head Neck Surg* 2013;34:236-8.
11 Gupta SK, Postma GN, Koufman JA. Laryngitis. In: Bailey BJ, Johnson JT, Newlands SD, eds. *Head and neck surgery—otolaryngology* . 4th ed. Lippincott Williams and Wilkins, 2006.
12 Chen HK, Thornley P. Laryngeal tuberculosis: a case of a non-healing laryngeal lesion. *Australas Med J* 2012;5:175-7.
13 Bhat VK, Latha P, Upadhya D, Hegde J. Clinicopathological review of tubercular laryngitis in 32 cases of pulmonary Kochs. *Am J Otolaryngol Head Neck Surg* 2009;30:327-30.
14 Wood N, Menzies R, McIntyre P. Epiglottitis in Sydney before and after the introduction of vaccination against Haemophilus influenzae type b disease. *Intern Med J* 2005;35:530-5.
15 Merati AL. Acute and chronic laryngitis. In: Flint PW, Haughey BH, Lund VL, Niparko JK, Richardson MA, Robbins KT, Thomas JR, eds. *Cummings otolaryngology head and neck surgery* . 5th ed. Mosby Elsevier, 2010.
16 Chandran SK, Lyons KM, Divi V, Geyer M, Sataloff RT. Fungal laryngitis. *Ear Nose Throat J* 2009;88:1026-7.
17 Ingle JW, Helou LB, Li NYK, Hebda PA, Rosen CA, Abbot KV. Role of steroids in acute phonotrauma: a basic science investigation. *Laryngoscope* 2014;124:921-7.

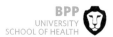

Viral meningitis

Sarah A E Logan, specialist registrar,
Eithne MacMahon, consultant

'Infection and Immunology, Guy's and St Thomas' NHS Foundation Trust, London SE1 7EH

Correspondence to: E MacMahon eithne.macmahon@gstt.nhs.uk

Cite this as: BMJ 2008;336:36

DOI: 10.1136/bmj.39409.673657.AE

http://www.bmj.com/content/336/7634/36

Viral meningitis is common and often goes unreported. In the absence of a lumbar puncture, viral and bacterial meningitis cannot be differentiated with certainty, and all suspected cases should therefore be referred. Lumbar puncture and analysis of cerebrospinal fluid may be done primarily to exclude bacterial meningitis, but identification of the specific viral cause is itself beneficial. Viral diagnosis informs prognosis, enhances care of the patient, reduces the use of antibiotics, decreases length of stay in hospital, and can help to prevent further spread of infection. Over the past 20 years, vaccination policies, the HIV epidemic, altered sexual behaviour, and increasing travel have altered the spectrum of causative agents. In this review we outline the changing epidemiology, discuss key clinical topics, and illustrate how identification of the specific viral cause is beneficial. Neonatal meningitis may be a component of perinatal infection and is not covered here.

How common is viral meningitis?

Viral meningitis can occur at any age but is most common in young children. In the largest reported study, a 1966 birth cohort of 12 000 children in Finland, the annual incidence of presumed viral meningitis was 219 per 100 000 in infants under 1 year and 27.8 per 100 000 overall in children under 14.[4] In a smaller retrospective study, the incidence of aseptic meningitis in people aged 16 and over was lower at 7.6 per 100 000.[5]

Viral meningitis is a notifiable disease in England and Wales, but many cases undoubtedly go unreported.[4][6][7] In 2005-6, 2898 people were admitted to hospital with a diagnosis of viral meningitis, 10 times the number of cases notified to the Health Protection Agency (233) for England and Wales over the same period (fig 1).[7][8]

SOURCES AND SELECTION CRITERIA

We searched PubMed with the terms "viral", "encephalitis", "HIV", "Herpes simplex", "Mumps", "Varicella", "Enterovirus", "Diagnosis", and "immunosuppression", in conjunction with meningitis. We also searched OVID, Embase, and Cochrane databases. We hand searched references from papers. For clinical guidelines, we accessed the websites of the UK Health Protection Agency, UK Department of Health, US Centers for Disease Control and Prevention, and World Health Organization. We also consulted several formal medical, infectious diseases, and virological textbooks.

SUMMARY POINTS

- Bacterial and viral meningitis cannot reliably be differentiated clinically, and all suspected cases should be referred to hospital
- Viral meningitis is most common in young children; the incidence decreases with age
- Enteroviruses are the most common cause at all ages
- Although most cases are self limiting, morbidity may be considerable
- Herpes simplex virus causes viral meningitis, which may recur
- Genital herpes infection may be acquired from a partner after many years within a monogamous relationship
- Meningitis is a feature of HIV seroconversion
- In the absence of associated encephalitis, the prognosis is usually good

What causes it?

As a consequence of mumps, measles, and rubella vaccination, enteroviruses have supplanted mumps as the most common cause of viral meningitis in children (box 1).[4][6] Enteroviruses are said to account for 80% of cases in adults, but a wider range of causes is increasingly implicated.[5][9] Often no cause is identified; among 144 consecutive adults with aseptic meningitis, only 72 had a confirmed diagnosis. Enteroviruses were most common, accounting for 46%, followed by herpes simplex virus type 2 (31%), varicella zoster virus (11%), and herpes simplex virus type 1 (4%).[5]

What is the initial approach to the patient?

Viral meningitis and bacterial meningitis are both characterised by acute onset of fever, headache, photophobia, and neck stiffness, often accompanied by nausea and vomiting.[1][9] Untreated patients with bacterial meningitis show progressive deterioration in mental status, whereas spontaneous recovery is usual in viral cases. At initial presentation, no reliable clinical indicators are available to differentiate between acute viral meningitis and bacterial meningitis, so all suspected cases should be referred to hospital.

Particular caution is warranted with young children, in whom meningitis is manifest as fever and irritability, without, as a rule, evidence of meningeal irritation.[9] Neck stiffness and photophobia may also be absent in adults.[1][10] Assessment should include evaluation for possible encephalitis, suggested by seizures, reduced Glasgow coma score, or focal neurological signs. Suspected encephalitis warrants empirical antiviral treatment with intravenous aciclovir. History and examination can yield clues as to viral causes (box 2).

How is it diagnosed?

Analysis of cerebrospinal fluid is needed, and lumbar puncture should be done unless it is contraindicated. Whether prior computed tomography imaging is needed is controversial, and guidance is now available (see box 2).[11][12] Viral meningitis in itself is not associated with abnormalities on imaging. C reactive protein concentration and peripheral blood white cell count can be helpful but

DEFINITIONS

- *Meningitis*—Inflammation of the meninges associated with an abnormal number of cells in the cerebrospinal fluid[1]
- *Aseptic meningitis*—A syndrome characterised by acute onset of meningeal symptoms and fever, with pleocytosis of the cerebrospinal fluid and no growth on routine bacterial culture[2]
- *Mononuclear pleocytosis*—An elevated white cell count in the cerebrospinal fluid, with predominant mononuclear cells (as opposed to polymorphonuclear leucocytes)
- *Encephalitis*—Inflammation of the brain parenchyma; cerebral cortex disease causes altered mental status early in the course, and focal or diffuse neurological signs may be present[1][3]
- *Meningoencephalitis*—Central nervous system infection with clinical features of both meningeal and parenchymal disease

do not reliably differentiate between possible causes. A blood glucose concentration is essential and should be collected immediately before lumbar puncture.[3] Cerebrospinal fluid needs to be processed promptly to avoid depletion of cell counts during transport or storage. Although characteristically associated with a mononuclear pleocytosis, neutrophils may predominate initially in viral meningitis (table 1). In 138 children with aseptic meningitis, 57% had a polymorphonuclear predominance that persisted beyond 24 hours.[14]

The usual initial approach to viral diagnosis (table 2) is to test the cerebrospinal fluid for enteroviruses, herpes simplex virus, and varicella zoster virus by using polymerase chain reaction technology, estimated to be threefold to 1000-fold more sensitive than routine viral culture.[15] Identification of a viral cause has been shown to be beneficial, facilitating reduced administration of antibiotics and decreased length of stay in hospital.[16]

Enteroviruses

Enteroviruses are by far the most common cause of viral meningitis; they account for most cases, at all ages, in which the cause is identified.[456 9] The term enteroviruses refers to the mode of transmission rather than the symptoms of infection. Indeed, infections with these ubiquitous viruses are mostly asymptomatic. They can cause systemic infections, however, and have a proclivity to be neuroinvasive. The enteroviruses encompass Coxsackie A and B viruses, echoviruses, polioviruses,

and the more recently identified viruses designated by number, such as enterovirus 71.[19] Almost any of the enterovirus types can give rise to neurological manifestations ranging from aseptic meningitis to meningoencephalitis and paralytic poliomyelitis. Coxsackie B viruses and echoviruses account for most cases of enterovirus meningitis. Enteroviral typing is essential to identify and monitor outbreaks.[19]

Who gets it?

Infants and young children with no immunity are most susceptible to enteroviruses, and the incidence decreases with age. Infection is seasonal in temperate climates—highest in summer and autumn—but high all year round in tropical and subtropical climates.[9]

Clinical features and management

Meningitis may be accompanied by mucocutaneous manifestations of enterovirus infection, including localised vesicles such as in hand, foot, and mouth disease; herpangina; and generalised maculopapular rash. Most cases that present clinically with meningitis are self limiting and carry a good prognosis. Nevertheless, enteroviral meningitis causes considerable morbidity, with moderate or high fever despite antipyretics and several days of severe headache warranting opiate analgesia.[10] Abrupt deterioration in mental status or seizures may be caused by progression from meningitis to meningoencephalitis.[9]

BOX 1 VIRAL MENINGITIS: CAUSES TO CONSIDER[1 3 9]

All patients
- Enteroviruses
- Herpes simplex viruses (HSV-2 and HSV-1)
- Varicella zoster virus (VZV)
- Human immunodeficiency virus (HIV)
- Epstein-Barr virus (EBV)

Unvaccinated/incomplete vaccination course
- Mumps virus

Immunocompromised host
- Cytomegalovirus (CMV)

Travel history
- West Nile virus (Americas, Africa, West Asia, Australia, mainland Europe)
- Saint Louis encephalitis virus (United States)
- Tick-borne encephalitis viruses (mainland Europe and Asia)

Contact with rodent droppings or urine
- Lymphocytic choriomeningitis virus (LCMV)

BOX 2 APPROACH TO THE PATIENT

History
- Classic symptoms—fever, headache, photophobia, neck stiffness
- Associated symptoms—rash, sore throat, swollen glands, vomiting, genitourinary symptoms
- Illness in contacts
- Sexual history
- Travel abroad
- Risk factors for HIV
- Mumps immunisation status
- Compromised immunity
- Exposure to rodents/ticks

Examination
- Classic signs:
  - Fever, nuchal rigidity
  - Absence of focal neurological signs; mental status intact
- Rash
- Lymphadenopathy
- Pharyngitis
- Parotid swelling
- Genital herpes

Imaging before lumbar puncture?
Recommended if any of the following are present[111213]
- Immunocompromised host:
- Immunosuppressive treatment
- Immunodeficiency (for example, HIV)
- History of central nervous system disease—mass lesion, stroke, focal infection
- New onset of seizure(s)—within one week of presentation
- Focal neurological deficit
- Abnormal level of consciousness manifest by:
- Glasgow coma score (GCS) <12 or
- Fluctuating conscious level (drop in GCS ≥2)
- Papilloedema

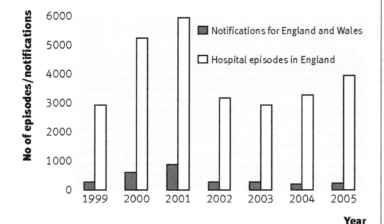

Fig 1 Notifications of viral meningitis for England and Wales compared with hospital episodes in England

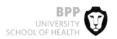

No specific antiviral treatment is available, and management is conservative. Immunoglobulin replacement has a role in patients with hypogammaglobulinaemia, who are prone to severe and chronic enteroviral disease.

Herpes simplex viruses (HSV-2, HSV-1)

Confusion sometimes arises when herpes simplex virus is detected in the cerebrospinal fluid of a patient with clinical meningitis. Recognising that herpes simplex virus meningitis and encephalitis are discrete entities in the immunocompetent host, rather than part of a continuous spectrum, is essential. Whereas herpes simplex virus encephalitis is a life threatening medical emergency warranting empiric antiviral treatment, herpes simplex virus meningitis is a self limiting condition in patients with normal immunity.[20]

Who gets it?

Herpes simplex virus now ranks second among the causes of viral meningitis in adolescents and adults in developed countries.[5] Herpes simplex virus meningitis is a complication of primary genital herpes, especially with HSV-2. By definition, primary herpes simplex virus infection is the first infection with either virus type in the absence of pre-existing antibodies to HSV-1 or HSV-2. In the most comprehensive study, 36% of 126 women and 13% of 63 men with primary genital HSV-2 infection had meningeal symptoms.[21]

Non-primary infection includes first episodes in the presence of pre-existing antibodies to HSV-1 or HSV-2 and recurrences. Unlike primary infection, non-primary genital infection with herpes simplex virus is rarely accompanied by aseptic meningitis. HSV-2 meningitis may also occur in the absence of clinical genital herpes. Of 69 patients with meningeal symptoms and HSV-2 detected in the cerebrospinal fluid, 82% had neither a history of genital herpes nor active genital lesions.[22]

As a consequence of the increasing incidence of genital herpes,[23] clinical cases of herpes simplex virus meningitis in the United Kingdom are set to increase. The rate of childhood infection with HSV-1 is declining; a documented drop in seropositivity rates among 10-14 year olds from 34% (1986-7) to 24% (1994-5) has occurred.[24] Thus, in the absence of previous oral herpes simplex virus infection, an increasing proportion of young people are likely to have symptomatic primary genital herpes simplex virus infections and hence meningitis.

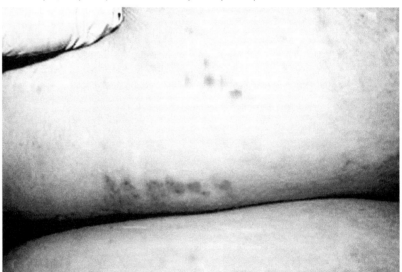

Fig 2 Patient 2—zoster associated with varicella zoster virus meningitis

Table 1 Typical cerebrospinal fluid (CSF) findings in infectious meningitis[1 3 14]

Cause of meningitis	White blood cell count (×10⁶ cells/l)	Predominant cell type	CSF:serum glucose (normal .0.5)	Protein (g/l) (normal 0.2-0.4)
Viral	50-1000	Mononuclear (may be neutrophilic early in course)	>0.5	0.4-0.8
Bacterial	100-5000	Neutrophilic (mononuclear after antibiotics)	<0.5	0.5-2.0
Tuberculous	50-300	Mononuclear	<0.3	0.5-3.0
Cryptococcal	20-500	Mononuclear	<0.5	0.5-3.0

Table 2 Diagnosing viral meningitis[1 15 17 18]

Cause	Key diagnostic test	Other potentially useful tests
Enteroviruses	CSF PCR*	Throat and rectal swabs—culture, PCR (positive for longer than CSF)
Herpes simplex virus (HSV)	CSF PCR*	HSV type specific serology. Detection in genital lesions—PCR, culture, immunofluorescence, electron microscopy, Tzanck smear
Varicella zoster virus	CSF PCR*	Detection in skin lesions—PCR, culture, immunofluorescence, electron microscopy, Tzanck smear
HIV	Serology*	Serial IgG or combined IgG and antigen tests—seroconversion? HIV viral load (plasma, CSF)
Mumps	Serology (serum, oral fluid)	PCR (throat swab, urine, EDTA blood, oral fluid)
Epstein-Barr virus (EBV)	EBV specific serology, VCA IgM and IgG, EBNA IgG	CSF PCR. Monospot test

CSF=cerebrospinal fluid; EBNA=Epstein-Barr nuclear antigen; PCR=polymerase chain reaction; VCA=viral capsule antigen.
*First line tests.

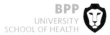

Clinical features and management

In addition to fever and symptoms of meningitis, constitutional symptoms of primary herpes infection may occur, with malaise and clinical features of genital herpes simplex virus infection. Whereas autonomic dysfunction occurs in 2% of cases of primary genital herpes, sacral radiculomyelitis (manifest as urinary retention, constipation, paraesthesias, and motor weakness) complicates one third of cases with primary HSV-2 meningitis.[21]

HSV-2 meningitis can recur, especially in women with primary genital infection.[21] Clinical recurrences have been described in 20-50% of cases, both with and without genital symptoms.[25][26] Indeed HSV-2 has been implicated in recurrent benign lymphocytic meningitis (including Mollaret's meningitis), a syndrome characterised by spontaneous recovery after each of at least three episodes of aseptic meningitis. HSV-2 (and occasionally HSV-1) DNA and herpes simplex virus type specific antibodies have been detected in the cerebrospinal fluid of up to 85% of patients.[26]

Although antiviral treatment with aciclovir, valaciclovir, or famciclovir is indicated for the treatment of first episode genital herpes, therapeutic trials have yet to be done in herpes simplex virus meningitis.[20] Evidence is lacking, but early treatment might decrease the viral burden, speed resolution of symptoms, and reduce the risk of recurrence.

Patients with herpes simplex virus meningitis should be referred to a sexual health clinic after recovery. However, the diagnosis of herpes simplex virus meningitis and possible associations with genital herpes may come as a shock to the patient, and this needs to be discussed sensitively at the earliest appropriate opportunity. Many people harbour genital herpes simplex virus infection and intermittently shed virus without ever having symptoms. Infection can thus be spread unknowingly to sexual contacts. The timing of transmission is unpredictable; it may occur only after several years within a monogamous sexual relationship.[27]

Varicella zoster virus

Aseptic meningitis is a recognised but rare complication of primary infection with varicella zoster virus (varicella). It is more commonly seen in association with reactivation of varicella zoster virus (zoster) and can also occur in the absence of cutaneous lesions. Among 21 patients with varicella zoster virus meningitis, more than 50% had no skin manifestations.[28] No specific recommendations for varicella zoster virus meningitis exist beyond the usual treatment for zoster.

Human immunodeficiency virus

Primary HIV infection is an important cause of aseptic meningitis. Symptoms occur in up to 17% of cases of HIV seroconversion and may be associated with faster disease progression.[29] Other features of primary HIV infection—lymphadenopathy, rash, dermatitis, gastrointestinal disturbances, oral candidiasis, and pharyngitis—should be sought. Atypical lymphocytes may be seen on the blood film in both primary HIV and Epstein-Barr virus infections (both are causes of viral meningitis). The neurological symptoms generally resolve over several weeks. Early diagnosis may benefit intimate contacts, as the risk of transmission of HIV is greater in the early stages of infection.[30]

Mumps

Meningitis is by far the most common neurological manifestation of mumps virus infection. Before widespread immunisation, mumps was a common cause of meningitis, which occurred in 15% of patients with mumps.[17] Mumps meningitis can precede or follow the parotid swelling, and 50% of cases occur in the absence of parotitis. Meningitis is more common in male than female patients.[17] The recent epidemic among young adults was associated with more than 100 cases of mumps meningitis in England in 2004-6.[8]

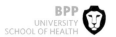

We thank William Tong and Mike Kidd for critical evaluation of the draft manuscript and Alice Gem for secretarial help.

Contributors: SAEL and EMM searched the literature and wrote the manuscript. EMM is the guarantor.

Competing interests: EMM received sponsorship from Aventis Pasteur MSD towards conference attendance in 2002.

1   Tunkel AR, Scheld WM. Acute meningitis. In: Mandell GL, Bennett JE, Dolin R, eds. *Mandell, Douglas, and Bennett's principles and practice of infectious diseases* . 6th ed. Philadelphia: Elsevier Churchill Livingstone, 2005:1083-126.

2   United States Department of Health and Human Services Centers for Disease Control and Prevention. Aseptic meningitis 1990 case definition. www.cdc.gov/epo/dphsi/casedef/asmeningitiscurrent.htm.

3   Cassady KA, Whitley RJ. Pathogenesis and pathophysiology of viral infections of the central nervous system. In: Scheld WM, Whitley RJ, Marra CM, eds. *Infections of the central nervous system* . 3rd ed. Philadelphia: Lippincott Williams & Wilkins, 2004:57-74.

4   Rantakallio P, Leskinen M, Von Wendt L. Incidence and prognosis of central nervous system infections in a birth cohort of 12,000 children. *Scand J Infect Dis* 1986;18:287-94.

5   Kupila L, Vuorinen T, Vainionpää R, Hukkanen V, Marttila RJ, Kotilainen P. Etiology of aseptic meningitis and encephalitis in an adult population. *Neurology* 2006;66:75-80.

6   Davison KL, Ramsay ME. The epidemiology of acute meningitis in children in England and Wales. *Arch Dis Child* 2003;88:662-4.

7   Health Protection Agency. Diseases notifiable (to Local Authority Proper Officers) under the Public Health (Infectious Diseases) Regulations 1988. www.hpa.org.uk/infections/topics_az/noids/noidlist.htm.

8   HESonline. Hospital episode statistics. www.hesonline.nhs.uk/Ease/servlet/ContentServer?siteID=1937&categoryID=537.

9   Sawyer MH, Rotbart H. Viral meningitis and aseptic meningitis syndrome. In: Scheld WM, Whitley RJ, Marra CM, eds. *Infections of the central nervous system* . 3rd ed. Philadelphia: Lippincott Williams & Wilkins, 2004:75-93.

10 Rotbart HA, Brennan PJ, Fife KH, Romero JR, Griffin JA, McKinlay MA, et al. Enterovirus meningitis in adults. *Clin Infect Dis* 1998;27:896-8.

11 Hasbun R, Abrahams J, Jekel J, Quagliarello VJ. Computed tomography of the head before lumbar puncture in adults with suspected meningitis. *N Engl J Med* 2001;345:1727-33.

12 Tunkel AR, Hartman BJ, Kaplan SL, Kaufman BA, Roos KL, Scheld WM, et al. Practice guidelines for the management of bacterial meningitis. *Clin Infect Dis* 2004;39:1267-84.

13 Meningitis Research Foundation. Early management of suspected bacterial meningitis and meningococcal septicaemia in immunocompetent adults. 2nd ed. www.meningitis.org/assets/pdf/health_professionals/Adult%20early%20management%20poster%20Dec%2004.pdf.

14 Negrini B, Kelleher KJ, Wald ER. Cerebrospinal fluid findings in aseptic versus bacterial meningitis. *Pediatrics* 2000;105:316-9.

15 Read SJ, Kurtz JB. Laboratory diagnosis of common viral infections of the central nervous system by using a single multiplex PCR screening assay. *J Clin Microbiol* 1999;37:1352-5.

16 Ramers C, Billman G, Hartin M, Ho S, Sawyer MH. Impact of a diagnostic cerebrospinal fluid enterovirus polymerase chain reaction test on patient management. *JAMA* 2000;283:2680-5.

17 Gupta RK, Best J, MacMahon E. Mumps and the UK epidemic 2005. *BMJ* 2005;330:1132-5.

18 Health Protection Agency. ERNVL reference and diagnostic testing services. www.hpa.org.uk/cfi/vrd/ernvl/testing.htm.

19 Pallansch MA, Roos RP. Enteroviruses: polioviruses, coxsackieviruses, echoviruses, and newer enteroviruses. In: Knipe DM, Howley PM, Griffin DE, Lamb RA, Martin MA, Roizman B, et al, eds. *Fields virology* . 4th ed. Philadelphia: Lippincott Williams & Wilkins, 2001:723-75.

20 Whitley RJ. Herpes simplex virus. In: Scheld WM, Whitley RJ, Marra CM, eds. *Infections of the central nervous system* . 3rd ed. Philadelphia: Lippincott Williams & Wilkins, 2004:123-44.

21 Corey L, Adams HG, Brown ZA, Holmes KK. Genital herpes simplex virus infections: clinical manifestations, course, and complications. *Ann Intern Med* 1983;98:958-72.

22 O'Sullivan CE, Aksamit AJ, Harrington JR, Harmsen WS, Mitchell PS, Patel R. Clinical spectrum and laboratory characteristics associated with detection of herpes simplex virus DNA in cerebrospinal fluid. *Mayo Clin Proc* 2003;78:1347-52.

23 Health Protection Agency. Trends in genital warts and genital herpes diagnoses in the United Kingdom. *Health Protection Report* 2007;1(35):4-9 (www.hpa.nhs.uk/hpr/archives/2007/hpr3507.pdf).

24 Vyse AJ, Gay NJ, Slomka MJ, Gopal R, Gibbs T, Morgan-Capner P, et al. The burden of infection with HSV-1 and HSV-2 in England and Wales: implications for the changing epidemiology of genital herpes. *Sex Transm Inf* 2000;76:183-7.

25 Bergstrom T, Vahine A, Alestig K, Jeansson S, Forsgren M, Lycke E. Primary and recurrent herpes simplex virus type 2-induced meningitis. *J Infect Dis* 1990;162:322-30.

26 Shalabi M, Whitley RJ. Recurrent benign lymphocytic meningitis. *Clin Infect Dis* 2006;43:1194-7.

27 Kulhanjian JA, Soroush V, Au DS, Bronzan RN, Yasukawa LL, Weylman LE, et al. Identification of women at unsuspected risk of primary infection with herpes simplex virus type 2 during pregnancy. *N Engl J Med* 1992;326:916-20.

28 Echevarría JM, Casas I, Tenorio A, de Ory F, Martínez-Martín P. Detection of varicella-zoster virus-specific DNA sequences in cerebrospinal fluid from patients with acute aseptic meningitis and no cutaneous lesions. *J Med Virol* 1994;43:331-5.

29 Boufassa F, Bachmeyer C, Carre N, Deveau C, Persoz A, Jadand C, et al. Influence of neurologic manifestations of primary human immunodeficiency virus infection on disease progression. *J Infect Dis* 1995;171:1190-5.

30 Brenner BG, Roger M, Routy JP, Moisi D, Ntemgwa M, Matte C, et al. High rates of forward transmission events after acute/early HIV-1 infection. *J Infect Dis* 2007;195:951-9.

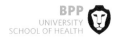
Spontaneous intracerebral haemorrhage

Rustam Al-Shahi Salman, MRC clinician scientist and honorary consultant neurologist[1],
Daniel L Labovitz, assistant professor[2], Christian Stapf, assistant professor of neurology[3]

[1]Division of Clinical Neurosciences, University of Edinburgh, Western General Hospital, Edinburgh EH4 2XU

[2]NYU Medical Center, Schwartz Health Care Center, Suite 5F, 530 First Avenue, New York, NY 10016, USA

[3]Stroke Unit, Service de Neurologie, Hôpital Lariboisière—APHP, 2 Rue Ambroise Paré, 75475 Paris cedex 10, France

Correspondence to: R Al-Shahi Salman
Rustam.Al-Shahi@ed.ac.uk

Cite this as: BMJ 2009;339:b2586

DOI: 10.1136/bmj.b2586

http://www.bmj.com/content/339/bmj.b2586

Spontaneous (non-traumatic) intracerebral haemorrhage accounts for at least 10% of all strokes in the United Kingdom,[1] but the incidence is higher in some ethnic groups.[w1] Intracerebral haemorrhage may present with a sudden focal neurological deficit or a reduced level of consciousness, after which it kills about half of those affected within one month and leaves most survivors disabled.[2]

Although early case fatality after spontaneous intracerebral haemorrhage has not changed over the past two decades,[1] [2] brain imaging has illuminated the pathophysiology of intracerebral haemorrhage and its various causes,[3] [w2] such that the term primary intracerebral haemorrhage now seems antiquated. Improving prevention of intracerebral haemorrhage in primary care and its outcome in secondary care is especially important in view of trends towards a rising incidence of intracerebral haemorrhage in an ageing population.[1]

How should intracerebral haemorrhage be distinguished from other causes of stroke?

No clinical scoring system has been shown to reliably differentiate intracerebral haemorrhage from ischaemic stroke.[w3] Timely brain imaging is the key to recognising intracerebral haemorrhage. Computed tomography detects symptomatic intracerebral haemorrhage within minutes of symptom onset and up to one week thereafter; magnetic resonance imaging with gradient-recalled echo sequences reliably differentiates infarction from haemorrhage more than one week after onset of stroke.[4] Diagnostic imaging distinguishes intracerebral haemorrhage from other types of intracranial haemorrhage (fig 1), although intracerebral haemorrhage may extend into other intracranial compartments. This distinction is important, because the causes, prognosis, and treatment vary according to the location of intracranial haemorrhage.[5]

What are the detectable causes of intracerebral haemorrhage?

The major risk factors for spontaneous intracerebral haemorrhage are systemic arterial hypertension, excess alcohol consumption, male sex, increasing age, and smoking.[6] [w4] [w5] These risk factors may lead to secondary

vascular changes, such as small vessel disease and arterial aneurysms, which may eventually cause intracerebral haemorrhage. Pioneer postmortem studies from the era when non-invasive brain imaging was not widely available suggested that many intracerebral haemorrhages, especially those in deep brain locations, were caused by deep perforating artery lipohyalinosis attributable to chronic hypertension.[w6] However, a systematic review found a much weaker association between hypertension before a stroke and deep intracerebral haemorrhage.[7]

Systematic investigation of selected patients with intracerebral haemorrhage identifies an underlying arteriovenous malformation in about 20% and an aneurysm in about 13%, so the focus should be on identifying these potentially treatable causes of recurrent intracerebral haemorrhage (table 1).[8]

As a result of the rising use of thrombolytic, antiplatelet, and anticoagulant drugs their association with intracerebral haemorrhage is also increasing,[1] such that many patients have several concurrent causes, none of which is either necessary or sufficient to have caused the intracerebral haemorrhage.[w7]

How should we investigate intracerebral haemorrhage?

After a radiological diagnosis of intracerebral haemorrhage, some routine investigations are essential (box 1), but international guidelines reflect the lack of consensus on which patients to image further, and how and when to do so.[9] [10] Doctors are most likely to further investigate younger patients with intracerebral haemorrhage.[8] But patient age, comorbidities, and location of intracerebral haemorrhage are unreliable means of predicting cause with certainty,[7] [8] so we recommend further imaging in all patients who can tolerate it and whose prognosis is not bleak (box 1).

Early computed tomography angiography is a quick and widely available first line investigation for an underlying aneurysm or arteriovenous malformation or fistula when these diagnoses are suspected (table 1), but only a few small studies have investigated its sensitivity (88-100%) and specificity (95-100%) compared with catheter angiography.[8] Arteriovenous malformations are likely to be under-ascertained in clinical practice because catheter angiography is not used systematically and needs to be repeated to show some arteriovenous malformations.[8] Magnetic resonance imaging is useful for detecting venous thrombosis acutely and for detecting underlying tumours and cavernous malformations at least two months after the intracerebral haemorrhage.[11] Magnetic resonance imaging may also detect some foci of haemosiderin, known as microbleeds, but the diagnostic importance of their detection and distribution is still under investigation.[12] [13]

What is the outcome after intracerebral haemorrhage?

The main predictors of death within one month are older age, low score on the Glasgow coma scale on admission, increasing volume of intracerebral haemorrhage,

SOURCES AND SELECTION CRITERIA

We referred to the Cochrane database of systematic reviews and the published guidelines in September 2008, and we used our personal reference collections.

SUMMARY POINTS

- Spontaneous intracerebral haemorrhage accounts for at least 10% of strokes in the United Kingdom
- Half of the patients die within the first month of onset
- Stroke unit care improves outcome
- Early neurosurgical haematoma evacuation can improve outcome
- Secondary prevention by lowering blood pressure is effective

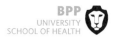

infratentorial intracerebral haemorrhage location, and intraventricular extension.[14] These five prognostic factors may help to assess the risk of death within one month for individual patients using the total intracerebral haemorrhage score (table 2),[14] which has been externally validated although it may not be as accurate as other scales.[w8] Intracerebral haemorrhage volume can be estimated easily using the "ABC/2" method. This method entails identifying the axial computed tomography slice with the largest area of intracerebral haemorrhage, and halving the product of its maximum width (A in figure 2), the width perpendicular to A (B in figure 2), and the depth (C, which is determined by multiplying the number of slices on which intracerebral haemorrhage was visible by the slice thickness of the relevant part(s) of the brain computed tomogram).[w9]

Early neurological deterioration is explained by various mechanisms, including perihaematomal oedema and haematoma expansion, which affects about a third of patients within the first 24 hours of onset (figure 2, C and D).[w10] However, withdrawal of care and "do not resuscitate" orders may have an equally powerful influence.[w11]

The location and underlying cause of an intracerebral haemorrhage partly determine the long term risk of recurrent haemorrhage, dependence in daily activities, and death.[3] The annual risk of recurrent intracerebral haemorrhage is about 2% for deep intracerebral haemorrhage without an identified cause and about 10% for lobar intracerebral haemorrhage.[w12] However, the annual risk of recurrent intracerebral

Table 1 Commonest causes of apparently spontaneous intracerebral haemorrhage

Cause*	Clues
Small vessel disease	Associated with risk factors such as hypertension; leukoaraiosis and lacunes on brain imaging are clues, but only pathological examination is definitive
Amyloid angiopathy	Older patients, without another detected cause for lobar intracerebral haemorrhage; lobar microbleeds are clues, but only pathological examination is definitive
Brain arteriovenous malformation	Extension of intracerebral haemorrhage into other compartments (fig 1); history of intracranial haemorrhage or epileptic seizure(s); calcified or enhancing vessels on imaging
Intracranial arterial aneurysm	Extension of intracerebral haemorrhage into other compartments (fig 1), or located near Sylvian or inter-hemispheric fissures
Cavernous malformation	Personal or family history of intracerebral haemorrhage or epileptic seizure(s); usually small, intracerebral haemorrhage without extension into other compartments
Intracranial venous thrombosis	Associated with pregnancy, thrombophilia, and inflammatory diseases. Intracerebral haemorrhage or haemorrhagic infarcts close to venous sinuses and cortical veins
Dural arteriovenous fistula	Pulsatile tinnitus; haematoma close to venous sinuses and cortical veins
Haemorrhagic transformation of cerebral infarction	Recent cerebral infarction, sometimes followed by a further deterioration
Clotting factor deficiency	Haemorrhages at other sites in the body (skin, joints)
Neoplasm (primary/metastasis)	History or current evidence of a tumour; recently pregnant
Vasculitis	Evidence of systemic vasculitis; lymphocytes in cerebrospinal fluid
Infective endocarditis	Septic embolism into brain arteries, leading to formation of "mycotic" aneurysms
Hypertensive encephalopathy	Evidence of accelerated phase hypertension
Undisclosed trauma	Scalp laceration or skull fracture; widespread contusions on imaging; extension of intracerebral haemorrhage into other compartments (fig 1)

*In descending order of frequency, although the likely cause is thought to depend on the age of the patient and his or her comorbidities and treatment, and on the location of the intracerebral haemorrhage.

BOX 1 TESTS TO INVESTIGATE INTRACEREBRAL HAEMORRHAGE*

Essential

- Full blood count
- Coagulation screen: prothrombin time, activated partial thromboplastin time, d-dimers
- Electrolytes, urea, creatinine, liver function tests
- Glucose
- Inflammatory markers (C reactive protein, erythrocyte sedimentation rate)
- Toxicology screen
- Electrocardiography
- Chest radiography
- Pregnancy test

Dependent on patient characteristics, prognosis, and characteristics of intracerebral haemorrhage

- Computed tomography angiography or venography
- Magnetic resonance imaging
- Catheter angiography

*Adapted from the American Heart Association's guidelines[9]

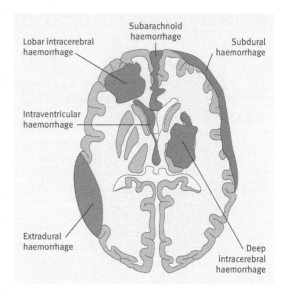

Fig 1 Axial illustration of the brain showing the subtypes of intracranial haemorrhage

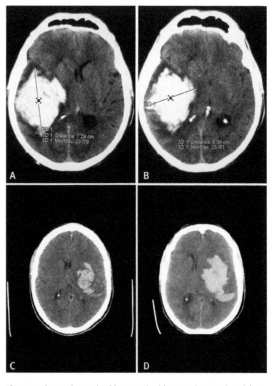

Fig 2 Location and growth of intracerebral haemorrhage. Lobar right temporoparietal haematoma (A and B, with diameter measurements); deep left basal ganglionic haematoma (C), which expanded in size 24 hours after onset (D)

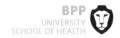

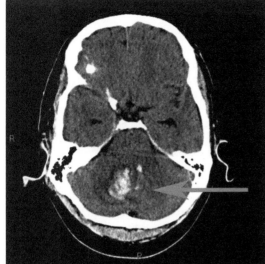

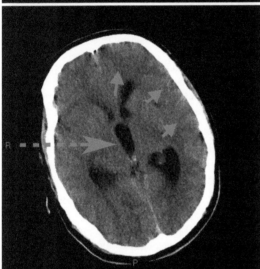

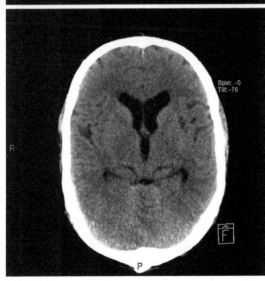

Fig 4 Infratentorial intracerebral haemorrhage. A 40 year old man presented with sudden headache, vomiting, and unsteadiness. On examination his score on the Glasgow coma scale was 15 and he had nystagmus, limb ataxia, bilateral retinal haemorrhages and papilloedema, a blood pressure of 315/180 mm Hg, and proteinuria. Blood tests showed acute renal failure, and he had immediate brain computed tomography, which showed a cerebellar haematoma adjacent to the fourth ventricle (top, arrow). Three days later, his consciousness level fell rapidly, and repeat brain computed tomography showed an increase in size of the third ventricle (centre, dashed arrow) and effacement of cortical sulci (centre, arrowheads) owing to obstructive hydrocephalus. His consciousness level improved rapidly after ventricular drainage and consequent resolution of hydrocephalus (bottom)

haemorrhage from a ruptured arteriovenous malformation varies from about 4% to about 34% according to its vascular anatomy, which is another reason for angiographic investigation of intracerebral haemorrhage.[3 15] People with intracerebral haemorrhage are also at risk of subsequent ischaemic stroke, at a rate of about 1% a year.[w13]

How should we treat intracerebral haemorrhage?

General management of stroke

Guidelines and systematic reviews recommend that patients with spontaneous intracerebral haemorrhage should be managed either in a stroke unit, or in an intensive care unit if they need ventilation or intracranial pressure monitoring.[9 10 16 w14] International guidelines are available for the management of hydration, nutrition, hyperglycaemia, and hyperthermia, prevention of complications, and early rehabilitation.[9 10] Although the risk of epileptic seizure(s) is higher within the first week of lobar than deep intracerebral haemorrhage (about 14% v about 4%),[w15] no evidence exists to support the use of prophylactic antiepileptic drugs after intracerebral haemorrhage.[9 10]

Because of the shortage of high quality evidence on how blood pressure should be managed after acute intracerebral haemorrhage, clinical guidelines recommend various blood pressure reduction regimens.[9 10] A recent, randomised pilot trial of adults who had a systolic blood pressure 150-220 mm Hg within six hours of onset of intracerebral haemorrhage found intensive blood pressure reduction to be feasible, well tolerated, and associated with a reduction in haematoma growth,[w16] although clinical benefit remains to be established in ongoing clinical trials (see web extra table on bmj.com). For now, the use of antihypertensive agents seems necessary if there is end organ damage (though the desirable parameters are uncertain),[10] but randomisation in relevant clinical trials is recommended if there is uncertainty.

Small randomised controlled trials have not found significant beneficial or harmful effects from the acute administration of corticosteroids,[w17] mannitol,[w18] glycerol,[w19] or a free radical-trapping neuroprotectant.[w20]

Haemostatic drugs

Because volume of intracerebral haemorrhage influences outcome and about a third of acute intracerebral haemorrhages enlarge within 24 hours of onset,[w10] early treatment with a haemostatic drug might improve outcome by limiting expansion of the haematoma. Phase II trials of intravenous recombinant activated factor VII were initially promising (fig 3), although their sample sizes were small and the outcomes for the placebo group were surprisingly poor. Recombinant activated factor VII did not improve clinical outcome in a larger phase III trial; the broader inclusion criteria, problems with randomisation, and preponderance of arterial thromboembolism after recombinant activated factor VII could all explain why this treatment shows no overall clinical benefit in a meta-analysis (risk ratio 0.91, 95% confidence interval 0.72 to 1.15; fig 3).[17]

Neurosurgical haematoma evacuation

Evacuation of the haematoma may show the underlying cause in the cavity or lead to the identification of amyloid angiopathy if cortical biopsy is performed, but the dilemma is whether surgery improves outcome.

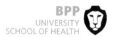

Infratentorial intracerebral haemorrhage

Guidelines recommend that neurosurgical intervention should be considered immediately for people with a cerebellar haemorrhage if it is causing deterioration in consciousness, brainstem compression, or hydrocephalus as a result of obstruction of the drainage pathways for cerebrospinal fluid (fig 4).[9] [10] Ventricular drainage may be sufficient to alleviate hydrocephalus, but further neurological deterioration requires evacuation of the haematoma.[9] [10] These recommendations are based on case series, in which outcome has been so good that randomised trials are unlikely to be undertaken.[w21]

Supratentorial intracerebral haemorrhage

One systematic review found that evacuation of spontaneous supratentorial intracerebral haemorrhage improves outcome (odds ratio 0.71, 95% confidence interval 0.58 to 0.88; fig 5),[18] although another did not.[w22] However, about 14 patients with supratentorial intracerebral haemorrhage would need to have neurosurgical evacuation for one to avoid death or dependence,[18] and these estimates are not robust because of the modest quality of most of the trials, methodological differences between them, and losses to follow up in the largest trial. A subgroup of patients with superficial lobar intracerebral haemorrhage within 1 cm of the cortical surface seemed to benefit in the STICH trial[w23] and is being studied further in the STICH 2 trial. Thrombolytic treatment of intraventricular extension from a spontaneous intracerebral haemorrhage is also the subject of ongoing randomised trials (see web extra table on bmj.com).

Treatments for specific causes

Some causes of intracerebral haemorrhage should not be missed because their treatment may improve outcome.

Aneurysms and arteriovenous malformations

One small randomised trial supports immediate evacuation of some intracerebral haematomas caused by aneurysm rupture, with concomitant clipping of the aneurysm.[19] A large randomised controlled trial of coiling versus clipping for ruptured arterial aneurysms that could be occluded by either of these treatments has shown that coiling is less likely to result in death at five years despite a higher risk of rebleeding after coiling.[20] Although a primary prevention trial for unruptured arteriovenous malformations is under way (www.arubastudy.org), there are no randomised trials of intervention for ruptured arteriovenous malformations[w24] or cavernous malformations.

Table 2 Scoring system to assess 30 day case fatality* after intracerebral haemorrhage (adapted from Hemphill et al[14])

Component	Score
Glasgow coma scale (at initial presentation or after resuscitation)	
3-4	2
5-12	1
13-15	0
Intracerebral haemorrhage volume (ml) (on initial computed tomography, using the ABC/2 method—see main text for definition)	
≥30	1
<30	0
Any intraventricular haemorrhage on initial computed tomography?	
Yes	1
No	0
Infratentorial origin of intracerebral haemorrhage?	
Yes	1
No	0
Patient's age (years)	
≥80	1
<80	0

*30 day case fatality as percentages (95% CI) as indicated by scores:
Score 1: 13 (5 to 28)
Score 2: 26 (13 to 45)
Score 3: 72 (55 to 84)
Score 4: 97 (83 to 99)
Score 5: 100 (61 to 100)
There were no patients with a score of 6.

Study	Events/total rFVIIa	Placebo	Risk ratio (random) (95% CI)	Risk ratio (random) (95% CI)
rFVIIa phase IIA USA	15/32	4/8		0.94 (0.43 to 2.06)
rFVIIa phase IIA EurAsia	16/36	5/11		0.98 (0.46 to 2.06)
rFVIIa phase IIB	160/303	66/96		0.77 (0.65 to 0.91)
rFVIIa phase III FAST	269/557	120/262		1.05 (0.90 to 1.23)
Total	460/928	195/377		0.91 (0.72 to 1.15)

0.2 0.5 1 2 5
Favours rFVIIa — Favours placebo

rFVIIa = recombinant activated factor VII

Fig 3 Forest plot of the effect of recombinant activated factor VII on death or dependence at 90 days after acute spontaneous intracerebral haemorrhage (dependence defined as score 4-5 on modified Rankin scale). Adapted with permission from a Cochrane review[17]

TIPS FOR NON-SPECIALISTS

- Computed tomography reliably distinguishes cerebral infarction from haemorrhage within minutes and for up to seven days after onset of symptoms
- Magnetic resonance imaging (including gradient-recalled echo sequences) is usually required to reliably detect haemorrhage more than one week after onset of stroke
- The early prognosis is poor, so seek specialist advice quickly
- Infratentorial haemorrhage causing a declining level of consciousness, brainstem compression, or hydrocephalus requires immediate neurosurgical referral
- Underlying causes meriting immediate consideration of specific treatment include anticoagulant drugs, uncontrolled hypertension, arterial aneurysms, and venous thrombosis

---

ADDITIONAL EDUCATIONAL RESOURCES (FOR PATIENTS)*

Europe
- Stroke Alliance For Europe (www.safestroke.org)
- Stroke Association (www.stroke.org.uk)
- Chest Heart and Stroke Scotland (www.chss.org.uk)
- Brain and Spine Foundation (www.brainandspine.org.uk)
- German Stroke Foundation (www.schlaganfall-hilfe.de)
- France AVC (www.franceavc.com)

North America
- National Stroke Association, USA (www.stroke.org)
- American Stroke Association (www.strokeassociation.org)
- Heart and Stroke Foundation, Canada (http://ww2.heartandstroke.ca/splash/)

Africa
- Heart and Stroke Foundation South Africa (www.heartfoundation.co.za)

Australasia
- National Stroke Foundation, Australia (www.strokefoundation.com.au)
- Stroke Foundation of New Zealand (www.stroke.org.nz)

Asia
- Japan Stroke Society (www.jsts.gr.jp)

*The organisations offer a range of services including support for patients, families, and carers; information leaflets and booklets; welfare grants; telephone and online advice lines; discussion groups

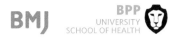

Intracranial venous thrombosis

Data from two randomised controlled trials show a reduction in the risk of death or severe disability after anticoagulation for cortical vein or venous sinus thrombosis.[21] Although the benefit of anticoagulation was based on relatively small trials, expert opinions favour immediate anticoagulation,[22] which does not seem to precipitate or worsen clinically important intracerebral haemorrhage.

Haemorrhage associated with antithrombotic drugs

Guidelines state that when intracerebral haemorrhage occurs in patients taking oral anticoagulants, these drugs should be stopped and their effects urgently reversed, although surprisingly little evidence exists about the best method of doing so.[9] [10] Although intravenous vitamin K is given in most circumstances, it is slow to act, so either prothrombin complex concentrate or fresh frozen plasma are given to immediately replenish vitamin K dependent coagulation factors.[10] The benefits of antiplatelet or even anticoagulant drugs may outweigh their risks after intracerebral haemorrhage for patients at very high risk of myocardial infarction or ischaemic stroke,[w11 w25] but for now, whether to restart these drugs at 7-10 days after an intracerebral haemorrhage should be decided on a patient by patient basis.

Infective endocarditis

Septic emboli may cause cerebral mycotic aneurysms, which may in turn lead to intracerebral haemorrhage if left untreated.

Other medical treatments

The enthusiasm for medical treatment of acute intracerebral haemorrhage has resulted in several ongoing trials to reduce haematoma expansion (blood pressure lowering, recombinant activated factor VII in subgroups, and platelet infusions for antiplatelet associated intracerebral haemorrhage) or to reduce adverse consequences of intracerebral haemorrhage (thrombolysis for intraventricular extension of intracerebral haemorrhage, anti-inflammatory drugs, statins, free radical scavengers, and iron chelators).

What about secondary prevention?

Guidelines recommend that survivors of intracerebral haemorrhage should stop smoking and limit their alcohol consumption.[9] [10] A large randomised controlled trial found that after the acute phase of intracerebral haemorrhage a reduction in blood pressure (with an angiotension converting enzyme and a diuretic, if tolerated) was beneficial in preventing future vascular events.[w26] For an average systolic blood pressure reduction of 12 mm Hg, the risk of recurrent intracerebral haemorrhage may fall by up to 76%.[23]

Conclusion

Randomised trials, systematic reviews, and international guidelines find that stroke units and secondary prevention with blood pressure reduction benefit people with intracerebral haemorrhage. Unfortunately, randomised trials of acute medical and surgical interventions do not conclusively support their routine use in clinical practice. Because the outcome after intracerebral haemorrhage is still extremely poor, ongoing trials are reason for optimism (see web extra table on bmj.com), and should be advocated in clinical practice.[24] [25]

Contributors: RA-SS searched the literature and drafted the article, and every author revised it critically for important intellectual content. All authors gave final approval of the final manuscript. RA-SS is the guarantor.

Competing interests: None declared.

Provenance and peer review: Commissioned; externally peer reviewed.

Patient consent obtained.

1   Lovelock CE, Molyneux AJ, Rothwell PM. Change in incidence and aetiology of intracerebral haemorrhage in Oxfordshire, UK, between 1981 and 2006: a population-based study. *Lancet Neurol* 2007;6:487-93.
2   Dennis MS. Outcome after brain haemorrhage. *Cerebrovasc Dis* 2003;16(suppl 1):9-13.
3   Van Beijnum J, Lovelock CE, Cordonnier C, Rothwell PM, Klijn CJ, Al-Shahi Salman R. Outcome after spontaneous and arteriovenous malformation-related intracerebral haemorrhage: population-based studies. *Brain* 2009;132(pt 2):537-43.
4   Wardlaw JM, Keir SL, Dennis MS. The impact of delays in computed tomography of the brain on the accuracy of diagnosis and subsequent management in patients with minor stroke. *J Neurol Neurosurg Psychiatry* 2003;74(1):77-81.
5   Al-Shahi R, White PM, Davenport RJ, Lindsay KW. Subarachnoid haemorrhage. *BMJ* 2006;333:235-40.
6   Ariesen MJ, Claus SP, Rinkel GJ, Algra A. Risk factors for intracerebral hemorrhage in the general population: a systematic review. *Stroke* 2003;34:2060-5.
7   Jackson CA, Sudlow CL. Is hypertension a more frequent risk factor for deep than for lobar supratentorial intracerebral haemorrhage? *J Neurol Neurosurg Psychiatry* 2006;77:1244-52.
8   Cordonnier C, Klijn CJM, van Beijnum J, Al-Shahi Salman R. Radiological investigation of spontaneous intracerebral hemorrhage: systematic literature review and tri-national survey. Unpublished data, 2009.
9   Broderick J, Connolly S, Feldmann E, Hanley D, Kase C, Krieger D, et al. Guidelines for the management of spontaneous intracerebral hemorrhage in adults: 2007 update: a guideline from the American Heart Association/American Stroke Association Stroke Council, High Blood Pressure Research Council, and the Quality of Care and Outcomes in Research Interdisciplinary Working Group. *Stroke* 2007;38:2001-23.
10   Steiner T, Kaste M, Forsting M, Mendelow D, Kwiecinski H, Szikora I, et al. Recommendations for the management of intracranial haemorrhage—part I: spontaneous intracerebral haemorrhage. The European Stroke Initiative Writing Committee and the Writing Committee for the EUSI Executive Committee. *Cerebrovasc Dis* 2006;22:294-316.
11   Al-Shahi Salman R, Berg MJ, Morrison L, Awad IA, Angioma Alliance Scientific Advisory Board. Hemorrhage from cavernous malformations of the brain: definition and reporting standards. *Stroke* 2008;39:3222-30.
12   Cordonnier C, Al-Shahi Salman R, Wardlaw J. Spontaneous brain microbleeds: systematic review, subgroup analyses and standards for study design and reporting. *Brain* 2007;130(pt 8):1988-2003.
13   Knudsen KA, Rosand J, Karluk D, Greenberg SM. Clinical diagnosis of cerebral amyloid angiopathy: validation of the Boston criteria. *Neurology* 2001;56:537-9.
14   Hemphill JC, III, Bonovich DC, Besmertis L, Manley GT, Johnston SC. The ICH score: a simple, reliable grading scale for intracerebral hemorrhage. *Stroke* 2001;32:891-7.
15   Stapf C, Mast H, Sciacca RR, Choi JH, Khaw AV, Connolly ES, et al. Predictors of hemorrhage in patients with untreated brain arteriovenous malformation. *Neurology* 2006;66:1350-5.

Study	Events/total		Odds ratio (random) (95% CI)	Odds ratio (random) (95% CI)
	Surgery + medical	Medical		
Auer 1989	28/50	37/50		0.45 (0.19 to 1.04)
Juvela 1989	25/26	22/27		5.68 (0.62 to 52.43)
Batjer 1990	6/8	11/13		0.55 (0.06 to 4.91)
Morgenstern 1998	8/15	11/16		0.52 (0.12 to 2.25)
Zuccarello 1999	4/9	7/11		0.46 (0.08 to 2.76)
Cheng 2001	86/263	98/231		0.66 (0.46 to 0.95)
Teernstra 2003	33/36	29/33		1.52 (0.31 to 7.35)
Hattori 2004	60/121	82/121		0.47 (0.28 to 0.78)
Mendelow 2005	378/468	408/496		0.91 (0.65 to 1.25)
Total	628/996	705/998		0.71 (0.58 to 0.88)

0.1 0.2   0.5 1   2   5   10

Favours surgery + medical   Favours medical

Fig 5 Forest plot of the effect of neurosurgical evacuation of acute spontaneous intracerebral haemorrhage on death or dependence at the end of follow up (dependence defined as Barthel index <60, score 3-5 on the Rankin scale, or 1-3 on the Glasgow outcome scale. Adapted with permission from a Cochrane review[18]

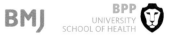

16   Stroke Unit Triallists' Collaboration. Organised inpatient (stroke unit) care for stroke. *Cochrane Database Syst Rev* 2007;(4):CD000197.

17   Al-Shahi Salman R, You H. Haemostatic drug therapies for acute spontaneous intracerebral haemorrhage. *Cochrane Database Syst Rev* 2009;(4):CD005951 (in press).

18   Prasad K, Mendelow AD, Gregson B. Surgery for primary supratentorial intracerebral haemorrhage. *Cochrane Database Syst Rev* 2008;(4):CD000200.

19   Heiskanen O, Poranen A, Kuurne T, Valtonen S, Kaste M. Acute surgery for intracerebral haematomas caused by rupture of an intracranial arterial aneurysm. A prospective randomized study. *Acta Neurochir (Wien)* 1988;90(3-4):81-3.

20   Molyneux AJ, Kerr RS, Birks J, Ramzi N, Yarnold J, Sneade M, et al. Risk of recurrent subarachnoid haemorrhage, death, or dependence and standardised mortality ratios after clipping or coiling of an intracranial aneurysm in the International Subarachnoid Aneurysm Trial (ISAT): long-term follow-up. *Lancet Neurol* 2009;8:427-33.

21   Stam J, de Bruijn SF, deVeber G. Anticoagulation for cerebral sinus thrombosis. *Cochrane Database Syst Rev* 2002;(4):CD002005.

22   Einhäupl K, Bousser MG, De Bruijn SF, Ferro JM, Martinelli I, Masuhr F, et al. EFNS guideline on the treatment of cerebral venous and sinus thrombosis. *Eur J Neurol* 2006;13:553-9.

23   Chapman N, Huxley R, Anderson C, Bousser MG, Chalmers J, Colman S, et al. Effects of a perindopril-based blood pressure-lowering regimen on the risk of recurrent stroke according to stroke subtype and medical history: the PROGRESS Trial. *Stroke* 2004;35:116-21.

24   Priorities for clinical research in intracerebral hemorrhage: report from a National Institute of Neurological Disorders and Stroke workshop. *Stroke* 2005;36(3):e23-41.

25   Stapf C, van der Worp HB, Steiner T, Rinkel GJ, Nedeltchev K, Mast H, et al. Stroke research priorities for the next decade—a supplement statement on intracranial haemorrhage. *Cerebrovasc Dis* 2007;23(4):318-9.

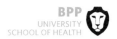

Cauda equina syndrome

Chris Lavy, honorary professor and consultant orthopaedic surgeon,
Andrew James, specialist registrar, James Wilson-MacDonald, consultant spine surgeon,
Jeremy Fairbank, professor of spine surgery

[1]Nuffield Department of
Orthopaedic Surgery, Nuffield
Orthopaedic Centre, Oxford OX3
7LD

Correspondence to: C Lavy
christopher.lavy@ndos.ox.ac.uk

Cite this as: *BMJ* 2009;338:b936

DOI: 10.1136/bmj.b936

http://www.bmj.com/content/338/
bmj.b936

An understanding of cauda equina syndrome is important not only to orthopaedic surgeons and neurosurgeons but also to general practitioners, emergency department staff, and other specialists to whom these patients present. Recognition of the syndrome by all groups of clinicians is often delayed as it presents with bladder, bowel, and sexual problems, which are common complaints and have a variety of causes. Patients may not mention such symptoms because of embarrassment or because the onset is slow and insidious.

Cauda equina syndrome is a clinical area that attracts a high risk of litigation. Although symptoms have poor predictive value on their own for the syndrome, it is important to document the nature and timing of bladder, bowel, and sexual symptoms (along with any associated clinical findings), particularly if they are new, especially in those with a history of back pain and associated leg pain, and to make a timely referral for appropriate investigation and expert treatment.

This review aims to highlight cauda equina syndrome as a possible clinical diagnosis, review the evidence for an emergency surgical approach, and maintain an awareness of the medicolegal issues that surround the condition.

What is cauda equina syndrome and how common is it?

Cauda equina syndrome results from the dysfunction of multiple sacral and lumbar nerve roots in the lumbar vertebral canal. Such root dysfunction can cause a combination of clinical features, but the term cauda equina syndrome is used only when these include impairment of bladder, bowel, or sexual function, and perianal or "saddle" numbness.[1][2] (box)

A retrospective review in Slovenia found an annual incidence of cauda equina syndrome resulting from intervertebral disc herniation of 1.8 per million population.[3] Using US data on annual incidence of symptomatic disc herniation (1500 per

---

SOURCES AND SELECTION CRITERIA

We searched Medline using the search term "cauda equina syndrome". In addition, we used our personal reference archives and consulted other experts.

---

million population), the author estimates that each year 0.12% of herniated discs are likely to cause cauda equina syndrome. We suspect this is an underestimate and are conducting our own review in the United Kingdom, but if these figures are even approximately correct then most UK general practitioners are unlikely to see even one true case caused by intervertebral disc herniation in their career.

How does cauda equina syndrome present and what symptoms suggest it?

A history of perianal sensory loss and sphincter disturbance, with or without urinary retention, suggests the presence of cauda equina syndrome (figure 1 illustrates the anatomy of the lower lumbar and sacral spine showing the cauda equina). Three classic patterns of presentation have been described.[4] It can present acutely as the first symptom of lumbar disc herniation (type 1); as the endpoint of a long history of chronic back pain with or without sciatica (type 2); or insidiously in a more chronic way with slow progression to numbness and urinary symptoms (type 3). Most clinicians now divide cauda equina syndrome into two clinical categories[4]: cauda equina syndrome with retention, in which there is established urinary retention; and incomplete cauda equina syndrome, in which there is reduced urinary sensation, loss of desire to void, or a poor stream, but no established retention or overflow.[5] Often the slower the presentation, the better tolerated the symptoms are and the less likely the patient is to be alarmed. Patients with pre-existing bladder and incontinence problems resulting from other disease may also present late.

What causes cauda equina syndrome?

The commonest cause of cauda equina syndrome in our practice and the focal causative condition in the literature[6] is compression arising from large central lumbar disc herniation at the L4/5 and L5/S1 level. Parke and colleagues suggest that there is an area of relative hypovascularity at the proximal portion of the cauda equina.[7] Blood supply alterations resulting from nerve root pressure may therefore be of greater importance in this region of the cauda equina than elsewhere, with rapid changes allowing less adaptation than those of a slower onset.

Patients may be predisposed to cauda equina syndrome if they have a congenitally narrow spinal canal or have acquired spinal stenosis arising from a combination of degenerative changes of the disc and the segmental posterior joints with consequent thickening of the ligamentum flavum and narrowing of the available canal cross section.

Numerous other less common causes of cauda equina syndrome have been reported—for example, spinal injury with fractures or subluxation. Spinal neoplasms of metastatic or primary origin can cause compression, usually accompanied by

---

CLINICAL DIAGNOSIS OF CAUDA EQUINA SYNDROME

- Dysfunction of bladder, bowel, or sexual function
- Sensory changes in saddle or perianal area

Other possible symptoms

- Back pain (with or without sciatic-type pains)
- Sensory changes or numbness in the lower limbs
- Lower limb weakness
- Reduction or loss of reflexes in the lower limbs
- Unilateral or bilateral symptoms

SUMMARY POINTS

- Cauda equina syndrome is rare, but devastating if symptoms persist
- Clinical diagnosis is not easy and even in experienced hands is associated with a 43% false positive rate
- The investigation of choice is magnetic resonance imaging
- Once urinary retention has occurred the prognosis is worse
- Good retrospective evidence supports urgent surgery especially in early cases
- Litigation is common when the patient has residual symptoms

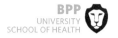

marked pain and often as part of a chronic condition. Infective causes with abscess formation or bony involvement, either within the spinal canal or impinging on it, may also cause cauda equina syndrome.[8] The spine is the most commonly affected skeletal site for tuberculosis, and Pott's paralysis is well documented.[9] A wide range of iatrogenic causes are reported, including manipulation,[10] spinal anaesthesia,[11] postoperative complications such as haematoma[12] or gelfoam implanted to protect the dura. Other space-occupying lesions, such as nerve derived tumours, schwannomas, ependymomas, facet joint cysts,[13] perineural Tarlov cysts, haemangiomas,[14] vena varix,[15] and hydatid cysts [16] are also recognised.

What features on examination suggest cauda equina syndrome?

When cauda equina syndrome is suspected a neurological examination of the legs should be performed, including perianal sensation and an assessment of anal tone (table). This is easily done in the lateral position: perineal sensation can be tested from the outside in towards the sphincter using a gentle gloved finger stroke and, if there is any uncertainty, a folded tissue and an unfolded paper clip. After this, a rectal examination can be performed. Loss or diminution of the bulbocavernosus reflex (whereby stimulation of the glans, penis, or clitoris causes reflex contraction of the anal sphincter) is suggestive of cauda equina syndrome as the reflex is mediated through the sacral roots.

How should suspected cauda equina syndrome be investigated?

Recently published guidelines for the management of patients with back pain and neurological signs recommend urgent surgical referral for suspected cauda equina syndrome.[17] Clinical diagnosis of cauda equina syndrome even by resident neurosurgeons has a 43% false positive rate,[18] so accurate confirmatory imaging is important. In the United Kingdom magnetic resonance imaging (MRI) is the imaging modality of choice. It does not define bone as clearly as computed tomography (CT) but is better at showing soft tissues such as intervertebral disc, ligamentum flavum, dural sac, and nerve roots. In resource poor settings where neither MRI nor CT is available myelography can be useful in showing the presence and site of compression of the cauda equina.[19] Figures 2 and 3 show examples of cauda equina on MRI scans.

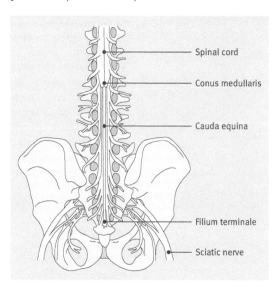

Fig 1 Anatomy of the lower lumbar and sacral spine showing the cauda equina

How is cauda equina syndrome treated?

When a patient has clinical features of cauda equina syndrome and an MRI scan shows a potentially reversible cause of pressure on the cauda equina then current consensus recommends surgical decompression.[6] This article will not review management of all the conditions leading to cauda equina syndrome, and some causes such as tumour clearly require detailed assessment of the nature and extent of the pathology. However, most cases of cauda equina syndrome are caused by herniation of the lumbar disc, for which the surgery indicated is decompression at the level of the herniation, usually involving discectomy. The operation can be very demanding technically, and great care is needed to avoid causing further damage to nerve roots or tearing tightly compressed dura.

Is surgery for cauda equina syndrome urgent?

The urgency of surgery remains controversial. When there is pressure on the cauda equina causing loss of sphincter control it would be understandable to think that the ideal treatment would be to remove the pressure as soon as possible with surgery. Ethical considerations will not allow this hypothesis to be tested by a randomised study, and it is very difficult to prove by literature review of retrospective and cohort studies (level 3 evidence) for two reasons. Firstly, the time of onset of symptoms is difficult to specify. Thus it is difficult to define the delay between symptoms and surgery. Secondly, any discussion is muddied by many published (mainly retrospective) series containing a mix of patients with both incomplete cauda equina syndrome and cauda equina syndrome with retention.

The authors of two recent reviews[20][21] argue that only incomplete cauda equina syndrome requires emergency surgery to try to stem the deterioration in bladder function. They conclude that in patients with cauda equina syndrome with retention the clinical outcome is poor anyway and bears no relation to timing of surgery. Thus these patients can wait until an elective surgical list the next morning rather than having a potentially difficult operation in the middle of the night, when circumstances are less than optimal.

Two other recently published UK series[22][23] have found that outcome is independent of the timing of surgery. Incontinence at presentation is a poor prognostic feature in the largest prospective series.[23]

A review that is widely quoted suggests that intervention less than 48 hours after the onset of symptoms will produce a better outcome than intervention delayed for longer than this.[6] These data have been selectively reanalysed[24] and suggest that the outcome for both types of cauda equina syndrome (with retention, or incomplete) is better with

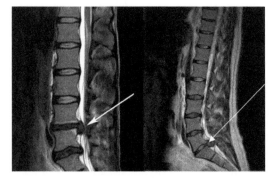

Fig 2 Left: MRI scan showing compression of the cauda equina (arrow) due to a large posterior disc herniation at L4/5. Right: MRI scan showing a large disc herniation at L5/S1 (arrow) bulging posteriorly and compressing the cauda equina syndrome

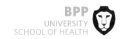

interventions within rather than after 24 hours. In a further analysis of the selected retrospective series, the authors noted that of 47 patients having surgery within 24 hours, 41 (87%) recovered normal bladder function, whereas of 46 patients having surgery later than 24 hours, only 20 (43%) recovered normal bladder function.[25]

A recent meta-analysis supports the view that early surgery is related to better results with incomplete cauda equina syndrome, but the case for cauda equina syndrome with retention is less certain.[4] We urge the establishment of a multicentre outcome study with clear clinical entry points and clear separation of incomplete cases and those with retention.

Motor sensory and reflex components of lumbar and sacral roots

Nerve level	Motor innervation	Sensory innervation	Reflexes
L2	Hip flexors, thigh adductors	Upper thigh	
L3	Quadriceps, knee extensors	Anterolateral thigh	
L4	Knee extensors and foot dorsiflexors	Anteromedial calf	Patella, knee
L5	Foot and toe dorsiflexors (extensor hallucis longus)	Lateral calf, dorsum of foot	
S1,2	Foot and toe plantar flexors	Lateral side of foot, sole of foot	Ankle
S2, S3, S4, S5	Sphincters	Perianal and saddle	Bulbocavernosus

---

QUESTIONS FOR FUTURE RESEARCH

- Multicentre outcome studies are needed to define which subgroups of cauda equina syndrome may benefit from emergency surgery and which do not need such urgent treatment
- Such studies may also develop prognostic indicators such as the length and degree of compression of the cauda equina
- Qualitative research is needed to determine appropriate questions and appropriate language to inquire about sensation in intimate areas

---

TIPS FOR NON-SPECIALISTS

- Be alert to the development of new symptoms of perianal sensory change or bladder symptoms in patients with an increase in back pain or sciatica
- Be aware that cauda equina syndrome can arise insidiously when patients who have had back and leg pain for a long time develop bladder symptoms gradually
- Establish the most appropriate channel for referral or further investigation in suspected cases in your specialty
- Make sure that clinical documentation is clear and well recorded

---

ADDITIONAL EDUCATIONAL RESOURCES*

- Cauda Equina Syndrome Resource Center (www.caudaequina.org)—Support group for people with cauda equina syndrome to share information about the condition
- BackPainExpert (www.backpainexpert.co.uk/CaudaEquinaSyndrome.html)—Patient information site with articles written by invited experts
- Wikipedia (http://en.wikipedia.org/wiki/Cauda_equina)—Part of the online editable encyclopedia wikipedia; anyone may post comments or make changes
- Cauda Equina (http://orthoinfo.aaos.org/topic.cfm?topic=A00362)—Information on the website of the American Academy of Orthopaedic surgeons

All these websites are free and do not need registration

A PATIENT'S PERSPECTIVE

I wasn't that concerned at first. I had just sneezed. I hadn't even lifted anything heavy. The sudden, searing lower back pain was unpleasantly familiar to me and it usually got better by itself. I didn't notice anything unusual until I started to get pins and needles in both my feet. And then, after painfully struggling to the toilet, I remember wiping myself with the toilet paper and it feeling decidedly odd—not completely numb but distant. It was my refusal to admit to numbness that fooled my general practitioner. He asked if I could feel him touching me, not whether his touch felt normal. He organised an urgent outpatient referral for three days later. Foolishly I just waited, not reporting the progressive loss of sensation, muscle fasciculation, creeping incontinence, and onset of a deep burning pain around my perineum. Unable to arrange ambulance transfer, a friend took me to the hospital lying in the back of his estate car. Within 90 minutes of arrival I had had an MRI scan and was in theatre undergoing an L4/5 discectomy. Two days later, the postoperative anxiety was replaced by euphoria when I managed to stand unaided and pass urine into a bottle.

What are the medicolegal implications of cauda equina syndrome?

Persisting cauda equina syndrome has a devastating effect on personal and social life, and its mismanagement is one of the commonest causes for litigation in spinal surgery. Most patients are young to middle aged and in work before they develop cauda equina syndrome, so the size of claims is large. The presence of residual symptoms means that many of these patients are unable to work and have genitourinary and bowel symptoms. From 1997 to 2006 the NHS Litigation Authority dealt with 107 cases in England in which care in hospital had been compromised (NHS Litigation Authority, personal communication, 2008). Extrapolating from previous data,[3] we would expect about 100 new cases of cauda equina syndrome annually in England, suggesting that at least 10% of cases involve litigation. The NHS Litigation Authority reported that between 1997 and 2006 in 35% of litigation cases the primary complaint was against the emergency department and in 52% it was against the inpatient management team (personal communication as above). In the remaining cases the primary complaints were against other clinical areas, such as outpatients. The responsible clinician in the litigation cases was in orthopaedics in 52% of cases, the emergency department in 27%, and neurosurgery in 8%; in the remaining cases the responsible clinician varied across various specialties.

JF and JW-MacD have prepared 22 medical negligence reports in cases of cauda equina syndrome over the past five years. The average delay to diagnosis was 67 hours and to treatment 6.14 days. These delays were attributed to orthopaedic surgeons in 32% of cases, general practitioners in 18%, and others in 14%, but in 34% of cases there was no clear case to answer. Fourteen per cent of patients had received their treatment within 24 hours and 32% within 48 hours. All patients had moderate or severe bowel and genitourinary symptoms. Most also had persisting back pain that would probably have occurred whatever the timing of surgery. Doctors who manage patients with spinal disorders need to be aware of cauda equina syndrome and its possible complications.

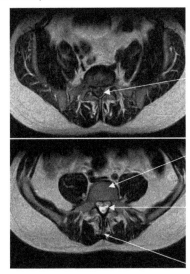

Fig 3 Top: Axial cross sectional MRI view at the level of L5/S1 of a patient with cauda equina syndrome showing a large irregular disc herniation (arrow) occupying most of the vertebral canal. Bottom: By contrast, a cross sectional MRI view at L5/S1 in a patient without cauda equina syndrome showing an unobstructed vertebral canal (arrows from top down: body of S1 vertebra; vertebral canal containing cauda equina with no compression; spine of S1)

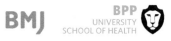

We acknowledge the help of our departmental colleagues in preparing this clinical review, in particular James Teh, Gavin Bowden, Nas Qureshi, Adi Zubovitch, David McKenna, David Mant, Elaine Buchanan, and Louise Hailey.

Contributors: This article was suggested after discussion at a departmental audit meeting. All authors contributed to the research and writing. CL is the guarantor.

Competing interests: None declared.

Provenance and peer review: Not commissioned; externally peer reviewed.

Patient consent obtained.

1   Kostuik JP. Medicolegal consequences of cauda equina syndrome: an overview. *Neurosurg Focus* 2004;16(6):e8.
2   Kostuik JP, Harrington I, Alexander D, Rand W, Evans D. Cauda equina syndrome and lumbar disc herniation. *J Bone Joint Surg Am* 1986;68:386-91.
3   Podnar S. Epidemiology of cauda equina and conus medullaris lesions. *Muscle Nerve* 2007;35:529-31.
4   DeLong WB, Polissar N, Neradilek B. Timing of surgery in cauda equina syndrome with urinary retention: meta-analysis of observational studies. *J Neurosurg Spine* 2008;8:305-20.
5   Gleave JR, Macfarlane R. Cauda equina syndrome: what is the relationship between timing of surgery and outcome? *Br J Neurosurg* 2002;16:325-8.
6   Ahn UM, Ahn NU, Buchowski JM, Garrett ES, Sieber AN, Kostuik JP. Cauda equina syndrome secondary to lumbar disc herniation: a meta-analysis of surgical outcomes. *Spine* 2000;25:1515-22.
7   Parke WW, Gammell K, Rothman RH. Arterial vascularization of the cauda equina. *J Bone Joint Surg Am* 1981;63:53-62.
8   Cohen DB. Infectious origins of cauda equina syndrome. *Neurosurg Focus* 2004;16(6):e2.
9   Nigam V, Chhabra HS. Easy drainage of presacral abscess. *Eur Spine J* 2007;16(suppl 3):322-5.
10 Haldeman S, Rubinstein SM. Cauda equina syndrome in patients undergoing manipulation of the lumbar spine. *Spine* 1992;17:1469-73.
11 Loo CC, Irestedt L. Cauda equina syndrome after spinal anaesthesia with hyperbaric 5% lignocaine: a review of six cases of cauda equina syndrome reported to the Swedish Pharmaceutical Insurance 1993-1997. *Acta Anaesthesiol Scand* 1999;43:371-9.
12 Jensen RL. Cauda equina syndrome as a postoperative complication of lumbar spine surgery. *Neurosurg Focus* 2004;16(6):e7.
13 Shaw M, Birch N. Facet joint cysts causing cauda equina compression. *J Spinal Disord Tech* 2004;17:442-5.
14 Ahn H, Jhaveri S, Yee A, Finkelstein J. Lumbar vertebral hemangioma causing cauda equina syndrome: a case report. *Spine* 2005;30:E662-4.
15 Moonis G, Hurst RW, Simon SL, Zager EL. Intradural venous varix: a rare cause of an intradural lumbar spine lesion. *Spine* 2003;28:E430-2.
16 Adilay U, Tugcu B, Gunes M, Gunaldi O, Gunal M, Eseoglu M. Cauda equina syndrome caused by primary lumbosacral and pelvic hydatid cyst: a case report. *Minim Invasive Neurosurg* 2007;50:292-5.
17 Haswell K, Gilmour J, Moore B. Clinical decision rules for identification of low back pain patients with neurologic involvement in primary care. *Spine* 2008;33:68-73.
18 Bell DA, Collie D, Statham PF. Cauda equina syndrome: what is the correlation between clinical assessment and MRI scanning? *Br J Neurosurg* 2007;21:201-3.
19 Akbar A, Mahar A. Lumbar disc prolapse: management and outcome analysis of 96 surgically treated patients. *J Pak Med Assoc* 2002;52(2):62-5.
20 Gleave JR, MacFarlane R. Prognosis for recovery of bladder function following lumbar central disc prolapse. *Br J Neurosurg* 1990;4:205-9.
21 Gleave J, MacFarlane R. Commentary. *Br J Neurosurg* 2005;19:307-8. [Commentary on: Todd NV. Cauda equina syndrome: the timing of surgery probably does influence outcome. *Br J Neurosurg* 2005;19:301-6.]
22 McCarthy MJ, Aylott CE, Grevitt MP, Hegarty J. Cauda equina syndrome: factors affecting long-term functional and sphincteric outcome. *Spine* 2007;32:207-16.
23 Qureshi A, Sell P. Cauda equina syndrome treated by surgical decompression: the influence of timing on surgical outcome. *Eur Spine J* 2007;16:2143-51.
24 Todd NV. Cauda equina syndrome: the timing of surgery probably does influence outcome. *Br J Neurosurg* 2005;19:301-6.
25 Jerwood D, Todd NV. Reanalysis of the timing of cauda equina surgery. *Br J Neurosurg* 2006;20:178-9.

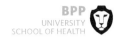

Ventilator associated pneumonia

John D Hunter, consultant in anaesthetics and intensive care

¹Department of Anaesthetics and Critical Care, Macclesfield District General Hospital, Macclesfield SK10 3BL, UK

Correspondence to: J D Hunter john. hunter4@nhs.net

Cite this as: BMJ 2012;344:e3325

DOI: 10.1136/bmj.e3325

http://www.bmj.com/content/344/ bmj.e3325

Ventilator associated pneumonia is the most common nosocomial infection in patients receiving mechanical ventilation, and it accounts for about half of all antibiotics given in the intensive care unit (ICU).[1] Its reported incidence depends on case mix, duration of mechanical ventilation, and the diagnostic criteria used. It occurs in 9-27% of mechanically ventilated patients, with about five cases per 1000 ventilator days.[2] The condition is associated with increased ICU and hospital stay and has an estimated attributable mortality of 9%.[3]

A number of evidence based strategies have been described for the prevention of ventilator associated pneumonia, and its incidence can be reduced by combining several in a care bundle.[4]

The purpose of this review is to update readers on the diagnosis, management, and prevention of this serious infection.

Ventilator associated pneumonia is a hospital acquired pneumonia that occurs 48 hours or more after tracheal intubation.[5] It can usefully be classified as early onset or late onset pneumonia. Early onset pneumonia occurs within four days of intubation and mechanical ventilation, and it is generally caused by antibiotic sensitive bacteria. Late onset pneumonia develops after four days and is commonly caused by multidrug resistant pathogens. However, patients who have been in hospital for two or more days before intubation will probably harbour organisms more commonly associated with late onset pneumonia, regardless of the duration of ventilation.

What causes ventilator associated pneumonia

The principal risk factor for the development of ventilator associated pneumonia is the presence of an endotracheal tube.[6] These tubes interfere with the normal protective upper airway reflexes, prevent effective coughing, and encourage microaspiration of contaminated pharyngeal contents. The importance of the endotracheal tube is emphasised by the incidence of pneumonia being significantly lower for non-invasive ventilation via a tight fitting facemask.[7] Reintubation after unsuccessful extubation also increases the risk of pneumonia.[8]

Most cases are caused by microaspiration of contaminated oropharyngeal secretions.[9] The oropharynx becomes rapidly colonised with aerobic Gram negative bacteria after illness, antibiotic treatment, or hospital admission

SOURCES AND SELECTION CRITERIA

I searched various sources to identify relevant evidence on the definition, epidemiology, and management of patients with ventilator associated pneumonia. These included PubMed, the Cochrane Library, and conference proceedings. I searched www. clinicaltrials.gov for current research.

as a result of alterations in host defences and subsequent changes in bacterial adherence to mucosal surfaces. These contaminated secretions pool above the cuff of the trachea or tracheostomy tube and slowly gain access to the airway via folds in the wall of the cuff.[6] A bacterial biofilm, which is impervious to systemic antibiotics, gradually forms on the inner surface of the endotracheal tube and serves as a nidus for infection.[10] Ventilator cycling propels pathogen rich biofilm and secretions to the distal airways. The size of the biofilm and the virulence of the bacteria within it contribute to the risk of infection, but it is the host's immune response that determines whether parenchymal infection and ventilator associated pneumonia will develop.

Critical illness is associated with immunosuppression, and this increases susceptibility to nosocomial infection.[11] Neutrophils are central to the body's response to most bacterial infections, and mechanically ventilated patients have neutrophil dysfunction and impaired phagocytosis. Recent work by Morris and colleagues examined neutrophil function in patients with a high clinical suspicion of ventilator associated pneumonia. They found that patients had significantly reduced phagocytic activity secondary to the overexpression of the inflammatory anaphylotoxin C5a, excess levels of which cause neutrophil dysfunction.[12] Further work by the same group suggests that this C5a driven immunosuppression precedes the acquisition of nosocomial infection and is not merely a coincidental finding.[13]

What are the risk factors for developing ventilator associated pneumonia?

Patients who are nursed in the supine position have an increased risk of pneumonia, presumably because of the increased likelihood of gastric aspiration.[14] Enteral feeding via a nasogastric tube may cause reflux of gastric contents and increase the risk of aspiration, but most intensive care physicians would agree that the benefits of providing adequate nutrition outweigh the increased risk of pneumonia.

Because the risk of developing pneumonia increases with duration of mechanical ventilation, modifiable factors associated with prolonged intubation such as oversedation or lack of protocol driven weaning increase the likelihood of pneumonia.[15]

How is ventilator associated pneumonia diagnosed?

Accurate diagnosis remains a challenge, with no consensus on a reference "gold standard" definition. Clinical diagnosis lacks sensitivity and specificity, leading to both overdiagnosis and underdiagnosis of the condition.[5] Despite

SUMMARY POINTS

- Ventilator associated pneumonia is the most common healthcare associated infection in intensive care
- The condition is associated with increased morbidity, mortality, length of stay, and costs
- Lack of a "gold standard" definition leads to both underdiagnosis and overdiagnosis
- A high clinical suspicion of pneumonia in a ventilated patient should prompt the immediate administration of an appropriate broad spectrum antibiotic(s)
- Implement evidence based interventions that reduce the incidence of pneumonia in all patients receiving mechanical ventilation

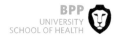

the difficulties of establishing an accurate diagnosis, a high clinical suspicion of pneumonia should lead to the immediate administration of appropriate antibiotics. Delays in antimicrobial treatment increase mortality.[16] [17]

Despite the lack of a universally agreed definition, ICU physicians generally agree that pneumonia should be suspected when there are new or persistent infiltrates on chest radiography plus two or more of the following[18]:

• Purulent tracheal secretions
• Blood leucocytosis (>12×10⁹ white blood cells/L) or leucopenia (<4×10⁹ white blood cells/L)
• Temperature greater than 38.3°C.

The Hospitals in Europe Link for Infection Control through Surveillance (HELICS) criteria are widely used for surveillance of ventilator associated pneumonia rates in Europe (fig 1). Ventilator associated pneumonia is categorised as pneumonia (PN) 1-5 depending on the microbiological method used to make the diagnosis.

Making the diagnosis can be a challenge because many conditions commonly encountered in critically ill patients—such as pulmonary oedema, pulmonary haemorrhage, and acute respiratory distress syndrome—can mimic the signs and symptoms of pneumonia. Many ventilated patients have infiltrates on chest radiography that are not attributable to infectious pathology (fig 2), and the presence of a new infiltrate only marginally increases the likelihood of ventilator associated pneumonia (summary likelihood ratio 1.7; 95% confidence interval 1.1 to 2.5).[5] Purulent tracheal secretions are often secondary to tracheobronchitis rather than parenchymal infection, and alterations in white cell count and fever symptoms can be caused by sepsis outside of the respiratory system.

Postmortem studies of patients suspected of having ventilator associated pneumonia suggest that using clinical criteria alone for diagnosis produces 30-35% false negative results and 20-25% false positive results.[5] Because of this lack of sensitivity and specificity, it is good practice to obtain microbiological samples of lower respiratory tract secretions before antibiotics are started. Samples can be obtained invasively or non-invasively. Invasive sampling methods include bronchoalveolar lavage (BAL), protected specimen brushing, and increasingly blind "mini-BAL." Mini-BAL, which is also referred to as non-bronchoscopic BAL or blind BAL, is performed using specially designed catheters that allow sampling of the distal airways via the tracheal tube. Because a bronchoscope is not needed it is quick and technically simple, with culture results that are comparable to other lavage methods.[19] Invasively obtained samples are analysed quantitatively to differentiate oropharyngeal contaminants (which are present at low concentrations) from higher concentrations of infecting organisms. The diagnostic threshold is 10³ colony forming units/mL for protected specimen brushing and 10⁴ colony forming units/mL for BAL. However, bronchoscopically directed sampling may miss the portion of lung worst affected by disease, so its sensitivity and specificity vary greatly (11-77% and 42-94%).[20] [21] Sampling can also be performed non-invasively, and the tracheal aspirates analysed quantitatively or qualitatively. This technique also misses many cases of pneumonia, with a reported sensitivity of 56-69% and a specificity of 75-95%.[21]

The relative benefits of non-invasive and invasive techniques for obtaining samples and differentiating between airway colonisation and true infection are still unclear. Although one French randomised uncontrolled study

showed a reduction in mortality when an invasive diagnostic strategy was used,[22] five other trials found no differences in hospital mortality, length of stay, or duration of mechanical ventilation when compared with non-quantitative culture of endotracheal aspirates.[23] A randomised trial by the Canadian Critical Care Trials Group randomised 740 patients with suspected ventilator associated pneumonia to undergo either BAL and quantitative culture or tracheal aspiration with non-quantitative culture of the specimens. No significant difference was seen between groups in the primary outcome (28 day mortality; 18.9% and 18.4%; P=0.94), days alive without antibiotics, or length of stay.[24] A recent systematic review of qualitative versus quantitative analysis concluded that quantitative analysis was not associated with reduced mortality, reduced length of stay in intensive care, or higher rates of antibiotic change.[25]

Several biomarkers have been investigated for diagnosing ventilator associated pneumonia, including procalcitonin, C reactive protein, and a glycoprotein known as soluble triggering receptor expressed on myeloid cells type 1 (sTREM-1).[26] The expression of sTREM-1 on phagocytes is strongly upregulated by exposure to bacteria. Although sTREM-1 concentrations are raised in BAL fluid from patients with ventilator associated pneumonia, the discriminatory value of this test is poor.[27] Procalcitonin, a calcitonin precursor hormone, is secreted in response to bacterial infection. Although it lacks sensitivity and specificity for the accurate diagnosis of pneumonia, its serial measurement may help reduce antibiotic exposure.[28] C reactive protein also lacks sufficient sensitivity and specificity for the diagnosis of pneumonia, but it can be useful for assessing the appropriateness of antibiotic treatment.[29]

Which organisms are associated with ventilator associated pneumonia?

To select the optimal antibiotic treatment it is essential to be aware of the organisms commonly associated with ventilator associated pneumonia. Most cases are bacterial in origin (table) and several organisms are often involved.[30] The clinical relevance of fungal and viral pneumonia is still poorly understood.

The duration of mechanical ventilation before the onset of pneumonia is an important determinant of the likely pathogen. Pneumonia that occurs within four days of intubation is typically caused by antibiotic sensitive community bacteria such as *Haemophilus* spp, streptococci including *Streptococcus pneumoniae*, and meticillin sensitive *Staphylococcus aureus*. Later infection is more commonly caused by multidrug resistant pathogens, including *Pseudomonas aeruginosa*, *Acinetobacter* spp, and meticillin resistant *S aureus*. However, it is increasingly recognised that patients who have been in recent close contact with the healthcare system are more likely to develop infection with multidrug resistant organisms. Hospital admission for two or more days during the 90 days before the development of ventilator associated pneumonia, chronic haemodialysis, residence in a nursing home, and intravenous antibiotics or chemotherapy within the past 30 days all increase the likelihood of extremely drug resistant bacterial infection.[31]

The pathogens associated with ventilator associated pneumonia also depend on case mix, underlying comorbidity, hospital, and type of ICU.[32] Each individual unit must collect continuous microbiological surveillance data to ensure optimal empirical antibiotic treatment of suspected pneumonia.

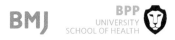

Which antibiotics are used to treat ventilator associated pneumonia?

A high clinical suspicion of pneumonia should lead to the immediate administration of appropriate empirical antibiotics. Ideally, airway samples for microbiological analysis should be taken before administration of antibiotics as long as this does not seriously delay treatment because delayed or inappropriate initial antimicrobial treatment is associated with excess mortality.[16 33]

Choose initial antibiotics on the basis of the results of local surveillance data and patient specific factors such as severity of illness, duration of hospital stay, and previous antibiotic exposure. Involvement of the local microbiologist is mandatory.

Although no optimal regimen has been identified, the chosen drug(s) should have a high degree of activity against aerobic Gram negative bacilli. Guidelines issues by the British Society for Antimicrobial Chemotherapy recommend co-amoxiclav or cefuroxime for patients with early onset infections who have not previously received antibiotics and have no other risk factors for multidrug resistant pathogens.[34] In those who have previously received antibiotics or who have other risk factors, a third generation cephalosporin (cefotaxime or ceftriaxone), a fluoroquinolone, or piperacillin-tazobactam would be appropriate. Late onset pneumonia is more commonly associated with drug resistant bacteria, particularly P aeruginosa. To date, no specific antibiotic or regimen has been proved to be superior in the management of patients with ventilator associated pneumonia secondary to P aeruginosa, and acceptable treatment options include ceftazidime, ciprofloxacin, meropenem, and piperacillin-tazobactam. When meticillin resistant S aureus is a possibility, vancomycin or linezolid should be included in the antibiotic regimen. Although linezolid penetrates lung tissue better than vancomycin, a recent meta-analysis of randomised controlled trials suggest that it is no better than vancomycin.[35]

Combination antibiotic treatment does not seem to be better than empirical broad spectrum monotherapy, which is cheaper and exposes patients to fewer antibiotics.[34] A de-escalation strategy should be used once the results of antimicrobial susceptibility tests are available. Antibiotics can be safely discontinued after eight days if an adequate clinical response is suggested by a resolution in the signs and symptoms of active infection (such as a reduction in C reactive protein, white cell count, and temperature, plus an improvement in oxygenation).[36]

Can ventilator associated pneumonia be prevented?

Although prevention of pneumonia is a vital part of the management of patients undergoing invasive mechanical ventilation, many studies of strategies and interventions that significantly reduce ventilator associated pneumonia rates fail to show a significant benefit in clinical outcomes, such as length of stay, duration of mechanical ventilation, or mortality.[37] This is probably because it is difficult to accurately diagnose ventilator associated pneumonia and many preventive measures simply reduce airway colonisation and not invasive infection.

The three main ways of preventing pneumonia are to reduce colonisation of the aerodigestive tract with pathogenic bacteria, prevent aspiration, and limit the duration of mechanical ventilation. Best results are seen by using various combinations (bundles) of interventions in all mechanically ventilated patients.[4] Recent guidance from the National Institute for Health and Clinical Excellence recommends that all bundles include oral antisepsis and nursing in the semirecumbent position.[38]

Reducing airway colonisation

Selective decontamination of the digestive tract and oral decontamination both aim to decrease the bacterial load of the digestive tract. Oral decontamination using antiseptics such as chlorhexidine seems to lower the risk of ventilator associated pneumonia (relative risk 0.61, 0.45 to 0.82),[39] especially when combined with thorough mechanical cleaning of the oral cavity. Selective decontamination involves the oral and gastric administration of non-absorbable oral antibiotics (usually polymyxin, tobramycin, and amphotericin B) plus the intravenous administration of a broad spectrum antibiotic. Despite large meta-analyses showing a reduction in the incidence of pneumonia,[40] selective decontamination is not widely used in the United Kingdom because of worries about the emergence of antibiotic resistance and increased incidence of Clostridium difficile infection. However, there is no evidence to support these concerns.

Microbial biofilms rapidly form on the luminal surface of endotracheal tubes and act as a reservoir for infection. Because silver has broad spectrum antimicrobial activity, coating the endotracheal tube with silver reduces bacterial colonisation and biofilm formation. A recent prospective randomised controlled study comparing traditional endotracheal tubes with silver coated ones showed a significant relative risk reduction of 35.9% (3.6% to 69%) in the occurrence of ventilator associated pneumonia with silver tubes.[41] However, no benefit was seen on the duration of intubation, duration of stay in intensive care, or mortality.

Preventing aspiration

All patients without specific contraindications should be nursed in the semirecumbent position, with the head raised at 45°.[42]

Secretions that have pooled above the cuff of the tracheal tube can be removed by subglottic secretion drainage using specially designed tubes with a separate dorsal lumen that opens directly above the cuff. A meta-analysis of five prospective studies found this technique to be effective in preventing ventilator associated pneumonia (relative risk 0.51, 0.37 to 0.71) in patients expected to need more than 72 hours of mechanical ventilation.[43]

Recently introduced endotracheal tubes feature an ultrathin polyurethane cuff membrane that has narrower longitudinal folds when inflated, which limits microaspiration.[44] A retrospective study reported a reduction in ventilator associated pneumonia rates from 5.3 per 1000 ventilator days to 2.8 per 1000 ventilator days after introduction of these tubes (P=0.0138),[45] although more robust studies are lacking.

Limiting duration of mechanical ventilation

The duration of mechanical ventilation is strongly associated with the development of pneumonia. Therefore, strategies aimed at reducing the duration of tracheal intubation may reduce the incidence of pneumonia. Oversedation prolongs mechanical ventilation and should be avoided by careful assessment of sedation status and daily interruption of sedation if appropriate.[15] Weaning protocols have also been shown to hasten discontinuation of mechanical ventilation.[46] Although tracheotomy is often advocated to aid earlier weaning from respiratory support, little evidence exists to suggest that early tracheotomy reduces the incidence of pneumonia.[47]

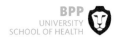

Radiography	Two or more serial chest radiographs or computed tomograms suggestive of pneumonia for patients with underlying cardiac or pulmonary disease. In patients without underlying cardiac or pulmonary disease one definitive chest radiograph or computed tomogram is sufficient

And at least one of the following

Symptoms	Fever >38°C with no other cause Leucopenia (<4x10^9 white blood cells/L) or leucocytosis (>12x10^9 white blood cells/L)

And at least one of the following (or at least two if clinical pneumonia only = PN4 and PN5)

New onset of purulent sputum or change in character of sputum (colour, odour, quantity, consistency)
Cough, dyspnoea, or tachypnoea
Suggestive auscultation (rales or bronchial breath sounds), rhonchi, wheezing
Worsening gas exchange (for example, oxygen desaturation, increased oxygen requirements, or increased ventilation demand)

And according to the used diagnostic method

Microbiology	PN1: Positive quantitative culture from minimally contaminated lower respiratory tract specimen – bronchoalveolar lavage specimen ≥10^4 colony forming units/mL PN2: Positive quantitative culture of lower respiratory tract (tracheal aspirate) with a threshold of 10^5 colony forming units/mL PN3: Positive culture related to no other source of infection – positive pleural fluid culture, pulmonary abcess with positive needle aspiration, positive histology, or positive exams for pneumonia with virus or particular organism (such as *Aspergillus*) PN4: Positive sputum culture or non-quantitative lower respiratory tract culture PN5: No positive microbiology

Fig 1 Hospitals in Europe Link for Infection Control through Surveillance (HELICS) criteria for ventilator associated pneumonia (PN)

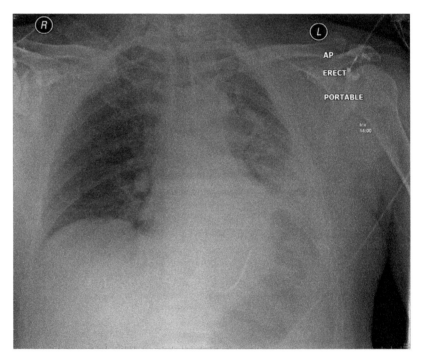

Fig 2 A typical chest radiograph from a critically ill patient with a tracheostomy showing patchy infiltration of the lower zone of the left lung, which may or may not be infective in origin

---

ADDITIONAL EDUCATIONAL RESOURCES FOR HEALTHCARE PROFESSIONALS

- Chastre J, Fagon JY. Ventilator-associated pneumonia. *Am J Respir Crit Care Med* 2002;165:867-903
- Masterton RG, Galloway A, French G, Street M, Armstrong J, Brown E, et al. Guidelines for the management of hospital-acquired pneumonia in the UK: report of the working party on hospital-acquired pneumonia of the British Society for Antimicrobial Chemotherapy. *J Antimicrob Chemother* 2008;62:5-34
- American Thoracic Society; Infectious Diseases Society of America. Guidelines for the management of adults with hospital-acquired, ventilator-associated, and healthcare-associated pneumonia. *Am J Respir Crit Care Med* 2005;171:388-416

UNANSWERED QUESTIONS AND ONGOING RESEARCH

- Is the incidence of ventilator associated pneumonia a useful quality indicator in intensive care? There is an increasing demand to use this parameter as such, but the lack of a gold standard definition and the paucity of studies showing a clinically meaningful improvement with apparent reduction in pneumonia suggest that this should be resisted
- Do aerosolised antibiotics have a role in the management of patients with ventilator associated pneumonia?
- Do probiotics prevent ventilator associated pneumonia?
- Do immunomodulatory agents have a role in the management of patients with ventilator associated pneumonia?

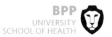

Distribution of organisms isolated from cases of ventilator associated pneumonia by bronchscopic techniques in 24 studies (1989-2000) including 1689 episodes and 2490 pathogens[30]

Pathogen	Frequency (%)
Pseudomonas aeruginosa	24.4
Acinetobacter spp	7.9
Stenotrophomonas maltophilia	1.7
Enterobacteriaceae*	14.1
Haemophilus spp	9.8
Staphylococcus aureus†	20.4
Streptococcus spp	8.0
Streptococcus pneumoniae	4.1
Coagulase negative staphylococci	1.4
Neisseria spp	2.6
Anaerobes	0.9
Fungi	0.9
Other (<1% each)‡	3.8

*Distribution when specified: Klebsiella spp 15.6%; Escherichia coli 24.1%; Proteus spp 22.3%; Enterobacter spp 18.8%; Serratia spp 12.1%; Citrobacter spp 5.0%; Hafnia alvei 2.1%.

†Distribution when specified: meticillin resistant S aureus 55.7%; meticillin sensitive S aureus 44.3%.

‡Including Corynebacterium spp, Moraxella spp, and Enterococcus spp.

Contributors: JDH conceived the article, performed the literature search, wrote the article, and is guarantor.

Funding: No funding received.

Competing interests: The author has completed the ICMJE uniform disclosure form at www.icmje.org/coi_disclosure.pdf (available on request from the corresponding author) and declares: no support from any organisation for the submitted work; no financial relationships with any organisations that might have an interest in the submitted work in the previous three years; no other relationships or activities that could appear to have influenced the submitted work.

Provenance and peer review: Not commissioned; externally peer reviewed.

1 Vincent JL, Bihari DJ, Suter PM, Bruining HA, White J, Nicolas-Chanoin MH, et al. The prevalence of nosocomial infection in intensive care units in Europe. Results of the European Prevalence of Infection in Intensive Care (EPIC) Study. EPIC International Advisory Committee. JAMA 1995;274:639-44.

2 Rello J, Ollendorf DA, Oster G, Vera-Llonch M, Bellm L, Redman R, et al. Epidemiology and outcomes of ventilator-associated pneumonia in a large US database. Chest 2002;122:2115-21.

3 Melsen WG, Rovers MM, Koeman M, Bonten MJ. Estimating the attributable mortality of ventilator-associated pneumonia from randomized prevention studies. Crit Care Med 2011;39:1-7.

4 Morris AC, Hay AW, Swann DG, Everingham K, McCulloch C, McNulty J, et al. Reducing ventilator-associated pneumonia in intensive care: impact of implementing a care bundle. Crit Care Med 2011;39:2218-24.

5 Klompas M. Does this patient have ventilator-associated pneumonia? JAMA 2007;297:1583-93.

6 Zolfaghari PS, Wyncoll DL. The tracheal tube: gateway to ventilator-associated pneumonia. Crit Care 2011;15:310.

7 Girou E, Schortgen F, Delclaux C, Brun-Buisson C, Blot F, Lefort Y, et al. Association of noninvasive ventilation with nosocomial infections and survival in critically ill patients. JAMA 2000;284:2361-7.

8 Torres A, Gatell JM, Aznar E, el-Ebiary M, Puig de la Bellacasa J, González J, et al. Re-intubation increases the risk of nosocomial pneumonia in patients needing mechanical ventilation. Am J Respir Crit Care Med 1995;152:137-41.

9 Estes RJ, Meduri GU. The pathogenesis of ventilator-associated pneumonia: I. Mechanisms of bacterial transcolonization and airway inoculation. Intensive Care Med 1995;21:365-83.

10 Adair CG, Gorman SP, Feron BM, Byers LM, Jones DS, Goldsmith CE, et al. Implications of endotracheal tube biofilm for ventilator-associated pneumonia. Intensive Care Med 1999;25:1072-6.

11 Boomer JS, To K, Chang KC, Takasu O, Osborne DF, Walton AH, et al. Immunosuppression in patients who die of sepsis and multiple organ failure. JAMA 2011;306:2594-605.

12 Morris AC, Kefala K, Wilkinson TS, Dhaliwal K, Farrell L, Walsh T, et al. C5a mediates peripheral blood neutrophil dysfunction in critically ill patients. Am J Respir Crit Care Med 2009;180:19-28

13 Morris AC, Brittan M, Wilkinson TS. C5a mediated neutrophil dysfunction is RhoA-dependent and predicts infection in critically ill patients. Blood 2011;117:5178-86

14 Torres A, Serra-Batlles J, Ros E, Piera C, Puig de la Bellacasa J, Cobos A, et al. Pulmonary aspiration of gastric contents in patients receiving mechanical ventilation: the effect of body position. Ann Intern Med 1992;116:540-3.

15 Kress JP, Pohlman AS, O'Connor MF, Hall JB. Daily interruption of sedative infusions in critically ill patients undergoing mechanical ventilation. N Engl J Med 2000;342:1471-7.

16 Iregui M, Ward S, Sherman G, Fraser VJ, Kollef MH. Clinical importance of delays in the initiation of appropriate antibiotic treatment for ventilator-associated pneumonia. Chest 2002;122:262-8.

17 Luna CM, Vujacich P, Niederman MS, Vay C, Gherardi C, Matera J, et al. Impact of BAL data on the therapy and outcome of ventilator-associated pneumonia. Chest 1997;111:676-85.

18 Fabregas N, Ewig S, Torres A, El-Ebiary M, Ramirez J, de La Bellacasa JP, et al. Clinical diagnosis of ventilator associated pneumonia revisited: comparative validation using immediate post-mortem lung biopsies. Thorax 1999;54:867-73.

19 Kollef MH, Bock KR, Richards RD, Hearns ML. The safety and diagnostic accuracy of minibronchoalveolar lavage in patients with suspected ventilator-associated pneumonia. Ann Intern Med 1995;122:743-8.

20 Papazian L, Thomas P, Garbe L, Guignon I, Thirion X, Charrel J, et al. Bronchoscopic or blind sampling techniques for the diagnosis of ventilator-associated pneumonia. Am J Respir Crit Care Med 1995;152:1982-91.

21 Marquette CH, Copin MC, Wallet F, Neviere R, Saulnier F, Mathieu D, et al. Diagnostic tests for pneumonia in ventilated patients: prospective evaluation of diagnostic accuracy using histology as a diagnostic gold standard. Am J Respir Crit Care Med 1995;151:1878-88.

22 Fagon JY, Chastre J, Wolff M, Gervais C, Parer-Aubas S, Stéphan F, et al. Invasive and noninvasive strategies for management of suspected ventilator-associated pneumonia. A randomized trial. Ann Intern Med 2000;132:621-30.

23 Muscedere J, Dodek P, Keenan S, Fowler R, Cook D, Heyland D. Comprehensive evidence-based clinical practice guidelines for ventilator-associated pneumonia: diagnosis and treatment. J Crit Care 2008;23:138-47.

24 Heyland D, Dodek P, Muscedere J, Day A; Canadian Critical Care Trials Group. A randomized trial of diagnostic techniques for ventilator-associated pneumonia. N Engl J Med 2006;355:2619-30.

25 Berton DC, Kalil AC, Teixeira PJZ. Quantitative versus qualitative cultures of respiratory secretions for clinical outcomes in patients with ventilator-associated pneumonia. Cochrane Database Syst Rev 2012;1:CD006482.

26 Palazzo SJ, Simpson T, Schnapp L. Biomarkers for ventilator-associated pneumonia: review of the literature. Heart Lung 2011;40:293-8.

27 Oudhuis GJ, Beuving J, Bergmans D, Stobberingh EE, ten Velde G, Linssen CF, et al. Soluble triggering receptor expressed on myeloid cells-1 in bronchoalveolar lavage fluid is not predictive for ventilator-associated pneumonia. Intensive Care Med 2009;3:1265-70.

28 Stolz D, Smyrnios N, Eggimann P, Pargger H, Thakkar N, Siegemund M, et al. Procalcitonin for reduced antibiotic exposure in ventilator-associated pneumonia: a randomised study. Eur Respir J 2009;34:1364-75.

29 Lisboa T, Seligman R, Diaz E, Rodriguez A, Teixeira PJ, Rello J. C-reactive protein correlates with bacterial load and appropriate antibiotic therapy in suspected ventilator-associated pneumonia. Crit Care Med 2008;36:166-71.

30 Chastre J, Fagon JY. Ventilator-associated pneumonia. Am J Respir Crit Care Med 2002;165:867-903.

31 American Thoracic Society; Infectious Diseases Society of America. Guidelines for the management of adults with hospital-acquired, ventilator-associated, and healthcare-associated pneumonia. Am J Respir Crit Care Med 2005;171:388-416.

32 Babcock HM, Zack JE, Garrison T, Trovillion E, Kollef MH, Fraser VJ. Ventilator-associated pneumonia in a multi-hospital system: differences in microbiology by location. Infect Control Hosp Epidemiol 2003;24:853-8.

33 Dupont H, Mentec H, Sollet JP, Bleichner G. Impact of appropriateness of initial antibiotic therapy on the outcome of ventilator-associated pneumonia. Intensive Care Med 2001;27:355-62.

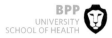

34 Masterton RG, Galloway A, French G, Street M, Armstrong J, Brown E, et al. Guidelines for the management of hospital-acquired pneumonia in the UK: report of the working party on hospital-acquired pneumonia of the British Society for Antimicrobial Chemotherapy. *J Antimicrob Chemother* 2008;62:5-34.

35 Walkey AJ, O'Donnell MR, Wiener RS. Linezolid vs glycopeptide antibiotics for the treatment of suspected methicillin-resistant Staphylococcus aureus nosocomial pneumonia: a meta-analysis of randomized controlled trials. *Chest* 2011;139:1148-55.

36 Chastre J, Wolff M, Fagon JY, Chevret S, Thomas F, Wermert D, et al. Comparison of 8 vs 15 days of antibiotic therapy for ventilator-associated pneumonia in adults: a randomized trial. *JAMA* 2003;290:2588-98.

37 Klompas M. The paradox of ventilator-associated pneumonia prevention measures *Crit Care* 2009;13:315.

38 National Institute for Health and Clinical Excellence. Technical patient safety solutions for ventilator-associated pneumonia in adults. PSG002. 2008. www.nice.org.uk/guidance/index. jsp?action=byId&o=12053.

39 Chan EY, Ruest A, Meade MO, Cook DJ. Oral decontamination for prevention of pneumonia in mechanically ventilated adults: systematic review and meta-analysis. *BMJ* 2007;334:889.

40 Kollef MH. The role of selective digestive tract decontamination on mortality and respiratory tract infections. A meta-analysis. *Chest* 1994;105:1101-8.

41 Kollef MH, Afessa B, Anzueto A, Veremakis C, Kerr KM, Margolis BD, et al. Silver-coated endotracheal tubes and incidence of ventilator-associated pneumonia: the NASCENT randomized trial. *JAMA* 2008;300:805-13.

42 Drakulovic MB, Torres A, Bauer TT, Nicolas JM, Nogue S, Ferrer M. Supine body position as a risk factor for nosocomial pneumonia in mechanically ventilated patients: a randomised trial. *Lancet* 1999;354:1851-8.

43 Dezfulian C, Shojania K, Collard HR, Kim HM, Matthay MA, Saint S. Subglottic secretion drainage for preventing ventilator-associated pneumonia: a meta-analysis. *Am J Med* 2005;118:11-8.

44 Dullenkopf A, Gerber A, Weiss M. Fluid leakage past tracheal tube cuffs: evaluation of the new Microcuff endotracheal tube. *Intensive Care Med* 2003;29:1849-53.

45 Miller MA, Arndt JL, Konkle MA, Chenoweth CE, Iwashyna TJ, Flaherty KR, et al. A polyurethane cuffed endotracheal tube is associated with decreased rates of ventilator-associated pneumonia. *J Crit Care* 2011;26:280-6.

46 Ely EW, Meade MO, Haponik EF, Kollef MH, Cook DJ, Guyatt GH, et al. Mechanical ventilator weaning protocols driven by nonphysician health-care professionals: evidence-based clinical practice guidelines. *Chest* 2001;120:454S-63S.

47 Terragni PP, Antonelli M, Fumagalli R, Faggiano C, Berardino M, Pallavicini FB, et al. Early vs late tracheotomy for prevention of pneumonia in mechanically ventilated adult ICU patients: a randomized controlled trial. *JAMA* 2010;303:1483-9.

Related links

bmj.com
- Get CME credits for this article

bmj.com/archive
Previous articles in this series
- Restless legs syndrome (2012;344:e3056)
- Pancreatic adenocarcinoma (2012;344:e2476)
- The modern management of incisional hernias (2012;344:e2843)
- Diagnosis and management of haemophilia (2012;344:e2707)

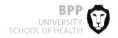

Spontaneous pneumothorax

Oliver Bintcliffe, clinical research fellow, Nick Maskell, consultant respiratory physician

¹Academic Respiratory Unit, School of Clinical Sciences, University of Bristol, Bristol BS10 5NB, UK

Correspondence to: N Maskell nick.maskell@bristol.ac.uk

Cite this as: BMJ 2014;348:g2928

DOI: 10.1136/bmj.g2928

http://www.bmj.com/content/348/bmj.g2928

Pneumothorax describes the presence of gas within the pleural space, between the lung and the chest wall. It remains a globally important health problem, with considerable associated morbidity and healthcare costs. Without prompt management pneumothorax can, occasionally, be fatal. Current research may in the future lead to more patients receiving ambulatory outpatient management. This review explores the epidemiology and causes of pneumothorax and discusses diagnosis, evidence based management strategies, and possible future developments.

How common is pneumothorax?

Between 1991 and 1995 annual consultation rates for pneumothorax in England were reported as 24/100 000 for men and 9.8/100 000 for women, and admission rates were 16.7/100 000 and 5.8/100 000, respectively, in a study analysing three national databases.[1] The overall incidence represents a rate of one pneumothorax a year in an average sized general practice population. Across the United Kingdom this equates to around 8000 admissions for pneumothorax each year, accounting for 50 000 bed days given an average length of stay of just under one week.[2] These admissions alone have estimated costs of £13.65m for the National Health Service. Annual costs in the United States have been estimated at $130m.[3]

What are the types of pneumothorax?

Pneumothorax is categorised as primary spontaneous, secondary spontaneous, or traumatic (iatrogenic or otherwise). Traumatic pneumothorax is out of the remit of this review and will not be discussed.

The distinction between primary and secondary pneumothoraxes is based on the absence or presence of clinically apparent lung disease. Primary and secondary pneumothoraxes are distinct groups regarding morbidity and mortality, rates of hypoxia at presentation, and recommended management.[4] Although primary pneumothorax is not associated with known lung disease, most affected patients have unrecognised lung abnormalities that may predispose to pneumothorax. A small case-control study found that emphysema-like changes were identified on computed tomography in 81% of 27 non-smokers with primary pneumothorax compared with 0% in the control group of 10 healthy volunteers who did not smoke.[5] Secondary pneumothorax is associated with considerably more morbidity and mortality than primary pneumothorax, in part resulting from the reduction in cardiopulmonary reserve in patients with pre-existing lung disease.

Tension pneumothorax is a life threatening complication that requires immediate recognition and urgent treatment. Tension pneumothorax is caused by the development of a valve-like leak in the visceral pleura, such that air escapes from the lung during inspiration but cannot re-enter the lung during expiration. This process leads to an increasing pressure of air within the pleural cavity and haemodynamic compromise because of impaired venous return and decreased cardiac output. Treatment is with high flow oxygen and emergency needle decompression with a cannula inserted in the second intercostal space in the midclavicular line. An intercostal drain is then inserted after decompression. Often emergency treatment must be based on a clinical diagnosis of tension pneumothorax before radiological confirmation, because of life threatening haemodynamic compromise. Radiographic features suggesting tension pneumothorax include cardiomediastinal shift away from the affected side and, in some cases, inversion of the hemidiaphragm and widening of intercostal spaces from the increased pressure within the affected hemithorax.

How is pneumothorax diagnosed?

Pneumothorax may be asymptomatic and diagnosed radiologically or may be suspected on the basis of typical clinical features. The most common symptoms are chest pain and breathlessness, characteristically with an acute onset, although these may be subtle or even absent. Patients with secondary pneumothorax tend to have more symptoms than those with primary pneumothorax as a result of coexistent lung disease. Clinical signs of pneumothorax include a reduction in lung expansion, a hyper-resonant percussion note, and diminished breath sounds on the affected side. The presence of hypotension and tachycardia may indicate tension pneumothorax.

SOURCES AND SELECTION CRITERIA

We searched the Cochrane database of systematic reviews for articles related to pneumothorax. We searched Medline using the search term "pneumothora*" appearing in relevant study types (clinical trials, literature reviews, and meta-analyses) as well as in recent conference proceedings. We limited studies to those in adults. We focused on randomised controlled trials, systematic reviews, and meta-analyses, and where possible used recent studies. The most up to date versions of relevant guidelines (British Thoracic Society, American College of Chest Physicians) were reviewed, as was information from clinicalevidence.bmj.com and uptodate.com.

SUMMARY POINTS

- Primary spontaneous pneumothorax is associated with smoking but defined as occurring in the absence of known lung disease
- Secondary spontaneous pneumothorax occurs in the presence of known lung disease and is associated with increased symptoms, morbidity, and rates of tension pneumothorax
- Immediate recognition and management of tension pneumothorax is required to prevent death
- Smoking increases the risk of pneumothorax and rates of recurrence, and smoking cessation is strongly advised
- Surgical intervention is warranted for patients with recurrent pneumothorax as the risk of further recurrence is high

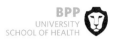

In most patients the diagnosis will be confirmed on a standard, inspiratory chest radiograph. Routine expiratory films are not recommended routinely as they do not improve diagnostic yield, contrary to historical recommendations.[4] The hallmark of a pneumothorax on a radiograph is a white visceral pleural line separated from the parietal pleura and chest wall by a collection of gas, resulting in a loss of lung markings in this space (fig 1).

Features of pneumothorax may be more subtle on supine radiographs, with more air needed within the pneumothorax to confidently make a diagnosis. The deep sulcus sign, caused by air collecting in the costophrenic sulcus, apparently deepening it, may indicate pneumothorax on a supine radiograph.

Computed tomography provides sensitive and specific imaging for pneumothorax and is particularly useful for complex disease processes, including pneumothoraxes that are loculated as a result of areas of lung remaining adherent to parietal pleura, as well as facilitating radiologically guided drain insertion in difficult cases. Additionally, computed tomography is useful in distinguishing a pneumothorax from large bullae, which may occur in severe emphysema and can mimic the appearance of pneumothorax due to the absence of lung markings within a bulla. Typically, on chest radiographs bullae are indicated by a concave appearance, whereas a pneumothorax is suggested by a visceral pleural line running parallel to the chest wall; however, this distinction may be made clearly with computed tomography, potentially avoiding the serious complication of inserting a drain into lung parenchyma.

What predisposes to pneumothorax?

Primary spontaneous pneumothorax

The most important risk factor contributing to risk of primary pneumothorax is tobacco smoking. A retrospective study over 10 years conducted in Stockholm assessed the smoking habits of 138 patients with primary pneumothorax and compared their rates of smoking with a contemporary random sample of over 15 000 people from the same geographical area. Within this study, 88% of the patients with primary pneumothorax smoked. Compared with non-smokers the relative risk of a first pneumothorax is increased by ninefold in women who smoke and by 22-fold in men who smoke.[6] In addition this study found a striking dose-response relation between number of cigarettes smoked a day and risk of pneumothorax.[6] Cannabis smoking is associated with pneumothorax, an effect that may be attributed to both parenchymal damage from smoke and the longer breath-holds or valsalva manoeuvres that may be associated with smoking cannabis.[7]

The risk of primary pneumothorax is greater in tall men, which has led to the hypothesis that a greater alveolar stretch at the lung apex in tall men contributes to the increased risk.[8] Pneumothorax as a whole has a biphasic age distribution with primary pneumothorax peaking in those between the ages of 15 and 34 and secondary pneumothorax in those aged more than 55.[1]

Secondary spontaneous pneumothorax

Chronic obstructive pulmonary disease is the most common lung disease causing secondary pneumothorax, accounting for around 57% of cases.[9] The risk of pneumothorax seems to increase with worsening chronic obstructive pulmonary

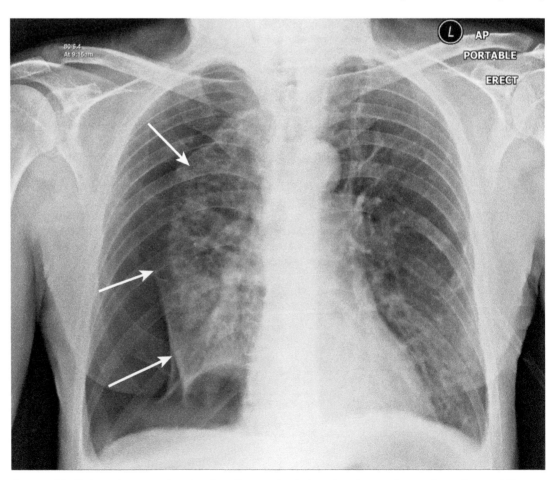

Fig 1 Large right sided secondary pneumothorax in patient with severe chronic obstructive pulmonary disease and acute dyspnoea. White arrows indicate visceral pleura surrounding collapsed lung

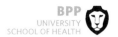

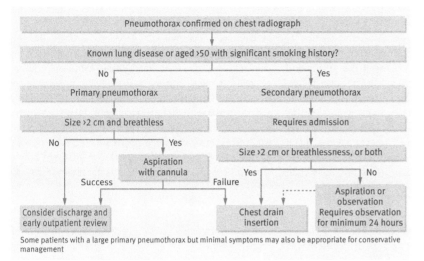

Some patients with a large primary pneumothorax but minimal symptoms may also be appropriate for conservative management

Fig 2 Initial management of pneumothorax. Adapted from British Thoracic Society guidelines, MacDuff et al[4]

disease; around 30% of patients with secondary pneumothorax have a forced expiratory volume in one second of less than 1 litre.[10] Other causes of secondary pneumothorax include asthma, *Pneumocystis jirovecii* pneumonia related to HIV infection, cystic fibrosis, lung cancer, tuberculosis, interstitial lung disease, and endometriosis.

Thoracic endometriosis seems to have been an under-recognised cause of pneumothorax; a prospective study evaluating 32 women with pneumothorax referred for surgery found that 25% (n=8) had features suggesting pneumothorax associated with menses and seven of these women had histopathological confirmation of diaphragmatic endometriosis.[11] Specifically evaluating women for this possibility may significantly alter management.

What predicts recurrence of pneumothorax?

Primary spontaneous pneumothorax
Smoking cessation is the only proved modifiable risk factor for recurrence of primary pneumothorax. In a retrospective study of patients with primary pneumothorax, including 99 smokers, the absolute risk of recurrent pneumothorax in the four year follow-up period was 40% in those who stopped smoking compared with 70% in those who continued to smoke.[12] Recurrence of primary pneumothorax is also associated with increased height in men[12] and is significantly reduced by open surgery or video assisted thoracic surgery.[13]

Secondary spontaneous pneumothorax
Patients with pre-existing lung disease are more likely to experience a recurrent pneumothorax than those with primary pneumothorax.[14][15] In a retrospective study of 182 patients, of whom around half had chemical pleurodesis, recurrence rates at one year were 15.8% for primary pneumothorax and 31.2% for secondary pneumothorax.[15] Rates of recurrence of secondary pneumothorax are noticeably lowered by thoracic surgery: after video assisted thoracic surgery or axillary minithoracotomy, recurrence rates of around 3% were reported in a study with a mean follow-up period of 30 months,[13] whereas a separate study, with a similar duration of follow-up, reported recurrence rates of 43% in a control group of 86 patients with secondary pneumothorax.[10]

What is the goal of management?

The goal of acute treatment in pneumothorax is to exclude a tension pneumothorax and to relieve any dyspnoea. These goals are reflected by the different treatment algorithms

in patients with primary or secondary pneumothorax, as patients with the latter are more likely to be symptomatic and more prone to associated cardiopulmonary compromise, in view of pre-existing disease. In contrast, patients with primary pneumothorax are often asymptomatic and tension pneumothorax is uncommon in this population.

Early studies evaluating treatment of pneumothorax focused on radiological resolution rather than patient centred outcomes, and this may have previously resulted in guidelines focused on intervention to remove air from the pleural space. Goals of treatment in pneumothorax are to exclude tension and reduce early morbidity and symptoms associated with pneumothorax, to limit inpatient management where possible, to reduce the risk of recurrence, and to identify patients who would benefit from a definitive surgical procedure.

What are the treatment options?

Surprisingly for such a common condition there is considerable disparity in societal guidelines and worldwide practice for the management of pneumothorax. Management options range from observation through aspiration or drainage to thoracic surgical intervention. The choice is largely determined by symptoms and haemodynamic compromise, the size and cause of the pneumothorax, whether an episode is the first or recurrent, and the success or failure of initial management. Major differences exist between guidelines relating to the management of primary and secondary pneumothorax, some of which are outlined below.[3][4] One key difference between guidelines is the method of measuring pneumothorax: the British Thoracic Society defines a pneumothorax as large with a >2 cm measurement from the lung margin to chest wall at the level of the hilum, whereas the American College of Chest Physicians define this as ≥ 3 cm from the lung apex to the thoracic cupola. The measurement used within the British guidelines may have the advantage of identifying those pneumothoraxes for which drain insertion in the "triangle of safety" is appropriate. Figure 2 summarises the current British Thoracic Society guidelines for the management of haemodynamically stable pneumothorax.

Primary spontaneous pneumothorax
Assuming that air leakage has stopped, a pneumothorax will gradually resolve as air is reabsorbed into pulmonary capillaries. The rate of resolution was calculated at 2.2% a day in a retrospective study assessing three dimensional estimates of pneumothorax size based on chest radiographs in patients treated conservatively.[16] The rate of reabsorption is increased fourfold when oxygen is administered[17] and therefore supplemental high flow oxygen is recommended when patients are admitted for observation.[4] A key difference between the American College of Chest Physicians Delphi consensus statement 2001[3] and the British Thoracic Society guidelines 2010[4] is the role of aspiration of air, as opposed to intercostal drain insertion. Whereas the British guidelines recommend aspiration for primary pneumothorax with a large (>2 cm) pneumothorax, the American consensus statement recommends inserting a chest drain or small bore catheter when intervention is required. Both the guidelines and consensus statement discourage the use of large bore "surgical" drains in uncomplicated pneumothorax in view of the similar success rate and lower levels of discomfort associated with smaller bore drains inserted with a seldinger technique (in which a guidewire is passed through a needle into the pleural space and a drain passed over the wire).[3][4]

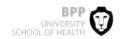

A randomised controlled trial of 56 patients assessed manual aspiration against intercostal drain insertion in patients with large primary pneumothorax.[18] Success and recurrence rates did not differ between the groups and manual aspiration was associated with significantly shorter hospital stays, suggesting that this strategy is appropriate in this group. An earlier Cochrane review, limited by the inclusion of only a single randomised controlled trial, also suggested that aspiration was no different from chest drain insertion in terms of early success or success at one year, and was associated with a reduction in the number of patients admitted to hospital.[19]

Secondary spontaneous pneumothorax

Management of secondary pneumothorax tends to involve a more interventional approach because of the associated increased morbidity, symptoms, and cardiorespiratory compromise. In reflection of this, both American College of Chest Physicians and British Thoracic Society guidelines recommend admission for all episodes of secondary pneumothorax.[3][4] Oxygen is indicated, but some caution may be required for patients at risk of carbon dioxide retention. Although most patients may ultimately require an intercostal drain, the British guidelines recommend attempting aspiration for asymptomatic secondary pneumothorax measuring 1-2 cm at the hilum, whereas the American consensus statement suggests that this is not appropriate.[3][4]

Air leakage in secondary pneumothorax is less likely to settle spontaneously than in primary pneumothorax[20] and patients with secondary pneumothorax have a longer average length of stay than those with primary pneumothorax: more than 10 days in some series.[21] Discussion with a thoracic surgeon is advised after 48 hours of persistent air leakage, offering an individualised approach to surgical management dependent on risks of recurrence and surgical morbidity. Some patients are unfit for a definitive surgical procedure and may require a longer trial of conservative management or a less invasive management strategy.

Suction

The use of suction through chest drains has been employed in patients with persistent air leak or incomplete lung re-expansion in whom the rate of air leakage from the lung may be greater than the removal of air from the pleural space through the drain. This is utilised to increase the air flow out through the drain in the hope that if the visceral and parietal pleura can be apposed then the defect in the visceral pleura may heal more readily. A small randomised study of 23 patients found no significant differences in rates of lung re-expansion and duration of hospital stay between suction and no suction.[22] British Thoracic Society guidelines recommend that suction is not routinely employed in the management of pneumothorax but can be used if the lung fails to re-expand; a pressure of −10 to −20 cm H_2O as part of a high-volume low-pressure system is the recommended method.[4] Such a system should minimise the risk of increasing air leak and "air-stealing"—a process by which a large volume of each breath is entrained out of the chest through the drain. The early application of suction after drainage of a pneumothorax should be avoided because of an increased risk of re-expansion pulmonary oedema precipitated by the rapid reinflation of the collapsed lung.

Surgery

Axillary minithoracotomy and video assisted thoracic surgery are both used for the treatment of recurrent pneumothorax. A recent randomised controlled trial of 66 patients with primary or secondary pneumothorax allocated to minithoracotomy or to video assisted thoracic surgery showed equivalent recurrence rates (2.7% and 3%, respectively) and postoperative pain.[13] Compared with minithoracotomy, video assisted thoracic surgery was associated with higher patient satisfaction (assessed by use of the ipsilateral arm postoperatively) and return to activity, albeit at the expense of a longer procedure time.[13]

Pleurodesis

Pleurodesis is a procedure that precipitates an inflammatory process leading to the adherence of parietal and visceral pleura, thereby obliterating the pleural space. This can be achieved through instillation of an agent such as talc or tetracycline derivatives through a chest drain (medical pleurodesis) or by mechanical abrasion of the pleura or instillation of a suitable agent during an operation (surgical pleurodesis). Because of the inflammatory nature of pleurodesis, it can be painful and requires the application of local anaesthesia into the pleural space as well as adequate analgesia.

A randomised controlled trial of 214 patients with primary pneumothorax in Taiwan assessed the effect of minocycline pleurodesis on recurrence of pneumothorax at one year. All the patients had pigtail catheters for aspiration of their pneumothorax and were randomised to minocycline pleurodesis or to no pleurodesis. Recurrence rates were significantly lower (P=0.003) in the minocycline pleurodesis group (29.2%) compared with the control group (49.1%).[23] This method of treatment, however, typically necessitated a two day hospital stay, and the rate of recurrence in the control group was higher than that reported in other studies (33% at one year in one study[15]). An earlier smaller randomised study including participants with primary and secondary pneumothorax compared simple drainage with tetracycline or talc pleurodesis and found that the rate of recurrence over a mean follow-up period of 4.6 years was only 8% in the talc pleurodesis group but 36% in the simple drainage group.[24] British Thoracic Society guidelines suggest that chemical pleurodesis should be considered only in patients with an ongoing air leak who are not fit for surgical intervention, rather than as a primary treatment, in view of the significantly lower recurrence rates (around 3%) after surgery.[13]

What advice do patients need after a pneumothorax?

Given the considerable recurrence rate for pneumothorax it is important that patients are advised of the symptoms that may indicate recurrence and the need to seek medical advice if this occurs.

British Thoracic Society guidelines suggest that all patients with a pneumothorax are followed up by a respiratory physician around 2-4 weeks after the initial episode to ensure resolution and to identify and treat underlying lung disease.[4] Patients can be advised to return to work and normal activity after resolution of symptoms, although extreme exertion and contact sports should be delayed for longer and until full radiological resolution.[4]

Smoking cessation significantly reduces the recurrence rate in patients after an initial primary pneumothorax, with a relative risk reduction of over 40%.[12] Therefore patients should be made aware of this and provided with support to successfully stop smoking. Aside from medical intervention,

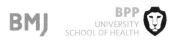

smoking is the only modifiable risk factor predicting recurrence. Unfortunately, smoking cessation rates seem to be low after pneumothorax; more than 80% of patients in a retrospective study of 142 patients with primary pneumothorax continued to smoke one year after the episode.[25]

Diving

British Thoracic Society guidelines advise that scuba diving should be avoided indefinitely after a pneumothorax unless a definitive procedure such as surgical pleurectomy has been performed.[4] This is because of the risk of recurrent pneumothorax underwater, the expansion of a pneumothorax that may develop during ascent, and the risk of resultant tension pneumothorax. For professional divers a decision to offer definitive surgical management after the first pneumothorax episode may allow safe reintroduction to diving.

Air travel

Air travel should not increase the risk of pneumothorax, but the consequences of a pneumothorax while airborne are such that patients should not travel on commercial flights with an undrained pneumothorax, and air travel should be delayed until after definitive intervention or until resolution has been confirmed radiologically.[26] The chances of recurrent pneumothorax and the degree to which patients would tolerate a recurrence will influence the decision on whether the risk of air travel is acceptable to an individual. The UK civil aviation authority suggests that it is safe to travel two weeks after successful drainage of a pneumothorax.

What new treatments can be expected?

Conservative treatment

British Thoracic Society guidelines recommend that conservative management should be considered in patients with a small pneumothorax (<2 cm to lung edge at level of hilum) who are not breathless and acknowledge that it may be appropriate in patients with a large pneumothorax and minimal symptoms. An Australian randomised controlled trial is currently recruiting patients with larger primary pneumothorax to compare conservative management (observation then discharge if clinically stable) with standard management (aspiration and chest drain insertion if unsuccessful) on lung re-expansion at eight weeks as well as the effect on symptoms, complications, and recurrence.[27]

Quantification of air leak

Digital thoracic drainage systems allow a quantification of air leak that is not possible with a conventional underwater seal. These systems have been studied predominantly in patients with air leakage after thoracic surgery, but they may allow earlier stratification in pneumothorax, distinguishing those patients who are likely to have a persistent air leak from those whose air leak will settle with continued intercostal tube drainage.

QUESTIONS FOR FUTURE RESEARCH

- Is conservative management safe, feasible and effective? The subject of a currently recruiting randomised controlled trial/Cochrane review
- Do Heimlich valves offer safe and effective ambulatory treatment?
- What is the current incidence of pneumothorax?
- Can we risk stratify patients with primary spontaneous pneumothorax at their first presentation according to their chance of recurrence, and therefore target surgical intervention at an earlier stage in this subgroup?

Endobronchial valves

Endobronchial valves have been utilised as a non-surgical means of achieving a reduction in lung volume in emphysema and have also been studied as a treatment for persistent air leak in pneumothorax. These one-way valves may be inserted during a bronchoscopy, and when placed in segmental or subsegmental bronchi allow collapse of the distal lung and reduction in air leak while allowing drainage of secretions from distal airways. Endobronchial valves have been studied in 40 patients with varying causes of ongoing air leak, 25 of whom had spontaneous pneumothorax. Of the total, 93% (n=37) had a reduction or resolution in air leak, with 48% (n=19) achieving a complete resolution of leak.[28] This technique may allow a non-surgical method of managing patients who do not respond to conventional treatment, and prospective trials may help elucidate its role.

Blood patch

The effect of intrapleural injection of autologous blood was assessed in a small randomised controlled trial of 44 patients with advanced chronic obstructive pulmonary disease, secondary pneumothorax, and a persistent air leak after seven days of intercostal tube drainage.[29] This intervention was associated with a statistically significant reduction in ongoing air leak at 13 days. The air leak stopped in 9% (n=1) of those administered placebo and 73% (n=16) administered 1-2 mL/kg of blood, with greater success rates seen in those with a smaller air leak. Fourteen per cent of patients who were administered this dose of blood developed a low grade fever, which in all cases settled quickly with antibiotics. This study suggests that this technique may be useful as an alternative to chemical pleurodesis in patients with a significant risk from surgery.[29]

Ambulatory treatment

Heimlich valves are one-way flutter valves that may be attached to an intercostal drain in place of an underwater seal. They offer an outpatient treatment option for the management of pneumothorax, which may have an increasing role in the future. A randomised controlled trial of 48 patients with primary pneumothorax presenting to emergency departments compared Heimlich valves with needle aspiration and detected non-significantly lower rates of admission of 44% (n=11) in the valve group compared with 61% (n=14) in the needle aspiration group. At first outpatient review, full re-expansion of the lung occurred in 24% (n=6) of participants in the valve group compared with only 4% (n=1) in the needle aspiration group. Both procedures appeared safe, were well tolerated, and the intercostal drain was removed at a mean of 3.5 days in participants in the valve group.[30]

A subsequent systematic review (n=1235 cases) assessed available evidence for the use of Heimlich valves.[31] Despite being limited by a large proportion of unrandomised data with potential sources of bias, the review suggested an overall success rate of 85.8% with Heimlich valves, with successful treatment as an outpatient in 77.9% of cases. This treatment may offer benefits related to comfort and the avoidance of admissions with acceptable complication rates of 1.7%.[31] A larger well designed randomised controlled trial evaluating the use of Heimlich valves is required to evaluate the utility of this device.

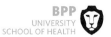

TIPS FOR NON-SPECIALISTS

- Pneumothorax is associated with a sudden onset of breathlessness and pleuritic chest pain, although in some patients it can be asymptomatic
- The diagnosis can usually be made on chest radiographs, but computed tomography is sometimes required
- Management depends on whether the episode is a primary or secondary pneumothorax
- The presence of haemodynamic compromise with pneumothorax may indicate tension pneumothorax, which requires urgent decompression with a cannula through the second intercostal space in the midclavicular line
- Smoking cessation reduces the risk of recurrence of primary spontaneous pneumothorax
- After pneumothorax, air travel should be delayed until after definitive intervention or until resolution has been confirmed radiologically—the UK civil aviation authority recommends delaying air travel until two weeks after resolution

---

ADDITIONAL EDUCATIONAL RESOURCES

Resources for healthcare professionals

- British Thoracic Society Guidelines (www.brit-thoracic.org.uk/guidelines-and-quality-standards/pleural-disease-guideline/)—the pleural disease guideline (2010) includes evidence based recommendations related to the management of spontaneous pneumothorax and pleural procedures. Free resource; registration not required
- BMJ Clinical evidence bmj.com (http://clinicalevidence.bmj.com/x/index.html)—provides systematic reviews of interventions for the management of spontaneous pneumothorax. Subscription required

Resources for patients

- British Lung Foundation (www.blf.org.uk/Conditions/Detail/Pneumothorax)—patient information sheet for pneumothorax detailing symptoms, treatment, and recurrence rates. Free resource; registration not required
- Patient.co.uk (www.patient.co.uk/doctor/pneumothorax)—information on the epidemiology of pneumothorax, risk factors, treatment, and prognosis. Free resource, registration not required

Contributors: Both authors jointly prepared the manuscript. NM is the guarantor.

Competing interests: We have read and understood the BMJ Group policy on declaration of interests and declare the following interests: none.

Provenance and peer review: Commissioned; externally peer reviewed.

1. Gupta D, Hansell A, Nichols T, Duong T, Ayres JG, Strachan D. Epidemiology of pneumothorax in England. Thorax 2000;55:666-71.
2. Data from Health & Social Care Information Centre. 2013. www.hscic.gov.uk.
3. Baumann MH, Strange C, Heffner JE, Light R, Kirby TJ, Klein J, et al. Management of spontaneous pneumothorax: an American College of Chest Physicians Delphi consensus statement. Chest 2001;119:590-602.
4. MacDuff A, Arnold A, Harvey J, Group BTSPDG. Management of spontaneous pneumothorax: British Thoracic Society Pleural Disease Guideline 2010. Thorax 2010;65(Suppl 2):ii18-31.
5. Bense L, Lewander R, Eklund G, Hedenstierna G, Wiman LG. Nonsmoking, non-alpha 1-antitrypsin deficiency-induced emphysema in nonsmokers with healed spontaneous pneumothorax, identified by computed tomography of the lungs. Chest 1993;103:433-8.
6. Bense L, Eklund G, Wiman LG. Smoking and the increased risk of contracting spontaneous pneumothorax. Chest 1987;92:1009-12.
7. Feldman AL, Sullivan JT, Passero MA, Lewis DC. Pneumothorax in polysubstance-abusing marijuana and tobacco smokers: three cases. J Subst Abuse 1993;5:183-6.
8. Withers JN, Fishback ME, Kiehl PV, Hannon JL. Spontaneous pneumothorax: suggested etiology and comparison of treatment methods. Am J Surg 1964;108:772-6.
9. Chen CH, Liao WC, Liu YH, Chen WC, Hsia TC, Hsu TH, et al. Secondary spontaneous pneumothorax: which associated conditions benefit from pigtail catheter treatment? Am J Emerg Med 2012;30:45-50.
10. Light RW, O'Hara VS, Moritz TE, McElhinney AJ, Butz R, Haakenson CM, et al. Intrapleural tetracycline for the prevention of recurrent spontaneous pneumothorax. Results of a Department of Veterans Affairs cooperative study. JAMA 1990;264:2224-30.
11. Alifano M, Roth T, Broet SC, Schussler O, Magdeleinat P, Regnard JF. Catamenial pneumothorax: a prospective study. Chest 2003;124:1004-8.
12. Sadikot RT, Greene T, Meadows K, Arnold AG. Recurrence of primary spontaneous pneumothorax. Thorax 1997;52:805-9.
13. Foroulis CN, Anastasiadis K, Charokopos N, Antonitsis P, Halvatzoulis HV, Karapanagiotidis GT, et al. A modified two-port thoracoscopic technique versus axillary minithoracotomy for the treatment of recurrent spontaneous pneumothorax: a prospective randomized study. Surg Endosc 2012;26:607-14.
14. Lippert HL, Lund O, Blegvad S, Larsen HV. Independent risk factors for cumulative recurrence rate after first spontaneous pneumothorax. Eur Respir J 1991;4:324-31.
15. Guo Y, Xie C, Rodriguez RM, Light RW. Factors related to recurrence of spontaneous pneumothorax. Respirology 2005;10:378-84.
16. Kelly AM, Loy J, Tsang AY, Graham CA. Estimating the rate of re-expansion of spontaneous pneumothorax by a formula derived from computed tomography volumetry studies. Emerg Med J 2006;23:780-2.
17. Northfield TC. Oxygen therapy for spontaneous pneumothorax. BMJ 1971;4:86-8.
18. Parlak M, Uil SM, van den Berg JWK. A prospective, randomised trial of pneumothorax therapy: manual aspiration versus conventional chest tube drainage. Respir Med 2012;106:1600-5.
19. Wakai A, O'Sullivan RG, McCabe G. Simple aspiration versus intercostal tube drainage for primary spontaneous pneumothorax in adults. Cochrane Database Syst Rev 2007;1:CD004479.
20. Chee CB, Abisheganaden J, Yeo JK, Lee P, Huan PY, Poh SC, et al. Persistent air-leak in spontaneous pneumothorax—clinical course and outcome. Respir Med 1998;92:757-61.
21. Schoenenberger RA, Haefeli WE, Weiss P, Ritz RF. Timing of invasive procedures in therapy for primary and secondary spontaneous pneumothorax. Arch Surg 1991;126:764-6.
22. So SY, Yu DY. Catheter drainage of spontaneous pneumothorax: suction or no suction, early or late removal? Thorax 1982;37:46-8.
23. Chen JS, Chan WK, Tsai KT, Hsu HH, Lin CY, Yuan A, et al. Simple aspiration and drainage and intrapleural minocycline pleurodesis versus simple aspiration and drainage for the initial treatment of primary spontaneous pneumothorax: an open-label, parallel-group, prospective, randomised, controlled trial. Lancet 2013;381:1277-82.
24. Almind M, Lange P, Viskum K. Spontaneous pneumothorax: comparison of simple drainage, talc pleurodesis, and tetracycline pleurodesis. Thorax 1989;44:627-30.
25. Smit HJ, Chatrou M, Postmus PE. The impact of spontaneous pneumothorax, and its treatment, on the smoking behaviour of young adult smokers. Respir Med 1998;92:1132-6.
26. Ahmedzai S, Balfour-Lynn IM, Bewick T, Buchdahl R, Coker RK, Cummin AR, et al. Managing passengers with stable respiratory disease planning air travel: British Thoracic Society recommendations. Thorax 2011;66(Suppl 1):i1-30.
27. Perrin K. Trial ID: ACTRN12611000184976. A randomised controlled trial of conservative versus interventional treatment of primary spontaneous pneumothorax. 2013. www.anzctr.org.au/Trial/Registration/TrialReview.aspx?ID=336270.
28. Travaline JM, McKenna RJ Jr, De Giacomo T, Venuta F, Hazelrigg SR, Boomer M, et al. Treatment of persistent pulmonary air leaks using endobronchial valves. Chest 2009;136:355-60.
29. Cao G, Kang J, Wang F, Wang H. Intrapleural instillation of autologous blood for persistent air leak in spontaneous pneumothorax in patients with advanced chronic obstructive pulmonary disease. Ann Thorac Surg 2012;93:1652-7.
30. Ho KK, Ong ME, Koh MS, Wong E, Raghuram J. A randomized controlled trial comparing minichest tube and needle aspiration in outpatient management of primary spontaneous pneumothorax. Am J Emerg Med 2011;29:1152-7.
31. Brims FJ, Maskell NA. Ambulatory treatment in the management of pneumothorax: a systematic review of the literature. Thorax 2013;68:664-9.

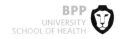

Diagnosis and management of pulmonary embolism

S Takach Lapner, research fellow and haematologist, C Kearon, professor of medicine

¹Department of Medicine, McMaster University, Hamilton, Ontario, Canada

Correspondence to: C Kearon, Hamilton Health Sciences, Juravinski Hospital Division, 711 Concession Street, Hamilton, Ontario L8V 1C3, Canada kearonc@mcmaster.ca

Cite this as: BMJ 2013;346:f757

DOI: 10.1136/bmj.f757

http://www.bmj.com/content/346/bmj.f757

Pulmonary embolism is one manifestation of venous thromboembolism, the other being deep vein thrombosis. Pulmonary embolism occurs when a deep vein thrombosis breaks free, passes through the right side of the heart, and lodges in the pulmonary arteries. About 90% of pulmonary emboli come from the legs, with most involving the proximal (popliteal or more central) veins. Prevention of pulmonary embolism therefore requires both prevention of venous thromboembolism and effective treatment of deep vein thrombosis when it occurs. There is a wealth of high quality individual studies and meta-analyses to guide the diagnosis and treatment of pulmonary embolism, and we provide an overview and synthesis of that evidence in this review.

Why is pulmonary embolism important?

Symptomatic venous thromboembolism occurs in 1-2 per 1000 adults each year, with about a third presenting with pulmonary embolism.[1][2] Pulmonary embolism is the most common cause of vascular death after myocardial infarction and stroke, and the leading preventable cause of death in hospital patients.[2] About 10% or more of cases of symptomatic pulmonary embolism are thought to be rapidly fatal, and another 5% of patients die after starting treatment. About a third of patients are left with some residual symptoms, and 2% develop thromboembolic pulmonary hypertension due to unresolved pulmonary embolism.[3]

Who is at risk?

Presentation of venous thromboembolism as pulmonary embolism rather than deep vein thrombosis is more common in elderly people and in those with cardiorespiratory disease,

SOURCES AND SELECTION CRITERIA

We searched Medline and the Cochrane Collaboration for up to date systematic reviews, meta-analyses, and high quality randomised controlled trials pertaining to the epidemiology, diagnosis, and treatment of pulmonary embolism. We also drew on the recently published guidelines on diagnosis and treatment of pulmonary embolism from the National Institute for Health and Clinical Excellence (NICE) and on treatment for venous thromboembolism from the American College of Chest Physicians.

SUMMARY POINTS

- Assessment of clinical pre-test probability (CPTP) is the first step in the diagnosis of pulmonary embolism
- Combinations of CPTP and test results are usually needed to identify patients who require, and do not require, anticoagulant therapy
- Thrombolytic therapy is usually reserved for patients with hypotension and without major risk factors for bleeding
- Pulmonary embolism associated with a reversible risk factor is usually treated for three months
- Pulmonary embolism associated with active cancer, or a second unprovoked pulmonary embolism, is usually treated indefinitely
- The decision to treat an unprovoked pulmonary embolism for three months or indefinitely is sensitive to an individual patient's preference and risk of bleeding

and less common in those with factor V Leiden. Three quarters of venous thromboembolisms are first events, while a quarter are recurrences, mainly after stopping treatment. Incidence doubles with each decade of age, and is about one per 1000 at 60 years. First episodes of venous thromboembolism occur with similar frequency in men and women, except for an increase in younger women associated with oestrogen therapy. Compared with white people, the incidence of venous thromboembolism is about 20% higher with African ethnicity and 33% lower with Asian ethnicity.

Virchow identified hypercoagulability, vessel wall injury, and stasis as the pathogenic triad for thrombosis (box 1). About 25% of patients with venous thromboembolism have no apparent provoking risk factor ("unprovoked" or "idiopathic" venous thromboembolism), 50% have a temporary provoking risk factor such as recent surgery or oestrogen therapy, and 25% have cancer.[1][2] Half of venous thromboembolism episodes are associated with hospitalisation, and about half of these are in surgical patients and half occur after hospital discharge. Therefore, preventive measures in hospitalised patients who are at high risk have the potential to markedly reduce pulmonary embolism.

How does pulmonary embolism present?

The symptoms and signs are non-specific and vary with the extent of pulmonary embolism and underlying cardiopulmonary impairment. Extensive pulmonary embolism may present with syncope, due to acute lowering of cardiac output, and patients may be found to have hypotension, evidence of poor perfusion (such as confusion), and elevated jugular venous pressure. Breathlessness occurs in most patients. Pleuritic chest pain is caused by pulmonary infarction, which occurs more often with non-massive pulmonary embolism and may be associated with haemoptysis. Although symptoms are usually present for days or weeks, they may be longstanding. Less than a quarter of patients have symptoms or signs of deep vein thrombosis, even though deep vein thrombosis is present in most patients with pulmonary embolism. Unexplained tachycardia, tachypnoea, or low arterial oxygen saturation may also suggest pulmonary embolism

With the widespread use of computed tomography, particularly for the assessment of cancer progression, diagnosis of incidental pulmonary embolism has become increasingly common. Incidental pulmonary embolism was reported in 2.6% of thoracic scans in one meta-analysis, with higher prevalence among hospitalised and cancer patients.[4] In retrospect, many of these patients had symptoms such as fatigue or breathlessness.

How is pulmonary embolism diagnosed?

Before describing the specific test results, or combinations of test results, that "rule in" and "rule out" pulmonary embolism, we will first quantify the level of diagnostic certainty that is required for each of these goals. The primary goal of diagnostic testing for pulmonary embolism

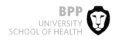

is to identify patients who would benefit from treatment. We suggest that a pulmonary embolism probability of ≥85% is the threshold that "rules in" pulmonary embolism and justifies anticoagulant therapy; this corresponds to a moderate or high clinical suspicion for pulmonary embolism and a "high probability" ventilation-perfusion lung scan.[5] Conversely, the threshold that "rules out" pulmonary embolism and justifies withholding anticoagulant therapy is a ≤2% probability of progressive venous thromboembolism in the next three months.[5][6] We emphasise that the threshold for withholding anticoagulant therapy focuses on the risk of continuing or progressive symptoms from pulmonary embolism, or of a new episode of venous thromboembolism (that is, progressive thrombosis) during follow-up, rather than the probability that pulmonary embolism is present and has been missed; it is acceptable not to treat a patient with test results possibly associated with pulmonary embolism provided we are confident, based on the findings of previous prospective studies, that patients with those test results have a very low risk for progressive venous thromboembolism. If the probability of pulmonary embolism lies between these two thresholds the patient requires further testing. If, despite further testing, findings remain non-diagnostic, the options are to (a) withhold treatment while performing serial ultrasound imaging of the proximal deep veins of the leg over a two week period and to treat only if deep vein thrombosis is detected (usually the preferred option),[5] or (b) treat despite a pulmonary embolism probability of <85% (less preferable).

Clinical pre-test probability

Diagnosis of pulmonary embolism starts with an assessment of clinical pre-test probability. This is based on assessment of whether symptoms and signs are typical for pulmonary embolism, if there are risk factors for pulmonary embolism, if pulmonary embolism is thought to be the most likely diagnosis, and if there is evidence of deep vein thrombosis.

BOX 1: RISK FACTORS FOR PULMONARY EMBOLISM*

Major risk factors

Intrinsic factors
- Previous venous thromboembolism
- Age >70 years

Acquired factors
- Malignancy
- Cancer chemotherapy
- Paralysis
- Major or lower limb trauma
- Lower limb orthopaedic surgery
- General anaesthesia for >30 minutes
- Heparin induced thrombocytopenia
- Antiphospholipid antibodies

Minor risk factors

Intrinsic factors
- Inherited hypercoagulable state

Acquired factors
- Obesity
- Pregnancy or puerperium
- Oestrogen therapy
- Prolonged immobility

**Combinations of factors have at least an additive effect on the risk of venous thromboembolism*

CPTP assessment is facilitated by use of a clinical prediction rule, of which the Wells score (table 1) is most widely used and extensively validated.[7][9] Although CPTP alone cannot diagnose pulmonary embolism, and generally does not exclude pulmonary embolism, it guides the selection of diagnostic tests (for example, a confirmatory test with high CPTP, an exclusionary test with low CPTP) and may be diagnostic in combination with these test results (box 2).[5][10] Every patient for whom pulmonary embolism is initially considered does not need to be tested for pulmonary embolism; a convincing alternative diagnosis may subsequently be found.

D-dimer testing

D-dimer is formed when cross linked fibrin is broken down by plasmin. Levels are almost always increased in venous thromboembolism, and consequently a normal D-dimer level helps to rule out pulmonary embolism (that is, it has a high negative predictive value).[7][11] However, because D-dimer levels are commonly increased by other conditions, an abnormal result has low positive predictive value for pulmonary embolism. D-dimer tests vary in terms of the measurement method and the D-dimer level that is used to categorise a test as positive or negative; consequently, negative predictive value differs among D-dimer tests, and this influences how a negative D-dimer result is used to rule out pulmonary embolism in combination with CPTP or other test results. D-dimer tests can be divided into those that are highly, or only moderately, sensitive for venous thromboembolism.

Highly sensitive tests have sensitivity ≥95%, but specificity is only about 40% in outpatients (lower in inpatients, see below). A negative highly sensitive test has very high negative predictive value and therefore rules out pulmonary embolism in patients with low or moderate CPTP (box 2); however, a negative test is obtained in only about 30% of outpatients because of the low specificity.

Moderately sensitive tests have a sensitivity of 80–94%, and a specificity of up to 70% in outpatients. A negative test has lower negative predictive value than a very sensitive D-dimer test and therefore rules out pulmonary embolism only in patients with low CPTP (box 2); however, most outpatients with low CPTP who do not have pulmonary embolism have a negative test, which increases the value of testing.

Specificity of D-dimer testing decreases with age, pregnancy, inflammatory conditions, cancer, trauma, and recent surgery. If it is very probable that a patient will have a positive D-dimer test in the absence of pulmonary embolism, such as after major surgery, D-dimer testing should not be performed. It is also of limited value in patients with high CPTP because about half will have a positive test due to pulmonary embolism and, if a negative test is obtained, its negative predictive value is reduced by the high prevalence of disease. D-dimer testing should not be ordered to "screen out" pulmonary embolism in patients who have yet to be evaluated clinically because the high frequency of false positive results will increase, rather than decrease, the need for additional testing.

Computed tomographic pulmonary angiography

Computed tomographic (CT) pulmonary angiography, which outlines thrombi in the pulmonary arteries with intravenous contrast medium, has become the primary diagnostic test for pulmonary embolism. Its positive predictive value varies with the extent of pulmonary embolism and CPTP: the positive predictive value is (a) 97% with main or lobar, 68%

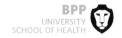

with segmental, but only 25% with isolated subsegmental pulmonary artery abnormalities, and (b) 96% with high CPTP, 92% with moderate CPTP, but only 58% with low CPTP (box 2).[12] Management studies have established that it is safe to withhold anticoagulant therapy in patients with a good quality negative CT pulmonary angiogram, with only about 1% of such patients returning with progressive venous thromboembolism during three months of follow-up (box 2).[13] [14]

Isolated subsegmental abnormalities, which are reported in 10–20% of CT pulmonary angiograms, may be due to pulmonary embolism that is causing symptoms or incidental pulmonary embolism that is not responsible for the patient's symptoms (such as after knee replacement surgery[15]), or may be false positive findings. Consequently, it is uncertain if patients with these findings should be treated (box 2).[16] We treat patients with isolated subsegmental abnormalities if there is persuasive evidence for pulmonary embolism (clear, usually multiple, defects on CT pulmonary angiography; moderate or high CPTP) and the risk of bleeding is not high,[17]

Table 1 Clinical prediction rule—Wells model for pulmonary embolism

Variables	No of points	Proportion of patients	Prevalence of pulmonary embolism
Clinically suspected deep vein thrombosis	3		
Alternative diagnosis is less likely than pulmonary embolism	3		
Heart rate >100 beats/min	1.5		
Immobilisation or surgery in previous 4 weeks	1.5		
History of venous thromboembolism	1.5		
Haemoptysis	1		
Malignancy or treatment for it in previous 6 months	1		
Score interpretation			
High probability*	≥6.5	10%	60%
Moderate probability*	4.5–6.0	30%	25%
Low probability†	≤4.0	60%	5%

*A score of ≥4.5 (moderate and high probability groups combined) has been termed "pulmonary embolism likely." This group makes up about 40% of patients and has a prevalence of pulmonary embolism of about 33%.
†Has also been termed "pulmonary embolism unlikely." In the original derivation of the Wells pulmonary embolism model, patients were required to have a score of ≤1.5 to be categorised as low probability, but a score of ≤4 has subsequently been used for low probability.[7 8]

BOX 2: TEST RESULTS THAT CONFIRM OR EXCLUDE PULMONARY EMBOLISM (ADAPTED FROM KEARON[5])

Diagnostic for pulmonary embolism (≥85% probability of pulmonary embolism)
- Computed tomography (CT) pulmonary angiogram:
- Intraluminal filling defect in a lobar or main pulmonary artery
- Intraluminal filling defect in a segmental pulmonary artery *and* moderate or high CPTP
- Ventilation-perfusion scan: High probability scan* *and* moderate or high CPTP
- Positive diagnostic test for deep vein thrombosis (with a non-diagnostic ventilation-perfusion scan or CT pulmonary angiogram)

Excludes pulmonary embolism (≤2% probability of progressive venous thromboembolism during 3 months' follow-up†)
- CT pulmonary angiogram: Normal
- Perfusion scan: Normal
- D-dimer test:
- Negative test which has high sensitivity (>95%) *and* low or moderate CPTP
- Negative test which has moderately high sensitivity (>85%) *and* low CPTP
- Non-diagnostic ventilation-perfusion scan or suboptimal CT pulmonary angiogram *and* normal venous ultrasound of the proximal veins *and*
- Low CPTP *or*
- Negative D-dimer test which has moderately high sensitivity (≥85%) *or*
- Normal repeat venous ultrasound scans of the proximal veins after 7 and 14 days
CPTP=clinical pre-test probability.
*Presence of two large (each ≥0.75 segments) perfusion defects with normal ventilation.
†Patients should be told there is still a small chance that pulmonary embolism is present and instructed to return for further evaluation if symptoms persist or deteriorate.

and we conduct serial ultrasound scans of the deep veins of the legs over two weeks in those who we do not treat, similar to how we manage patients with non-diagnostic ventilation-perfusion scans (see below). Less than 10% of CT pulmonary angiograms are technically inadequate.

CT pulmonary angiography can lead to contrast induced nephropathy and is associated with substantial radiation exposure. Its use should therefore be minimised, particularly in women under the age of 40 because of the associated increased risk of breast cancer.

Ventilation-perfusion lung scanning

Ventilation-perfusion lung scanning has largely been supplanted by CT pulmonary angiography. A "high probability scan," in which there is ≥1.5 segmental perfusion defects with normal ventilation ("ventilation-perfusion mismatch"), is associated with a prevalence of pulmonary embolism of ≥85% and is seen in about half of patients with pulmonary embolism (box 2).[5 18] A normal perfusion scan rules out pulmonary embolism, but is found in only 25% of patients. More than half of patients, therefore, have a non-diagnostic scan and require further testing. CT pulmonary angiography can then be performed, but ventilation-perfusion scanning is often done when CT pulmonary angiography is contraindicated (for example, with renal insufficiency). Consequently, it is usually preferable to do venous ultrasound scans of the proximal deep veins of both legs on the day of presentation and twice during the next two weeks, and to treat patients only if deep vein thrombosis is detected. The specificity of ventilation-perfusion scanning is lower if there is respiratory disease, and higher in younger patients.

Diagnosis of pulmonary embolism in pregnancy

Diagnosis of pulmonary embolism is similar in pregnant and non-pregnant patients, although there are some differences, and many diagnostic strategies have not been well validated in pregnant women.[19] Although the specificity of D-dimer testing decreases in later pregnancy, it is expected to retain most of its negative predictive value. Ultrasound scans of the leg veins, particularly if there are leg symptoms, may identify deep vein thrombosis. Ventilation-perfusion scanning with a lower radiation dose and longer imaging period for the perfusion component, or CT pulmonary angiography modified for physiological changes in pregnancy, can be used. Ventilation-perfusion scanning is probably associated with higher fetal radiation that CT pulmonary angiography, but this is still below the level considered harmful. CT pulmonary angiography is associated with much higher maternal radiation. Non-diagnostic ventilation-perfusion scans are also much less common during pregnancy (young patients without comorbidity) than in the general population. For these reasons, if imaging is necessary, we usually prefer ventilation-perfusion scanning to CT pulmonary angiography in pregnant patients, and prefer to do serial ultrasound testing rather than CT pulmonary angiography in patients with non-diagnostic ventilation-perfusion scans. CT pulmonary angiography is preferred to ventilation-perfusion scanning in sicker patients and particularly if there is haemodynamic instability or if the results of chest radiography suggest that a ventilation-perfusion scan is likely to be non-diagnostic. Isolated iliac deep vein thrombosis is more common in pregnant patients, which, if the iliac veins are not part of the initial and follow-up examinations, may undermine the role of serial venous ultrasonography.

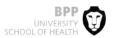

How is pulmonary embolism treated?

Anticoagulant therapy before diagnostic testing

This decision depends on the probability that pulmonary embolism is present, how soon diagnostic testing can be performed, how sick the patient is, and the patient's risk of bleeding. A pragmatic approach is to start anticoagulant therapy if (*a*) CPTP is high, (*b*) CPTP is moderate and testing will not be completed within four hours, or (*c*) CPTP is low and testing will be delayed for over 24 hours.[17]

Treating patients with incidental pulmonary embolism

Incidental pulmonary embolism, detected on a CT scan that has been done for another reason, is often reported after an outpatient has left the hospital. If it would be difficult for patients to return the same evening, it is usually reasonable to defer further evaluation and treatment until the next day because, if pulmonary embolism is confirmed, it has usually been present for some time.[17] The decision whether to treat long term will be influenced by the certainty that pulmonary embolism is present (addition diagnostic testing, such as dedicated CT pulmonary angiography, may be required), whether the abnormality has gone unnoticed on previous CT scans, and the patient's risk of bleeding. However, because incidental pulmonary embolism seems to carry a similar risk of recurrence and poor long term prognosis as symptomatic pulmonary embolism, we treat most the same way as symptomatic episodes.

When are thrombolytic therapy and mechanical thrombus removal used?

Active removal of thrombus is mostly reserved for the roughly 5% of patients with pulmonary embolism who have hypotension (systolic blood pressure <90 mm Hg; usually with other features of shock).[3][17] Systemic thrombolytic therapy is most commonly used, often as 100 mg of tissue plasminogen activator given as a two hour infusion.[17] Alternatively, if expertise is available, thrombus removal may be achieved by infusion of lower doses of thrombolytic drug directly into the thrombus, by catheter based fragmentation and aspiration of thrombus, by use of these two modalities together, or by surgical embolectomy.[3][17][20] These techniques may be preferred if there is a high risk of bleeding,[17] a poor response to systemic thrombolysis, or concern that the patient will die before systemic thrombolytic

therapy has a chance to work.[17] Surgical embolectomy is indicated if there is impending paradoxical embolism, with thrombus present in a septal defect.

While there is strong evidence from randomised trials that systemic thrombolysis accelerates resolution of pulmonary embolism, its ability to save lives or reduce long term cardiopulmonary impairment remains uncertain.[21] Fewer than 800 patients have been included in trials that have randomised patients with acute pulmonary embolism to receive or not receive thrombolytic therapy, and these trials were usually not designed to assess clinical outcomes, did not follow up patients to assess long term disability, and had other important methodological limitations that undermine confidence in their findings.[8][21] Systemic thrombolytic therapy, however, is known to markedly increase risk of bleeding, and particularly intracranial bleeds.

Use of thrombus removal interventions in patients with pulmonary embolism and hypotension is based on the expectation that these patients, who otherwise are expected to have a mortality of up to 30%, will derive net benefit.[3][17] Right ventricular dysfunction on echocardiography and elevated biomarkers of right ventricular injury are predictive of short term mortality from pulmonary embolism; two ongoing large trials are testing if, in the absence of hypotension, patients with these findings benefit from systemic thrombolytic therapy (NCT00639743; NCT00680628).

Anticoagulant therapy

Anticoagulant therapy can be divided into two overlapping phases.[17][22] The first is treatment of the presenting episode of pulmonary embolism, which takes about three months. The second, which is optional, is extended therapy designed to prevent new episodes of venous thromboembolism.

Standard initial therapy is with subcutaneous low molecular weight heparin, fondaparinux, or unfractionated heparin, or intravenous unfractionated heparin.[17] There is no strong evidence that any one method is superior. Subcutaneous low molecular weight heparin and fondaparinux do not require intravenous infusion or laboratory monitoring, whereas intravenous unfractionated heparin is preferred if there is shock, severe renal impairment (low molecular weight heparin and fondaparinux are renally excreted), thrombolytic therapy is being considered, or it may be necessary to reverse anticoagulation rapidly. These treatments should be overlapped with a vitamin K antagonist (such as warfarin) and stopped after a minimum of five days provided the international normalised ratio (INR) has been above 2.0 for at least a day.

Alternatively, low molecular weight heparin can be continued long term, a treatment strategy that is generally preferred in patients with cancer associated pulmonary embolism because of superior efficacy of low molecular weight heparin, difficulty in controlling vitamin K antagonist therapy, and greater compatibility of low molecular weight heparin with chemotherapy and the need for invasive procedures.[17][23] Long term low molecular weight heparin is also used to treat venous thromboembolism during pregnancy because vitamin K antagonists are teratogenic. Observational studies and a recent randomised trial have shown that, with appropriate selection (less acutely ill, good social supports, patient preference), about half of outpatients with acute pulmonary embolism can be treated at home.[24][25]

The new oral anticoagulants rivaroxaban and dabigatran (apixaban is at an earlier stage of assessment in the treatment of venous thromboembolism) are as effective

Table 2 | Duration of anticoagulant therapy for venous thromboembolism

Category of VTE	Duration of treatment*
Provoked by a transient risk factor†	3 months
Unprovoked VTE‡	Minimum of 3 months and then reassess
First unprovoked proximal DVT or PE with no or minor risk factors for bleeding	Indefinite therapy with annual review§
Isolated distal DVT as a first unprovoked event	3 months
Second unprovoked VTE	Indefinite therapy with annual review¶
Cancer associated VTE	Indefinite treatment

VTE= venous thromboembolism. DVT=deep vein thrombosis. PE=pulmonary embolism.

*Treatment with a vitamin K antagonist (VKA) or low molecular weight heparin (LMWH) are currently considered first line therapy. VKA therapy is suggested in preference to LMWH in patients without cancer (avoids injection, less costly). LMWH is preferred in patients with cancer (more effective, dosing and reversal more flexible if there is severe thrombocytopenia or invasive procedures are required, VKA is difficult to control in sicker patients). The choice between VKA and LMWH is also sensitive to patient preference. New oral anticoagulants (such as rivaroxaban, dabigitran) are considered second line therapy as they are not yet widely available or approved for extended therapy of VTE, and there is limited post-marketing experience with these agents.[17]

†Transient risk factors include surgery, hospitalisation, or plaster cast immobilisation in the previous three months; oestrogen therapy, pregnancy, prolonged travel (>8 hours), lesser leg injuries, or more recent (≤6 weeks) immobilisations. The greater the provoking reversible risk factor (such as recent major surgery), the lower the expected risk of recurrence after stopping anticoagulant therapy.

‡Absence of a transient risk factor or active cancer.

§This decision is sensitive to patient preference.

¶Indefinite therapy is suggested if there is moderate risk of bleeding, and three months is suggested if there is a high risk of bleeding; both of these decisions are sensitive to patient preference.

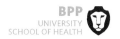

as conventional anticoagulant therapy, do not require laboratory monitoring, and are associated with a lower risk of intracranial bleeding but a higher risk of gastrointestinal bleeding.[17 26 27 28 29 30] Dabigatran is preceded by heparin therapy, whereas rivaroxaban does not require initial heparin therapy but requires a higher dose for the first three weeks of treatment. Both are contraindicated if there is severe renal impairment and are contraindicated or must be used cautiously with some drugs, and there is little experience of using them to treat venous thromboembolism in patients with advanced cancer or receiving cancer chemotherapy. The decision to use one of these drugs for the acute or long term treatment of venous thromboembolism is also influenced by local availability and licensing, whether their cost is covered by state or private insurance plans, and patient and physician satisfaction with current therapy. Because they are emerging therapies, these factors differ among jurisdictions and are rapidly changing.

How long should anticoagulant therapy be continued?
When the presenting episode of pulmonary embolism has been effectively treated, there is the option of continuing anticoagulants indefinitely to prevent new episodes of venous thromboembolism. Extended therapy reduces the risk of recurrent venous thromboembolism by over 90% but increases the risk of bleeding twofold to threefold.[17] If anticoagulant treatments are extended and then stopped the risk of recurrent venous thromboembolism is similar to that if they had been stopped at three months, with the highest risk occurring in the first six months after stopping.[22 31] The risk of recurrent venous thromboembolism is similar after a pulmonary embolism or a proximal deep vein thrombosis, but the recurrent episode is about three times as likely to be a pulmonary embolism after an initial pulmonary embolism, so is more likely to be fatal.[32] The decision to treat indefinitely therefore depends on balancing the increased risk of recurrence with stopping therapy against the increased risk of bleeding with continued therapy, while also considering patient preference and associated costs.

Most patients with active cancer or a second unprovoked venous thromboembolism should receive extended therapy because of a high risk of recurrence (table 2).[17] Most patients with pulmonary embolism associated with a reversible provoking risk factor, such as surgery or oestrogen therapy, should stop treatment after three months because of the low risk of recurrence.[17 31] In patients with a first unprovoked pulmonary embolism, who are estimated to have a risk of recurrence of 10% at one year and 30% at five years if they stop treatment, the decision whether to extend treatment is sensitive to patients' preferences and their individual risk of bleeding.[17] There is a lower risk of recurrence in women than in men, and in those who have a normal D-dimer level a month after stopping therapy. Therefore, extended therapy may not be justified in women with a first unprovoked pulmonary embolism who have a negative D-dimer test a month after stopping anticoagulants.[33 34] Thrombophilia testing has little influence on the treatment of venous thromboembolism.[10 35]

Antiplatelet therapy
Results from two recent placebo controlled randomised trials support that aspirin reduces risk of recurrent venous thromboembolism by about a third in patients with a first unprovoked venous thromboembolism who have completed at least three months of anticoagulant therapy.[36] Therefore, if patients are not candidates for extended anticoagulant therapy, this reduction in recurrent venous thromboembolism can be included in the overall assessment of benefit to risk for indefinite aspirin therapy.

Inferior vena cava filters
Vena cava filters block emboli from reaching the lungs.[3 17 37] We limit use of filters to patients with acute proximal deep vein thrombosis or pulmonary embolism who cannot be given anticoagulants. Observational studies, however, suggest that filters may also benefit patients with pulmonary embolism and hypotension who do receive anticoagulants.[38 39] Removable filters can be used in patients with short term contraindications to anticoagulation, but only about 25% are removed and the long term safety of those that remain is uncertain.[17]

Contributors: Both authors contributed to writing the manuscript and take responsibility for its integrity. CK is guarantor.

FUTURE RESEARCH QUESTIONS

- Should systemic thrombolytic therapy or other thrombus removal techniques be used to treat pulmonary embolism associated with right ventricular dysfunction?
- Which patients with a first unprovoked pulmonary embolism should receive anticoagulant therapy for three months rather than indefinitely?
- Do all patients with asymptomatic incidental pulmonary embolism require treatment?
- Which patients with CT pulmonary angiography findings suggestive of isolated subsegmental pulmonary embolism should receive anticoagulant therapy?

TIPS FOR NON-SPECIALISTS

- Anticoagulant therapy should be started before diagnostic testing if there is high clinical suspicion for pulmonary embolism or if testing will be delayed
- Pulmonary embolism is ruled out without further testing by low clinical suspicion for pulmonary embolism (such as Wells pulmonary embolism score ≤4) and a negative D-dimer test
- D-dimer testing should not be performed if it is very probable that patients will have a positive result even if pulmonary embolism is not present (such as after major surgery)
- Computed tomography (CT) pulmonary angiography is associated with substantial radiation so it should be used selectively, particularly in younger patients (<40 years old)
- Anticoagulant therapy is not invariably indicated in patients who have an isolated subsegmental pulmonary embolism on CT pulmonary angiography or an incidental pulmonary embolism on a CT scan that was done for another reason
- Low molecular weight heparin is often the preferred long term anticoagulant for patients with cancer

---

ADDITIONAL EDUCATIONAL RESOURCES

Resources for healthcare professionals

- National Institute for Health and Clinical Excellence. Venous thromboembolic diseases (clinical guidelines CG144). http://guidance.nice.org.uk/CG144. (No registration required, free resource)
- American College of Chest Physicians. Antithrombotic therapy and prevention of thrombosis, 9th ed: American College of Chest Physicians evidence-based clinical practice guidelines. *Chest* 2012;141(2 suppl). http://journal.publications.chestnet.org/issue.aspx?journalid=99&issueid=23443. (Registration required, payment may be required)

Resources for patients (no registration required, free resources)

- NHS Choices. Pulmonary embolism. http://www.nhs.uk/conditions/pulmonary-embolism/pages/introduction.aspx. (UK National Health Service pati
- ent resources)
- US Department of Health and Human Services. Your guide to preventing and treating blood clots. www.ahrq.gov/consumer/bloodclots.pdf
- Investigators Against Thromboembolism (INATE). About thrombosis. www.inate.org/en/1/2/

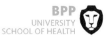

Competing interests: Both authors have completed the ICMJE uniform disclosure form (www.icmje.org/coi_disclosure.pdf) and declare: CK has been a consultant to Boehringer Ingelheim, Bayer, Diagnostica Stago, and Alere; he was supported by the Heart and Stroke Foundation of Ontario; and he is an author of the current American College of Chest Physician's guidelines on the treatment of venous thromboembolism.

Provenance and peer review: Commissioned; externally peer reviewed.

1   Naess IA, Christiansen SC, Romundstad P, Cannegieter SC, Rosendaal FR, Hammerstrom J. Incidence and mortality of venous thrombosis: a population-based study. J Thromb Haemost 2007;5:692-9.
2   Heit JA. The epidemiology of venous thromboembolism in the community. Arterioscler Thromb Vasc Biol 2008;28:370-2.
3   Jaff MR, McMurtry MS, Archer SL, Cushman M, Goldenberg N, Goldhaber SZ, et al. Management of massive and submassive pulmonary embolism, iliofemoral deep vein thrombosis, and chronic thromboembolic pulmonary hypertension: a scientific statement from the American Heart Association. Circulation 2011;123:1788-830.
4   Dentali F, Ageno W, Becattini C, Galli L, Gianni M, Riva N, et al. Prevalence and clinical history of incidental, asymptomatic pulmonary embolism: a meta-analysis. Thromb Res 2010;125:518-22.
5   Kearon C. Diagnosis of pulmonary embolism. CMAJ 2003;168:183-94.
6   Bates SM, Jaeschke R, Stevens SM, Goodacre S, Wells PS, Stevenson MD, et al. Diagnosis of DVT: antithrombotic therapy and prevention of thrombosis, 9th ed: American College of Chest Physicians Evidence-Based Clinical Practice Guidelines. Chest 2012;141(2 Suppl):e351-418S.
7   Geersing GJ, Erkens PM, Lucassen WA, Buller HR, Cate HT, Hoes AW, et al. Safe exclusion of pulmonary embolism using the Wells rule and qualitative D-dimer testing in primary care: prospective cohort study. BMJ 2012;345:e6564.
8   Kearon C, Ginsberg JS, Douketis J, Turpie AG, Bates SM, Lee AY, et al. An evaluation of D-dimer in the diagnosis of pulmonary embolism: a randomized trial. Ann Intern Med 2006;144:812-21.
9   Lucassen W, Geersing GJ, Erkens PM, Reitsma JB, Moons KG, Buller H, et al. Clinical decision rules for excluding pulmonary embolism: a meta-analysis. Ann Intern Med 2011;155:448-60.
10   Chong LY, Fenu E, Stansby G, Hodgkinson S. Management of venous thromboembolic diseases and the role of thrombophilia testing: summary of NICE guidance. BMJ 2012;344:e3979.
11   Di Nisio M, Squizzato A, Rutjes AW, Buller HR, Zwinderman AH, Bossuyt PM. Diagnostic accuracy of D-dimer test for exclusion of venous thromboembolism: a systematic review. J Thromb Haemost 2007;5:296-304.
12   Stein PD, Fowler SE, Goodman LR, Gottschalk A, Hales CA, Hull RD, et al. Multidetector computed tomography for acute pulmonary embolism. N Engl J Med 2006;354:2317-27.
13   Van Belle A, Buller HR, Huisman MV, Huisman PM, Kaasjager K, Kamphuisen PW, et al. Effectiveness of managing suspected pulmonary embolism using an algorithm combining clinical probability, D-dimer testing, and computed tomography. JAMA 2006;295:172-9.
14   Mos IC, Klok FA, Kroft LJ, A DER, Dekkers OM, Huisman MV. Safety of ruling out acute pulmonary embolism by normal computed tomography pulmonary angiography in patients with an indication for computed tomography: systematic review and meta-analysis. J Thromb Haemost 2009;7:1491-8.
15   Gandhi R, Salonen D, Geerts WH, Khanna M, McSweeney S, Mahomed NN. A pilot study of computed tomography-detected asymptomatic pulmonary filling defects after hip and knee arthroplasties. J Arthroplasty 2012;27:730-5.
16   Carrier M, Righini M, Wells PS, Perrier A, Anderson DR, Rodger MA, et al. Subsegmental pulmonary embolism diagnosed by computed tomography: incidence and clinical implications. A systematic review and meta-analysis of the management outcome studies. J Thromb Haemost 2010;8:1716-22.
17   Kearon C, Akl EA, Comerota AJ, Prandoni P, Bounameaux H, Goldhaber SZ, et al. Antithrombotic therapy for VTE disease: Antithrombotic therapy and prevention of thrombosis, 9th ed: American College of Chest Physicians evidence-based clinical practice guidelines. Chest 2012;141(2 suppl):e419-94S.
18   The PIOPED Investigators. Value of the ventilation/perfusion scan in acute pulmonary embolism. Results of the prospective investigation of pulmonary embolism diagnosis (PIOPED). JAMA 1990;263:2753-9.
19   Chan WS, Ray JG, Murray S, Coady GE, Coates G, Ginsberg JS. Suspected pulmonary embolism in pregnancy: clinical presentation, results of lung scanning, and subsequent maternal and pediatric outcomes. Arch Intern Med 2002;162:1170-5.
20   Kuo WT, Gould MK, Louie JD, Rosenberg JK, Sze DY, Hofmann LV. Catheter-directed therapy for the treatment of massive pulmonary embolism: systematic review and meta-analysis of modern techniques. J Vasc Interv Radiol 2009;20:1431-40.
21   Dong B, Jirong Y, Wang Q, Wu T. Thrombolytic treatment for pulmonary embolism. Cochrane Database Syst Rev 2006;(2):CD004437.
22   Kearon C. A conceptual framework for two phases of anticoagulant treatment of venous thromboembolism. J Thromb Haemost 2012;10:507-11.
23   Akl EA, Labedi N, Barba M, Terrenato I, Sperati F, Muti P, et al. Anticoagulation for the long-term treatment of venous thromboembolism in patients with cancer. Cochrane Database Syst Rev 2011;(6):CD006650.
24   Aujesky D, Roy PM, Verschuren F, Righini M, Osterwalder J, Egloff M, et al. Outpatient versus inpatient treatment for patients with acute pulmonary embolism: an international, open-label, randomised, non-inferiority trial. Lancet 2011;378:41-8.
25   Vinson DR, Zehtabchi S, Yealy DM. Can selected patients with newly diagnosed pulmonary embolism be safely treated without hospitalization? A systematic review. Ann Emerg Med 2012;60:651-62.
26   Schulman S, Kearon C, Kakkar AK, Mismetti P, Schellong S, Eriksson H, et al. Dabigatran versus warfarin in the treatment of acute venous thromboembolism. N Engl J Med 2009;361:2342-52.
27   Buller HR, Prins MH, Lensin AW, Decousus H, Jacobson BF, Minar E, et al. Oral rivaroxaban for the treatment of symptomatic pulmonary embolism. N Engl J Med 2012;366:1287-97.
28   Fox BD, Kahn SR, Langleben D, Eisenberg MJ, Shimony A. Efficacy and safety of novel oral anticoagulants for treatment of acute venous thromboembolism: direct and adjusted indirect meta-analysis of randomised controlled trials. BMJ 2012;345:e7498.
29   Agnelli G, Buller HR, Cohen A, Curto M, Gallus AS, Johnson M, et al. Apixaban for extended treatment of venous thromboembolism. N Engl J Med 2013;368:699-708.
30   Schulman S, Kearon C, Kakkar AK, Mismetti P, Schellong S, Eriksson H, et al. Extended use of dabigatran, warfarin, or placebo in venous thromboembolism. N Engl J Med 2013;368:709-18.
31   Boutitie F, Pinede L, Schulman S, Agnelli G, Raskob G, Julian J, et al. Influence of preceding length of anticoagulant treatment and initial presentation of venous thromboembolism on risk of recurrence after stopping treatment: analysis of individual participants' data from seven trials. BMJ 2011;342:d3036.
32   Baglin T, Douketis J, Tosetto A, Marcucci M, Cushman M, Kyrle P, et al. Does the clinical presentation and extent of venous thrombosis predict likelihood and type of recurrence? A patient level meta-analysis. J Thromb Haemost 2010;8:2436-42.
33   Douketis J, Tosetto A, Marcucci M, Baglin T, Cosmi B, Cushman M, et al. Risk of recurrence after venous thromboembolism in men and women: patient level meta-analysis. BMJ 2011;342:d813.
34   Douketis J, Tosetto A, Marcucci M, Baglin T, Cushman M, Eichinger S, et al. Patient-level meta-analysis: effect of measurement timing, threshold, and patient age on ability of D-dimer testing to assess recurrence risk after unprovoked venous thromboembolism. Ann Intern Med 2010;153:523-31.
35   Kearon C. Influence of hereditary or acquired thrombophilias on the treatment of venous thromboembolism. Curr Opin Hematol 2012;19:363-70.
36   Becattini C, Agnelli G, Schenone A, Eichinger S, Bucherini E, Silingardi M, et al. Aspirin for preventing the recurrence of venous thromboembolism. N Engl J Med 2012;366:1959-67.
37   Eight-year follow-up of patients with permanent vena cava filters in the prevention of pulmonary embolism: the PREPIC (Prevention du Risque d'Embolie Pulmonaire par Interruption Cave) randomized study. Circulation 2005;112:416-12.
38   Kucher N, Rossi E, De Rosa M, Goldhaber SZ. Massive pulmonary embolism. Circulation 2006;113:577-82.
39   Stein PD, Matta F, Keyes DC, Willyerd GL. Impact of vena cava filters on in-hospital case fatality rate from pulmonary embolism. Am J Med 2012;125:478-84.

Related links

bmj.com
- Respiratory medicine updates from BMJ Group

bmj.com/archive

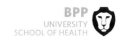

Diagnosis and management of supraventricular tachycardia

Zachary I Whinnett, consultant cardiologist, S M Afzal Sohaib, British Heart Foundation clinical research training fellow and cardiology specialty registrar, D Wyn Davies, consultant cardiologist

[1]Waller Department of Cardiology, St Mary's Hospital, Imperial College Healthcare NHS Trust, London W2 1NY, UK

Correspondence to: D W Davies
dwyndavies@aol.com

Cite this as: *BMJ* 2012;345:e7769

DOI: 10.1136/bmj.e7769

http://www.bmj.com/content/345/
bmj.e7769

The term supraventricular tachycardia (SVT) encompasses many tachycardias in which atrial or atrioventricular nodal tissue are essential for sustaining the arrhythmia (box 1). In practice, however, the term SVT is generally used to refer to atrioventricular nodal re-entry tachycardia (AVNRT), atrioventricular re-entry tachycardia (AVRT), and atrial tachycardia[1]; in this review we follow that convention. We reviewed the literature to provide an up to date summary of our understanding of the mechanism for these arrhythmias, and we describe the approach to their diagnosis and management. Atrial fibrillation has been reviewed recently[2] so is not discussed in detail here. Much of the clinical evidence in this field is derived from observational and registry data, with a limited number of randomised control studies.

What is a supraventricular tachycardia?

SVTs are produced by disorders of impulse formation (causing generation of rapid electrical impulses from a small area) and/or disorders of impulse conduction, which result in re-entrant tachycardias, where tachycardia is produced because the electrical impulse repeatedly travels around a circuit. Re-entrant tachycardias typically require an extrasystole to initiate them. SVTs are among the few medical conditions that can be cured.

What are the different types of SVT?

AVNRT

AVNRT is caused by a re-entrant circuit involving the posterior and anterior inputs into the compact atrioventricular node.[3] A quarter of the population has two pathways that input into the compact atrioventricular node, one of which is a rapidly conducting pathway and the other a slower conducting pathway; these two pathways form the circuit for AVNRT (fig 1).

The extrasystole that triggers the tachycardia is critically timed so that the faster pathway is still refractory from the last sinus beat (that is, it is not yet ready to conduct an impulse because it is still recovering from depolarisation). The electrical impulse therefore propagates exclusively down

SOURCES AND SELECTION CRITERIA

As well as using our personal reference collections, we searched PubMed to identify peer reviewed original articles, meta-analyses, observational studies, and reviews, as well as searching Clinical Evidence (http://clinicalevidence.bmj.com) and the Cochrane Collaboration databases. We used the search terms supraventricular tachycardia, atrioventricular nodal re-entry tachycardia, atrioventricular re-entry tachycardia, atrial flutter, atrial tachycardia, Wolff-Parkinson-White syndrome. We selected randomised controlled studies or meta-analyses when available; if none were available, we used observational studies and registry data.

the slow pathway, which has a shorter refractory period (that is, it takes less time to recover from depolarisation) and then returns up the fast pathway, which has by then recovered. The circuit for typical AVNRT is thus formed.

Less commonly, activation travels anterogradely down the fast pathway and returns up the slow pathway, forming atypical AVNRT. These different mechanisms result in very different appearances on the surface electrocardiogram (ECG). In the typical form, atrial and ventricular activation occur virtually simultaneously (because the impulse returns up the fast pathway at the same time as travelling down the His-Purkinje system), so the P waves are invisible in the QRS complexes (a pseudo-RSR' pattern in lead V1 often provides a clue to the presence of the P wave), whereas the delayed atrial activation via the slow pathway in atypical AVNRT produces inverted P waves typically in the middle of or late in the RR interval.

Typical AVNRT presents as a short RP tachycardia (the ECG during tachycardia has a RP interval shorter than PR interval) while atypical AVNRT produces a long RP tachycardia (RP interval longer than PR interval) (fig 2).

AVRT (including Wolff-Parkinson-White syndrome)

AVRT is also a re-entrant tachycardia; it requires the presence of an accessory pathway, a small strand of myocardium that bridges the normal insulation between atria and ventricles (fig 3).

Some pathways can conduct impulses only from the ventricle to the atrium and are known as concealed accessory pathways. Others can conduct in both directions and usually produce pre-excitation of the ventricle because they conduct more rapidly than the atrioventricular node. This early ventricular activation shows on the 12 lead ECG as a delta wave at the start of the QRS (fig 3). The terminal portion of the QRS complex is narrow, reflecting the rapid conduction via the His-Purkinje system once the atrioventricular node has been crossed. The degree of pre-excitation varies depending on the time required to cross the atrioventricular node and the location of the accessory pathway.

The diagnosis of Wolff-Parkinson-White syndrome describes patients with a delta wave on the surface ECG who also experience palpitations.

SUMMARY POINTS

- Supraventricular tachycardia comprises a group of conditions in which atrial or atrioventricular nodal tissues are essential for sustaining the arrhythmia
- Common symptoms include palpitations, chest pain, anxiety, light headedness, pounding in the neck, shortness of breath, and uncommonly syncope
- They are produced either by disorders of impulse formation and/or disorders of impulse conduction
- For patients presenting with a regular narrow complex tachycardia, initial management is usually to slow atrioventricular node conduction, using either vagal manoeuvres or adenosine
- Drug treatment may reduce the frequency of symptoms, but complete suppression is uncommon
- Catheter ablation, a procedure done under local anaesthesia in the cardiac catheter laboratory, is usually curative

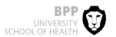

AVRT is usually triggered by a critically timed atrial extrasystole that finds the accessory pathway refractory, therefore antegrade conduction occurs exclusively down the atrioventricular node. The accessory pathway is no longer refractory by the time the wave front reaches its ventricular insertion and it therefore conducts retrogradely to the atrium— the re-entrant circuit is thus formed (fig 3); this activation pattern is termed orthodromic AVRT, and produces a narrow complex tachycardia. Rarely, anterograde conduction travels down the accessory pathway returning to the atrium via the atrioventricular node, producing antidromic AVRT, which has broad QRS complexes that exaggerate the pattern of pre-excitation seen in sinus rhythm because ventricular activation occurs exclusively via the accessory pathway.

Atrial tachycardia

Atrial tachycardia may result from either abnormal impulse formation or a re-entrant mechanism. Atrial tachycardias are commonly classified according to whether they originate from a small localised area in the atrium (focal atrial tachycardia) or involve a larger re-entrant circuit (macro re-entry).

Focal atrial tachycardia

In focal atrial tachycardia there is generation of rapid electrical impulses from a small localised area in the atria (fig 4).

Multifocal atrial tachycardia

Multifocal atrial tachycardia is less common than focal atrial tachycardia and occurs most often in acutely unwell patients and those with pulmonary disease and/or digoxin toxicity. At least three different morphologies of P wave are usually present.[4]

Macro re-entrant atrial tachycardia

The re-entrant circuit involves a large area of the atrium. The commonest is "typical" atrial flutter where the re-entrant loop circles the right atrium (fig 5). Other re-entrant atrial tachycardias are seen in patients who have structural heart disease and in those who have had previous surgery (increasingly in those who have had catheter ablation procedures to treat atrial fibrillation).[5]

Who gets SVT?

People of all ages, either sex, and any ethnicity can develop SVT. In a large retrospective observational study in the United States the peak incidence of SVT presentation was in the middle decades of life (AVNRT at 48 (range 30-66) years; AVRT at 36 (18-64) years; and atrial fibrillation at 50 (31-69) years).[6]

A higher proportion of AVNRT cases occur in women, and AVRT is more likely to affect men.[7] No sex difference was observed for atrial fibrillation.

SVTs usually manifest themselves as recurrent palpitations, can seriously impair quality of life,[8] and often prompt visits to

Fig 1 Mechanism for atrioventricular nodal re-entry tachycardia

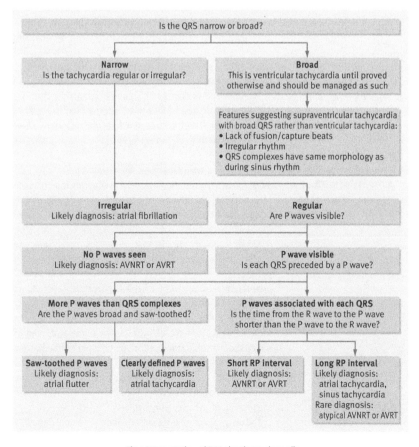

Fig 2 Interpretation of ECG showing tachycardia

BOX 1 DIFFERENTIAL DIAGNOSIS OF A NARROW COMPLEX TACHYCARDIA

Common causes

- Sinus tachycardia
- Atrioventricular nodal re-entry tachycardia (AVNRT)
- Atrioventricular re-entry tachycardia (AVRT)
- Atrial tachycardia
- Atrial flutter
- Atrial fibrillation

Rare causes

- Inappropriate sinus tachycardia
- Sinus node re-entry
- Permanent junctional reciprocating tachycardia
- Non-paroxysmal junctional tachycardia
- Focal junctional tachycardia

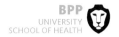

primary care doctors and acute medical units. The incidence in a large cohort in the United States was found to be 35/100 000 patient years, with a prevalence of 0.2%.[9] An estimated prevalence for atrial fibrillation is 0.4% to 1% in the general population.[10]

How does SVT present?

Common symptoms include palpitations, chest pain, anxiety, lightheadedness, pounding in the neck, shortness of breath, and uncommonly syncope.[11]

Sudden onset and offset of palpitations is typical for a re-entrant arrhythmia, while for sinus tachycardia onset and offset is usually gradual. Patients with AVNRT or AVRT may be able to terminate palpitations with vagal manoeuvres such as the Valsalva manoeuvre, breath holding, or coughing.

Some patients can identify triggers such as caffeine or alcohol intake, which can initiate re-entrant tachycardia by increasing the frequency of extrasystoles.

In the absence of an acute episode the examination is usually normal. In a patient with tachycardia, prominent jugular venous A waves caused by atrial contraction against the closed tricuspid valve may be seen.[12]

What investigations are needed?

Electrocardiography

Attempts should always be made to capture the arrhythmia during an episode of palpitations. We recommend giving the patient a copy to ensure it is never lost and is easily available to health professionals. A rhythm strip should be recorded if 12 lead electrocardiography is not available, and every effort should be made to capture the termination of the tachycardia.

For patients with non-sustained episodes of palpitations, an ambulatory electrocardiograph or an event monitor can be useful in capturing an ECG during an episode.

Narrow complex tachycardia is most frequently seen (QRS <120 ms), but less commonly the QRS complexes are broad during tachycardia. Even though supraventricular tachycardias can present with broad QRS complexes, in the initial evaluation, a broad complex tachycardia should be treated as a ventricular tachycardia until proven otherwise.

A 12 lead ECG in sinus rhythm should also be recorded and carefully examined for the presence of a delta wave. In figure 2 we suggest how to analyse the 12 lead ECG during tachycardia.

Echocardiography

Echocardiography is an important investigation for patients presenting with palpitations. The presence of structural heart disease such as left ventricular impairment should prompt urgent referral and investigation. Left ventricular impairment is associated with an increased risk of sudden cardiac death,[13] and patients are less likely to tolerate tachycardia. Such patients should not be prescribed class 1 antiarrhythmic drugs, such as flecainide.[1]

Most patients with SVT have a structurally normal heart. In a series of 145 patients referred for ablation, only 4% had heart failure.[14] However, certain types of structural heart disease are associated with particular SVTs. Patients with Ebstein's anomaly (congenital displacement of the septal tricuspid valve leaflet into the right ventricle) have an increased frequency of right sided accessory pathways.[15] Incisional atrial tachycardia occurs as a result of re-entry around surgical scars and is a major source of morbidity in the growing population of survivors of congenital heart disease.[16]

What are the acute management options in SVT?

Non-drug treatment

Patients presenting with sustained tachycardia should be assessed for haemodynamic stability; rarely, the arrhythmia is so poorly tolerated that immediate electrical cardioversion is needed. With the important exception of pre-excited atrial fibrillation (in which case the ECG shows an irregular, broad complex tachycardia, with variation of

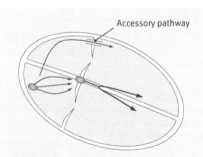

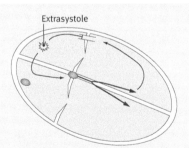

Delta wave:
Anterograde conduction via an accessory pathway usually produces pre-excitation of the ventricle, because the accessory pathway conducts more rapidly than the atrioventricular node. This early ventricular activation is manifest as a delta wave, which is a slurred upstroke at the start of the QRS complex. The terminal portion of the QRS complex is narrow, reflecting the rapid conduction via the His-Purkinje system once the atrioventricular node has been crossed

AVNRT:
Tachycardia is typically initiated by an extrasystole which occurs early and therefore cannot conduct via the accessory pathway but is able to conduct via the atrioventricular node (accessory pathway has a longer refractory period than the atrioventricular node). By the time the impulse reaches the accessory pathway from the ventricular side it is no longer refractory and can conduct retrogradely to the atrium

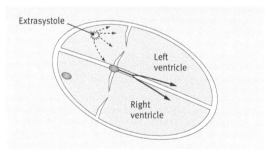

Fig 4 Mechanism for focal atrial tachycardia. Generation of rapid electrical impulses from a small localised area in the atria (in this example, the left atrium)

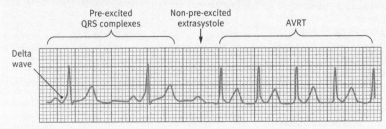

Fig 3 Mechanism for atrioventricular re-entry tachycardia

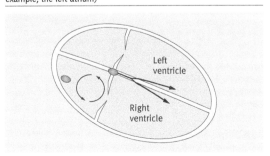

Fig 5 Mechanism for atrial flutter, an example of a macro re-entrant circuit. The electrical activation circles the right atrium

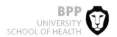

the QRS morphology (fig 6)), the first line manoeuvre is usually to slow conduction through the atrioventricular node. This may either terminate the tachycardia if the mechanism is dependent on the atrioventricular node (AVNRT, AVRT) or provide diagnostic information in the case of atrial tachycardia (P wave morphology exposed and lack of dependence on the atrioventricular node to maintain the tachycardia). A continuous 12 lead ECG recording should be made during these manoeuvres (fig 7).

Atrioventricular node conduction can be slowed by vagal stimulation with carotid sinus massage or the Valsalva manoeuvre.

Pre-excited atrial fibrillation should be managed with electrical cardioversion, or by flecainide infusion if the tachycardia is haemodynamically well tolerated and the heart is normal.

Drug treatment

If vagal manoeuvres are unsuccessful in slowing atrioventricular conduction then, unless the patient is asthmatic, the ACC/AHA/ESC guidelines[1] recommend intravenous adenosine as first line medication. Adenosine is preferred owing to its rapid onset of action and short half life. In a randomised double blinded placebo trial in participants with SVT, tachycardia was terminated in 91% of those who received adenosine (at a dose of either 6 mg or 12 mg) and in 16% of those receiving placebo.[17] When administering adenosine, ensure that resuscitation equipment is available in case the rare complications of bronchospasm or ventricular fibrillation occur.

The effectiveness of intravenous verapamil seems similar to that of adenosine in terminating SVT. In a randomised controlled trial, intravenous verapamil (2.5-7.5 mg) resulted in termination of tachycardia in 91% of patients, compared with termination in 93% of those receiving adenosine (6 mg dose followed by a 12 mg dose if required).[17] A meta-analysis of eight trials with a total of 605 patients, found similarly high rates of termination with both adenosine and verapamil (91% v 90%), with slightly higher rates of minor adverse effects and lower rates of hypotension described with adenosine.[18] β blockers are a further option and are effective in lowering heart rate, but in a small randomised study intravenous esmolol converted only 6% of SVTs to sinus rhythm.[19] Amiodarone[20] and flecainide are further options. Acute administration of flecainide successfully restored sinus rhythm in 72% of patients with AVRT and 83% with AVNRT.[21]

Macro re-entrant atrial tachycardias are not usually responsive to antiarrhythmic drugs and usually require electrical cardioversion (or overdrive atrial pacing, where tachycardia is terminated by rapid pacing of the atrium using either an existing pacemaker or temporary pacing lead in the right atrium) to restore sinus rhythm. The ACC/AHA/ESC guidelines recommend that before cardioversion the same guidelines for thromboembolic prophylaxis are followed for atrial flutter as for atrial fibrillation (international normalised ratio 2-3, or arrhythmia duration <48 hours, or no evidence of atrial thrombus on transoesophageal echocardiography).[1]

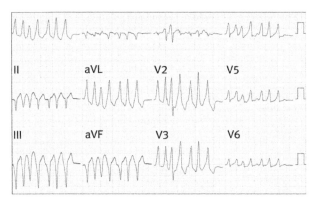

Fig 6 Pre-excited atrial fibrillation

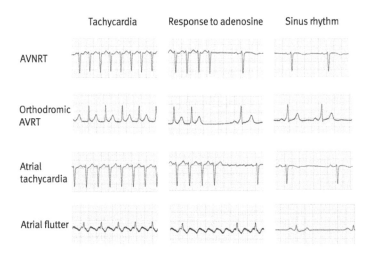

Fig 7 Typical electrocardiographic recordings for four common SVTs during tachycardia, administration of adenosine, and sinus rhythm. AVNRT: As atrial and ventricular activation occurs virtually simultaneously in typical AVNRT, the retrograde P waves are either hidden in the QRS complex or produce a pseudo r' in V1. Tachycardia is usually terminated with adenosine. Orthodromic AVRT: During tachycardia ventricular activation occurs exclusively via the atrioventricular node and His-Purkinje system; tachycardia is therefore narrow complex. Typically, the RP interval is short; less commonly, if the accessory pathway conducts slowly, a long RP interval is observed. Adenosine usually terminates the tachycardia and in sinus rhythm a delta wave is commonly seen. Atrial tachycardia: Often the RP interval is long. Tachycardia is not dependent on the atrioventricular node so it usually continues even after the administration of adenosine (though adenosine may terminate focal atrial tachycardia). When atrioventricular conduction is blocked the underlying P waves can be clearly seen. Atrial flutter: The characteristic flutter waves are seen clearly after administration of adenosine, and tachycardia continues because it does not depend on the atrioventricular node.

What are the long term management options?

In general, improvement of quality of life is the major therapeutic goal for SVTs, and treatment strategies should be guided according to symptoms and patient preference. Patients troubled by recurrent symptomatic episodes should be offered treatment; options include medication or catheter ablation. Patients can be taught the Valsalva manoeuvre and some find this helpful in controlling their symptoms. This can be described to the patient as simulating straining on the toilet, or trying to breathe out forcefully while keeping the mouth closed and nose pinched.

BOX 2 WHICH PATIENTS SHOULD YOU REFER TO AN ELECTROPHYSIOLOGIST?

Urgent referral
Patients with:

- Syncope with palpitations on exertion
- Broad complex tachycardia
- Pre-excitation (delta wave) on a 12 lead ECG
- Structural heart disease
- Severe symptoms

Routine referral
Those with:

- Drug resistance or intolerance
- Preference not to take medication
- Diagnostic uncertainty

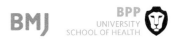

There have been no large scale randomised studies comparing these treatments. However, data from prospective non-randomised studies suggest that catheter ablation results in a greater reduction in symptoms and higher quality of life scores compared with medical treatment.[22] [23]

Patients with pre-excitation (delta wave on ECG) warrant special consideration. Such patients are at risk of sudden cardiac death from ventricular fibrillation induced by rapidly conducted atrial fibrillation. The findings from a recent meta-analysis suggest that in patients who do not have palpitations, this risk seems to be relatively low (1.25 per 1000 person years, 95% confidence interval 0.57 to 2.19 per 1000 person years).[24] Symptoms of palpitations appear to be associated with an increased risk of ventricular fibrillation.[25]

We advise referring patients with pre-excitation to an electrophysiologist for further assessment. Patients with documented broad complex tachycardia (QRS duration >120 ms and heart rate >100 beats/min), even if they have only had a single episode, are also best referred early. Box 2 outlines which patients to refer to an electrophysiologist.

Drug treatment

In general drug treatment is reserved for minimising symptoms while awaiting catheter ablation or for long term management of patients who decline catheter ablation or in whom the procedure carries an unacceptably high risk. Drug treatment may be effective in reducing the frequency of symptoms but complete suppression is uncommon.[26]

A major limitation in evaluating antiarrhythmic agents for treatment of SVTs is the absence of large, multicentre, randomised, placebo controlled studies.

For AVNRT and AVRT without pre-excitation, agents to block atrioventricular node conduction are commonly used as first line medication, although only limited data are available on the long term efficacy of these medications. Data from a small, randomised, double blind trial, showed that verapamil, propranolol, and digoxin all reduced the frequency of symptoms, with all equally effective.[26]

For patients who do not respond to these drugs, alternatives include flecainide and sotalol.[27] Although only relatively small numbers of patients have been included in randomised studies of flecainide and sotalol, the available data suggest they can be effective in reducing symptoms. In one small placebo controlled study 79% of patients in the flecainide group and 15% in the placebo group did not experience symptoms, though the follow-up period was only eight weeks.[28] Proarrhythmia, including ventricular tachycardia, has been reported in 6% of

patients.[29] Agents to slow atrioventricular node conduction are often co-administered, as flecainide may predispose to atrial flutter with 1:1 atrioventricular conduction.[29]

Flecainide is not recommended in patients with structural or ischaemic heart disease, in whom it is associated with an increased risk of sudden cardiac death.[30] Amiodarone is generally not recommended owing to the potential for serious adverse effects in patients with a benign condition. However, it may be used to treat atrial tachycardias resistant to other treatments, particularly in patients with structural heart disease and in elderly people.

Catheter ablation

Catheter ablation provides a definitive management option for SVT and is usually done under local anaesthesia as a day case. Catheters capable of recording electrical activation in the heart are inserted via the femoral vessels and manipulated under x ray guidance. Radiofrequency energy delivered via a catheter is used to create small localised areas of scar.

In AVNRT, the slow pathway is targeted with the aim of modifying conduction so that re-entrant tachycardia can no longer be sustained. Both acute and long term success rates for this procedure are high. In a large observational study acute success was achieved in 98% of cases.[31] A meta-analysis of 10 observational studies comprising 1204 patients reported a 4.3% recurrence rate.[32] Serious complications are uncommon, the most serious being atrioventricular block requiring pacemaker therapy (affecting 1% of patients in early series).[31] [33] [34]

AVRT is also amenable to catheter ablation. No randomised prospective studies have been conducted, but observational studies and registries have observed acute success rates of more than 95% and recurrence rates less than 5%.[33] [35] Atrioventricular block is a risk in cases where the accessory pathway is close to the atrioventricular node and the His bundle; the use of cryothermal energy may reduce this risk.[36] Other complications are reported to occur in less than 2-3% of patients and include vascular injury, bleeding, venous thrombosis, pulmonary embolism, myocardial perforation, systemic embolism (in the case of a left sided accessory pathway), and rarely, death (0-0.2%).[33] [34] [35]

Focal atrial tachycardia can also be successfully treated with catheter ablation, although randomised control trials are lacking, and evidence is limited to small observational studies. Acute success rates of 85%[37] [38] with recurrence rates of 8% have been reported.[39]

For re-entrant atrial tachycardias, radiofrequency ablation has high success rates and is often used as first line treatment.[5] [40] Radiofrequency ablation is the treatment of choice for typical atrial flutter. This practice is supported by the findings from a medium sized randomised study which found that, compared with medical treatment, as first line treatment ablation produced higher rates of sinus rhythm (80% v 36%), fewer hospital admissions, and a lower occurrence of atrial fibrillation.[40]

After the procedure, most patients can return to their normal activities very quickly. We recommend they avoid heavy lifting for two weeks after the procedure. In the UK, the Driver and Vehicle Licensing Agency states that car drivers (group 1 entitlement) may not drive for two days after successful catheter ablation (vocational drivers (group 2) for two weeks afterwards) if the arrhythmia was not or did not have the potential to be incapacitating. If the arrhythmia was or had the potential to be incapacitating, the restriction is six weeks after successful ablation.[41]

QUESTIONS FOR FUTURE RESEARCH

- Uncertainty remains about the optimal management of patients with asymptomatic pre-excitation (delta wave on the ECG)—in particular, whether sufficiently sensitive risk stratification is possible or whether most patients should be managed with catheter ablation of their accessory pathway
- There is ongoing development of invasive and non-invasive methods for mapping complex arrhythmias, such as atrial tachycardias occurring after ablation for atrial fibrillation. These have the potential to help with diagnosis and to guide the catheter ablation procedure

---

TIPS FOR NON-SPECIALISTS

- If a patient presents with tachycardia always record an ECG and give the patient a copy; this can be helpful for future management
- Broad complex tachycardia is ventricular tachycardia until proved otherwise
- For narrow complex tachycardia, the first step is usually to slow AV node conduction with either a Valsalva manoeuvre or adenosine. This provides diagnostic information and will usually terminate AVNRT and AVRT
- For patients with recurring symptoms, catheter ablation has high acute and long term success rates

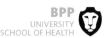

ADDITIONAL EDUCATIONAL RESOURCES

For healthcare professionals

- The Resuscitation Council provides free algorithms for the acute management of tachycardia: www.resus.org.uk/pages/glalgos.htm
- ACC/AHA/ESC guidelines for the management of patients with supraventricular arrhythmias. 2003. www.escardio.org/guidelines-surveys/esc-guidelines/Pages/supraventricular-arrhythmias.aspx
- Fox DJ, Tischenko A, Krahn AD, Skanes AC, Gula LJ, Yee RK, et al. Supraventricular tachycardia: diagnosis and management. *Mayo Clin Proc* 2008;83:1400-11.
- Delacrétaz E. Clinical practice: supraventricular tachycardia. *N Engl J Med* 2006;354:1039-51.

For patients (free web based resources)

- Arrhythmia Alliance (www.heartrhythmcharity.org.uk)—The patient pages give information on the full range of rhythm disturbances and treatments available, and downloadable single sheet summaries for different arrhythmias
- British Heart Foundation (www.bhf.org.uk)—The "Heart Health" pages give information on different cardiac conditions and investigations including electrophysiology studies; telephone advice line (Heart Helpline) is also available.
- NHS Choices (www.nhs.uk/conditions/supraventricular-tachycardia)—Simple overview of supraventricular tachycardia
- Patient.co.uk website (www.patient.co.uk/health/Supraventricular-Tachycardia-(SVT).htm)—Brief overview of SVT in lay terms

Contributors: All authors contributed fully to all stages of the planning, researching, and preparation of the manuscript. DWD and ZIW are the guarantors.

Competing interests: All authors have completed the ICMJE uniform disclosure form at www.icmje.org/coi_disclosure.pdf (available on request from the corresponding author) and declare: SMAS is funded by the British Heart Foundation; no financial relationships with any organisations that might have an interest in the submitted work in the previous three years; no other relationships or activities that could appear to have influenced the submitted work.

Provenance and peer review: Commissioned; externally peer reviewed.

1 Blomström-Lundqvist C, Scheinman MM, Aliot EM, Alpert JS, Calkins H, Camm AJ, et al. ACC/AHA/ESC guidelines for the management of patients with supraventricular arrhythmias—executive summary. A report of the American College of Cardiology/American Heart Association Task Force on practice guidelines and the European Society of Cardiology committee for practice guidelines (writing committee to develop guidelines for the management of patients with supraventricular arrhythmias) developed in collaboration with NASPE-Heart Rhythm Society. *J Am Coll Cardiol* 2003;42:1493-531.
2 Lafuente-Lafuente C, Mahé I, Extramiana F. Management of atrial fibrillation. *BMJ* 2009;339:b5216.
3 McGuire MA, Bourke JP, Robotin MC, Johnson DC, Meldrum-Hanna W, Nunn GR, et al. High resolution mapping of Koch's triangle using sixty electrodes in humans with atrioventricular junctional (AV nodal) reentrant tachycardia. *Circulation* 1993;88:2315-28.
4 Kastor JA. Multifocal atrial tachycardia. *N Engl J Med* 1990;322:1713-7.
5 Wasmer K, Mönnig G, Bittner A, Dechering D, Zellerhoff S, Milberg P, et al. Incidence, characteristics, and outcome of left atrial tachycardias after circumferential antral ablation of atrial fibrillation. *Heart Rhythm* 2012;9:1660-6.
6 Porter MJ, Morton JB, Denman R, Lin AC, Tierney S, Santucci PA, et al. Influence of age and gender on the mechanism of supraventricular tachycardia. *Heart Rhythm* 2004;1:393-6.
7 Tada H, Oral H, Greenstein R, Pelosi F Jr, Knight BP, Strickberger SA, et al. Analysis of age of onset of accessory pathway-mediated tachycardia in men and women. *Am J Cardiol* 2002;89:470-1.
8 Walfridsson U, Strömberg A, Janzon M, Walfridsson H. Wolff-Parkinson-White syndrome and atrioventricular nodal re-entry tachycardia in a Swedish population: consequences on health-related quality of life. *Pacing Clin Electrophysiol* 2009;32:1299-306.
9 Orejarena LA, Vidaillet H Jr, DeStefano F, Nordstrom DL, Vierkant RA, Smith PN, et al. Paroxysmal supraventricular tachycardia in the general population. *J Am Coll Cardiol* 1998;31:150-7.
10 Fuster V, Rydén LE, Cannom DS, Crijns HJ, Curtis AB, Ellenbogen KA, et al. 2011 ACCF/AHA/HRS focused updates incorporated into the ACC/AHA/ESC 2006 Guidelines for the management of patients with atrial fibrillation: a report of the American College of Cardiology Foundation/American Heart Association Task Force on Practice Guidelines developed in partnership with the European Society of Cardiology and in collaboration with the European Heart Rhythm Association and the Heart Rhythm Society. *J Am Coll Cardiol* 2011;57:e101-98.
11 Delacretaz E. Supraventricular tachycardia. *N Engl J Med* 2006;354:1039-51.
12 Gursoy S, Steurer G, Brugada J, Andries E, Brugada P. The hemodynamic mechanism of pounding in the neck in atrioventricular nodal reentrant tachycardia. *N Engl J Med* 1992;327:772-4.
13 Myerburg RJ, Kessler KM, Castellanos A. Sudden cardiac death: epidemiology, transient risk, and intervention assessment. *Ann Intern Med* 1993;119:1187-97.
14 Wood KA, Drew BJ, Scheinman MM. Frequency of disabling symptoms in supraventricular tachycardia *Am J Cardiol* 1997;79:145-9..
15 Ho S, Goltz D, McCarthy K, Cook A, Connell M, Smith A, et al. The atrioventricular junctions in Ebstein malformation. *Heart* 2000;83:444-9.
16 Walsh EP. Arrhythmias in patients with congenital heart disease. *Card Electrophysiol Rev* 2002;6:422-30.
17 DiMarco JP, Miles W, Akhtar M, Milstein S, Sharma AD, Platia E, et al. Adenosine for paroxysmal supraventricular tachycardia: dose ranging and comparison with verapamil: assessment in placebo-controlled, multicenter trials. *Ann Intern Med* 1990;113:104-10.
18 Delaney B, Loy J, Kelly AM. The relative efficacy of adenosine versus verapamil for the treatment of stable paroxysmal supraventricular tachycardia in adults: a meta-analysis. *Eur J Emerg Med* 2011;18:148-52.
19 Anderson S, Blanski L, Byrd RC, Das G, Engler R, Laddu A, et al. Comparison of the efficacy and safety of esmolol, a short-acting beta blocker, with placebo in the treatment of supraventricular tachyarrhythmias. *Am Heart J* 1986;111:42-8.
20 Holt P, Crick JC, Davies DW, Curry P. Intravenous amiodarone in the acute termination of supraventricular arrhythmias. *Int J Cardiol* 1985;8:67-79.
21 Hohnloser SH, Zabel M. Short- and long-term efficacy and safety of flecainide acetate for supraventricular arrhythmias. *Am J Cardiol* 1992;70:3-9A.
22 Bathina MN, Mickelsen S, Brooks C, Jaramillo J, Hepton T, Kusumoto FM. Radiofrequency catheter ablation versus medical therapy for initial treatment of supraventricular tachycardia and its impact on quality of life and healthcare costs. *Am J Cardiol* 1998;82:589-93.
23 Goldberg AS, Bathina MN, Mickelsen S, Nawman R, West G, Kusumoto FM. Long-term outcomes on quality-of-life and health care costs in patients with supraventricular tachycardia (radiofrequency catheter ablation versus medical therapy). *Am J Cardiol* 2002;1;89:1120-3.
24 Obeyesekere MN, Leong-Sit P, Massel D, Manlucu J, Modi S, Krahn AD, et al. Risk of arrhythmia and sudden death in patients with asymptomatic preexcitation: a meta-analysis. *Circulation* 2012;125:2308-15.
25 Klein GJ, Bashore TM, Sellers TD, Pritchett EL, Smith WM, Gallagher JJ. Ventricular-fibrillation in the Wolff-Parkinson-White Syndrome. *N Engl J Med* 1979;301:1080-5.
26 Winniford MD, Fulton KL, Hillis LD. Long-term therapy of paroxysmal supraventricular tachycardia: a randomized, double-blind comparison of digoxin, propranolol and verapamil. *Am J Cardiol* 1984;54:1138-9.
27 Kunze KP, Schlutter M, Kuck KH. Sotalol in patients with Wolff-Parkinson-White syndrome. *Circulation* 1987;75:1050-7.
28 Henthorn RW, Waldo AL, Anderson JL, Gilbert EM, Alpert BL, Bhandari AK, et al. Flecainide acetate prevents recurrence of symptomatic paroxysmal supraventricular tachycardia. *Circulation* 1991;83:119-125.
29 Benditt DG, Dunnigan A, Buetikofer J, Milstein S. Tachyarrhythmias. Flecainide acetate for long-term prevention of paroxysmal supraventricular. *Circulation* 1991;83:345-9.
30 Cardiac Arrhythmia Suppression Trial (CAST) Investigators. Preliminary report: effect of encainide and flecainide in a randomized trial of arrhythmia suppression after myocardial infarction. *N Engl J Med* 1989;321:406-12.
31 Feldman A, Voskoboinik A, Kumar S, Spence S, Morton JB, Kistler PM, et al. Predictors of acute and long-term success of slow pathway ablation for atrioventricular nodal reentrant tachycardia: a single center series of 1,419 consecutive patients. *Pacing Clin Electrophysiol* 2011;34:927-33.
32 Stern JD, Rolnitzky L, Goldberg JD, Chinitz LA, Holmes DS, Bernstein NE, et al. Meta-analysis to assess the appropriate endpoint for slow pathway ablation of atrioventricular nodal reentrant tachycardia. *Pacing Clin Electrophysiol* 2011;34:269-77.
33 Scheinman MM, Huang S. The 1998 NASPE prospective catheter ablation registry. *Pacing Clin Electrophysiol* 2000;23:1020-8.
34 Ganz LI, Friedman PL. Supraventricular tachycardia. *N Engl J Med* 1995;332:162-73.
35 Calkins H, Yong P, Miller JM, Olshansky B, Carlson M, Saul JP, et al. Catheter ablation of accessory pathways, atrioventricular nodal reentrant tachycardia, and the atrioventricular junction: final results of a prospective, multicenter clinical trial. The Atakr Multicenter Investigators Group. *Circulation* 1999;99:262-70.
36 Friedman PL, Dubuc M, Green MS, Jackman WM, Keane DT, Marinchak RA, et al. Catheter cryoablation of supraventricular tachycardia: results of the multicenter prospective "frosty" trial. *Heart Rhythm* 2004;1:129-38.
37 Kay GN, Epstein AE, Dailey SM, Plumb VJ. Role of radiofrequency ablation in the management of supraventricular arrhythmias: experience in 760 consecutive patients. *J Cardiovasc Electrophysiol* 1993;4:371-89.
38 Biviano AB, Bain W, Whang W, Leitner J, Dizon J, Hickey K, et al. Focal left atrial tachycardias not associated with prior catheter ablation for atrial fibrillation: clinical and electrophysiological characteristics. *Pacing Clin Electrophysiol* 2012;35:17-27.
39 Lesh MD, van Hare GF, Epstein LM, Fitzpatrick AP, Scheinman MM, Lee RJ, et al. Radiofrequency catheter ablation of atrial arrhythmias. Results and mechanisms. *Circulation* 1994;89:1074-89.

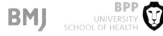

40 Natale A, Newby KH, Pisanó E, Leonelli F, Fanelli R, Potenza D, et al. Prospective randomized comparison of antiarrhythmic therapy versus first-line radiofrequency ablation in patients with atrial flutter. *J Am Coll Cardiol* 2000;35:1898-904.

41 Driver and Vehicle Licensing Agency (UK). For medical practitioners: at a glance guide to the current medical standards of fitness to drive. 2012. www.dft.gov.uk/dvla/medical/ataglance.aspx.

Related links

bmj.com
- All the latest BMJ Group articles on cardiovascular medicine

bmj.com/archive
Previous articles in this series
- Diagnosis and management of supraventricular tachycardia (2012;345:e7769)
- Generalized anxiety disorder: diagnosis and treatment (2012;345:e7500)
- Resistant hypertension (2012;345:e7473)
- Childhood constipation (2012;345:e7309)
- Preparing young travellers for low resource destinations (2012;345:e7179)

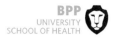

The diagnosis and management of aortic dissection

Sri G Thrumurthy, honorary research fellow,

Alan Karthikesalingam, specialist registrar in vascular surgery,

Benjamin O Patterson, clinical research fellow,

Peter J E Holt, clinical lecturer in vascular surgery and outcomes research,

Matt M Thompson, professor of vascular surgery

¹Department of Outcomes Research, St George's Vascular Institute, London SW17 0QT, UK

Correspondence to: P J E Holt
pholt@sgul.ac.uk

Cite this as: BMJ 2012;344:d8290

DOI: 10.1136/bmj.d8290

http://www.bmj.com/content/344/bmj.d8290

Aortic dissection is caused by an intimal and medial tear in the aorta with propagation of a false lumen within the aortic media. It is part of the "acute aortic syndrome"—an umbrella term for aortic dissection, intramural haematoma, and symptomatic aortic ulcer (table).[1] Acute dissection is the most common aortic emergency, with an annual incidence of 3-4 per 100 000 in the United Kingdom and United States, which exceeds that of ruptured aneurysm.[2w1] [w2] The prognosis is grave, with 20% preadmission mortality and 30% in-hospital mortality.[2]

The best treatment depends on the anatomical and temporal classification of the disease. Aortic dissection is therefore categorised according to the site of the entry tear and the time between the onset of symptoms and diagnosis. A dissection is considered "acute" when the diagnosis is made within 14 days of onset, and thereafter it is termed "chronic." The location of the entry tear plays a key role in treatment and outcome, and it is classified by being in the ascending aorta (Stanford type A dissection) or distal to the origin of the left subclavian artery (Stanford type B dissection) (fig 1).[3]

Type A dissection carries a far worse prognosis than type B dissection and urgent surgical intervention is often needed. By contrast, acute type B dissection is usually managed conservatively if uncomplicated and surgically if complicated.

We review the epidemiology, diagnosis, and management of aortic dissection drawing on evidence from population studies, randomised controlled trials, meta-analyses, and published guidelines.

SOURCES AND SELECTION CRITERIA

We searched the Medline, Embase, Web of Science, and Cochrane databases for "aortic dissection" and used reference lists to identify key studies. Two authors independently performed the searches and mutual consensus was reached. Because of the lack of large well designed randomised controlled trials, we gave priority to systematic reviews, meta-analyses, and studies from the International Registry of Acute Aortic Dissection.

SUMMARY POINTS

- Aortic dissection is diagnosed and managed according to its anatomical extent and chronicity
- White men aged over 40 years with hypertension, or those under 40 with Marfan's syndrome or bicuspid aortic valves, are at highest risk
- Patients often present with acute onset sharp chest pain, sometimes with loss of consciousness or poor perfusion of end organs
- Computed tomography aortography is the first line diagnostic investigation, followed by transoesophageal echocardiography; magnetic resonance angiography is preferred for surveillance
- Manage proximal (type A) dissection surgically if possible
- Uncomplicated distal (type B) dissection is best managed with intensive drug treatment; complicated type B dissection requires surgical intervention
- All patients need lifelong antihypertensive therapy and surveillance imaging

Who is at risk?

The causes of aortic dissection are multifactorial, and both inherited susceptibility and acquired degenerative disease have been implicated. Several modifiable and non-modifiable risk factors are recognised, the most important of which are discussed below.

Hypertension

Systemic hypertension is one of the most important risk factors for aortic dissection and is present in 40-75% of patients presenting with the condition.[3] Systolic hypertension exacerbates the differential haemodynamic forces acting on the relatively mobile aortic arch and the relatively fixed ascending and descending thoracic aorta. A cohort study of 175 patients identified physical exertion or emotional stress as the direct predecessor of acute pain in 66% of acute dissections, primarily as a result of acute changes in blood pressure during the event.[w3]

Race and sex

A cross sectional study of 951 patients by the International Registry of Acute Aortic Dissection, comprising data from 12 international referral centres, showed that 68% of all patients presenting with the condition were male and 79% were white.[5]

Connective tissue diseases

Various connective tissue diseases predispose to the inherent weakening of the aortic wall and subsequent dissection, and these diseases are especially important in patients under 40 years. These include Marfan's syndrome with fibrillin defects, which is seen in 15-50% of patients under 40 years[5w4]; Ehlers-Danlos type IV with abnormal synthesis of type III procollagen[w5]; and other connective tissue disorders associated with cystic medial necrosis.[w6]

Congenital cardiovascular abnormalities

A cross sectional study described a fivefold to 18-fold increased risk of dissection in 516 patients with bicuspid aortic valves.[5] This increased risk was attributed to a coinherited developmental defect of the proximal aorta, which conferred a predilection towards apoptosis of the cellular components of the aortic media, and subsequent medial weakening and aortic dilation. The presence of a bicuspid aortic valve was also associated with dissection in a greater proportion of patients under 40 years (9% under 40 v 1% over 40; P<0.001). A prospective study of 631 patients from the adult congenital heart disease database showed that the coexistence of coarctation of the aorta with a bicuspid aortic valve significantly increases the risk of acute aortic complications such as dissection (odds ratio

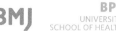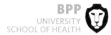

4.7, 95% confidence interval 1.5 to 15; P=0.01); this has been attributed largely to age, sex, aortic valve dysfunction, and the hypertension associated with coarctation.[w7] Several familial aneurysmal syndromes (such as congenital contractural arachnodactyly, familial thoracic aortic aneurysm or Erdheim's cystic medial necrosis, familial aortic dissection, familial ectopia lentis, and familial Marfan-like habitus) also predispose to aortic dissection.[6w8]

Miscellaneous risk factors

Prevalence studies have shown that aortic vasculitic disease,[w9] cocaine misuse,[w10] and pregnancy[7] are risk factors for aortic dissection. One report on 723 patients found a 5% rate of iatrogenic aortic dissection after cardiac interventions, including percutaneous revascularisation and coronary artery bypass grafting.[w11]

Although British national statistics show that dissection affects all ages (27% of patients aged 17-59 years, 40% aged 60-74 years,[w12] 33% aged >75 years), older patients (>40 years) are more likely to have concurrent hypertension or atherosclerosis, whereas younger patients are more likely to have Marfan's syndrome, a bicuspid aortic valve, or aortic intervention before presentation.[5]

How do patients present?

Patients typically present with the abrupt onset of sharp tearing or stabbing chest pain, which may improve slightly over time, although pain may be absent in 10% of patients.[8] Asymptomatic presentation is more common in patients with diabetes.[w13-w15] The pain may radiate to the neck in type A dissection or to the interscapular area in type B aortic dissection.[9] Acute rupture or inadequate perfusion—depending on the site and extent of the dissection—may cause a patient to become unconscious.[10] Interrupted perfusion may result in neurological deficits, symptomatic limb ischaemia, or visceral ischaemia. A cross sectional study of 617 patients with type A dissection found focal neurological deficits in 17% of patients.[11] One report from the International Registry of Acute Aortic Dissection showed that aortic regurgitation and pulse deficit were present in 32% and 15% of patients, respectively.[w15] Hypotension was seen in 25% of patients with type A dissection, whereas hypertension was typical in type B dissection.[w15]

Many differential diagnoses exist (box). Specific features, however, may alert clinicians to probable dissection. Consensus guidelines from the American Heart Association describe three categories of high risk features to identify patients at greatest risk: predisposing conditions, pain features, and examination findings.[12] High risk predisposing conditions include Marfan's syndrome, recent aortic manipulation, or a known thoracic aneurysm. High risk pain features include an abrupt onset of ripping, tearing, or stabbing pain in the chest, back, or abdomen. High risk features of the examination include a pulse or blood pressure discrepancy, neurological deficit, a new murmur of aortic regurgitation, and shock. Urgent aortic imaging is needed in patients who have one or more high risk feature,

but who present with no electrocardiographic changes of myocardial infarction and no history or examination findings that strongly suggest an alternative diagnosis. Although the specificity of this approach is unknown, a sensitivity of 95.7% has been reported.[13]

How are patients initially managed?

The emergency management of patients with suspected aortic dissection entails adequate resuscitation and optimisation for subsequent imaging and intervention. This includes ensuring adequate oxygenation and ventilation, with careful monitoring of respiratory function. Two large bore intravenous lines should be established for intravenous fluid resuscitation, with close monitoring of heart rate, heart rhythm, blood pressure, and urine output. β blockers may be given to reduce the rate of blood pressure changes and the shear forces on the aortic wall; aim for a heart rate of 60-80 beats/min and systolic blood pressure of 100-120 mm Hg.[w16] However, a careful balance must be maintained between suppressing tachycardia and hypertension and ensuring adequate end organ perfusion (by monitoring urine output; mental and neurological state; and peripheral vascular status, including the development or progression of carotid, brachial, and femoral bruits). Twelve lead electrocardiography is essential to exclude concurrent myocardial ischaemia, which would necessitate urgent discussion with cardiology colleagues about managing acute coronary syndrome in the context of a potential aortic dissection. Undertake definitive imaging and further intervention only once the patient is haemodynamically stable.

How is aortic dissection diagnosed?

Retrograde aortography was the gold standard for assessing patients in the 1970s and 1980s, but it has been superseded by cross sectional imaging, which performs better and has a better safety profile.[14]

Although chest radiography and electrocardiography are often ordered in the emergency care setting, these tests cannot establish or exclude the diagnosis of dissecting aortic aneurysm.[w17]

D-dimers are raised in aortic dissection and it has been suggested that a concentration below 500 ng/ml, which is already used to rule out pulmonary embolism, can exclude acute dissection (negative likelihood ratio of 0.07) in the first 24 hours.[w18 w19] However, these data were derived from a population of patients undergoing imaging for dissection in a tertiary centre. The high pre-test probability of dissection in this group limits the applicability of the study's findings,

---

DIFFERENTIAL DIAGNOSES

Patients with acute chest pain
- Myocardial infarction
- Pulmonary embolism
- Spontaneous pneumothorax

Patients with acute abdominal or back pain
- Ureteric colic
- Perforated viscus
- Mesenteric ischaemia

Patients with pulse deficit
- Non-dissection related embolic disease

Patients with focal neurological deficit
- Stroke
- Cauda equina syndrome

European Society of Cardiologists' classification of acute aortic syndrome

Classification	Pathology
Type 1	Classic dissection with true and false lumens separated by the dissecting membrane
Type 2	Intramural haematoma
Type 3	Discrete dissection with a bulge at the tear site but no haematoma
Type 4	Penetrating aortic ulcer
Type 5	Traumatic or iatrogenic dissection

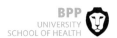

and the safety of using D-dimer testing to screen for dissection in all patients with non-coronary chest pain requires further study. Biomarkers such as smooth muscle myosin heavy chain protein have also proved to be less than useful in diagnosis.[w17]

Computed tomography can help the clinician rapidly confirm or exclude aortic dissection, classify its extent, and diagnose any complications. Correct categorisation of type A or type B dissection (fig 1) is imperative to plan treatment. Patients commonly need more than one non-invasive imaging test to acquire all necessary information. A cross sectional study of 464 patients reported computed tomography angiography as the initial investigation in 61% of cases, echocardiography in 33%, aortography in 4%, and magnetic resonance angiography in 2%.[w15]

Computed tomography angiography

Multidetector computed tomography angiography is recommended by the European Society of Cardiology as the first line of investigation for patients with suspected acute dissection.[1] This investigation can assess factors that are important in the planning of open or endovascular surgery, including the extent of dissection, the relative calibre of true and false lumens, and the involvement of aortic side branches. A meta-analysis of 1139 patients with aortic dissection found that multidetector computed tomography angiography had a sensitivity of 100%, specificity of 98%, and diagnostic odds ratio of 6.5.[w20] Outside the emergency setting, electrocardiogram gated computed tomography can provide dynamic information, although its spatial resolution is inferior to magnetic resonance imaging,[w21] which reduces its usefulness in planning complex aortic repairs. The disadvantages of computed tomography angiography include the need to use potentially nephrotoxic contrast media, exposure to ionising radiation, and inability to assess functional aortic insufficiency.

Echocardiography

A small prospective cohort study showed that in patients presenting in shock, transthoracic echocardiography had a 78.3% sensitivity and 83.0% specificity for diagnosing proximal dissection.[15] However, the role of this modality is limited because it cannot accurately visualise the descending aorta in most patients, despite its ability to diagnose aortic incompetence. The combined use of transthoracic echocardiography and computed tomography is useful in the absence of multidetector computed tomography functional imaging.[w22] A meta-analysis of cohort studies (1139 patients) found that transoesophageal echocardiography accurately visualised the entire thoracic aorta (sensitivity 98.0%, specificity 95.0%, diagnostic odds ratio 6.1) and, despite the requirement for oesophageal intubation, can be performed at the bedside.[w20] Unlike static imaging, transoesophageal echocardiography detects aortic regurgitation or pericardial effusion and can provide intraoperative assessment of operator position within the vessel lumen, although it cannot assess the abdominal aorta.[9] The operator dependency of transthoracic and transoesophageal echocardiography limits their accuracy and accessibility.

Magnetic resonance angiography

A meta-analysis of diagnostic studies showed magnetic resonance angiography to have a sensitivity of 98% and specificity of 98%, with diagnostic odds ratio of 6.8, in the diagnosis of dissecting aortic aneurysm.[w20] Gadolinium contrast agents used in magnetic resonance angiography are less nephrotoxic than iodinated substances used for computed tomography angiography and there is no associated ionising radiation.[w23] Disadvantages include its limited use in patients with claustrophobia or metal devices, although it can be used in those with nitinol aortic stent grafts.[1] Long acquisition times and limited availability reduce its usefulness in the emergency setting, for which computed tomography angiography is ideal. Magnetic resonance angiography offers greater potential for long term surveillance of treated dissection and for the assessment of stable patients presenting with chronic dissection.[1]

How is aortic dissection managed?

Owing to the paucity of evidence from randomised controlled trials, the management of aortic dissection is mainly guided by data from international registries, large series, and expert consensus.[1 16 17] The balance between medical and surgical management depends on the anatomical features of the lesion and its physiological sequelae.

Type A dissection

Cross sectional studies from the International Registry of Acute Aortic Dissection have suggested that, if left untreated, proximal (Stanford type A or DeBakey type I or II) dissection carries a one week mortality of 50-91% owing to complications such as aortic rupture, stroke, visceral ischaemia, cardiac tamponade, and circulatory failure.[w15] Drug treatment alone results in a mortality of nearly 20% by 24 hours and 30% by 48 hours (fig 2).[w15] Urgent cardiac surgical consultation is therefore imperative. Surgery involves replacing the affected ascending aorta, with or without the aortic arch, with a prosthetic graft; this procedure has an in-hospital mortality of 15-35%.[w24-w28] A variety of techniques may be needed. For example, proximal extension of the dissection to the aortic valve or ostia of the coronary arteries may require replacement or resuspension of the aortic valve,[1] or coronary artery bypass.[w29] The International Registry of Acute Aortic Dissection reported these techniques in 24% and 15% of type A dissections, respectively.[w30] Together with adjunctive measures such as hypothermic circulatory arrest and perfusion of the head vessels,[w31] surgery for proximal aortic dissection has three year and five year survival rates of 75% (standard deviation 5%) and 73% (6%), respectively.[14]

Acute type B dissection

The development of complicated dissection—defined by the presence of visceral or limb ischaemia, rupture, refractory pain, or uncontrollable hypertension—is the key factor that determines both intervention and outcome for patients with type B dissection.[1 w13 w15 w17 w20 w32 w33]

For uncomplicated acute type B dissection, series have shown that drug treatment alone can result in 78% three year survival after discharge from hospital.[18] Current guidelines deem this a difficult benchmark to surpass,[16] and medical management remains the gold standard. Careful regulation of systolic blood pressure at 100-120 mm Hg is needed to minimise haemodynamic shear stress and discourage rupture.[w17] β blockers (such as propranolol and metoprolol) are first line agents. Calcium channel blockers (such as non-dihydropyridine agents) are useful in patients with chronic obstructive pulmonary disease and those who cannot tolerate β blockers.[1 12] Endovascular treatment is increasingly possible

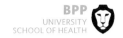

with low mortality,[19] and its role in uncomplicated acute type B dissection will be clarified by the results of the Acute Dissection Stent-grafting or Best Medical Treatment (ADSORB) trial (NCT00742274), which will randomise patients to best medical treatment, with and without stent grafting. Until these data are available, uncomplicated type B dissection should be medically managed.

Intervention, usually endovascular repair using a stent graft, is necessary for complicated acute type B dissection.[1] A prospective cohort study of 159 patients reported that, if untreated, this pathology carries a mortality of 50%.[w34] Conventional open surgery for complicated dissection has a 30 day mortality of 30%,[20] whereas meta-analysis has shown that endovascular treatment has a 30 day mortality of

9.8%.[21] Long term postoperative surveillance is mandatory: a prospective cohort study of 125 patients suggested that complete thrombosis of the false lumen may be achieved in only 44% of cases, with 20% of dissections rupturing within five years from continual aortic expansion.[w35] Multiple cohort studies have shown that even after complete false lumen thrombosis, 16% of patients develop evidence of dissection in the unstented distal aorta, which requires surgical reintervention.[w35-w37]

Chronic type B dissection

Uncomplicated chronic type B dissection can be managed conservatively, but many of these patients develop complications, the foremost of which is formation of an aneurysm, which may require surgical intervention. Data on the natural course of the disease suggest that 15% of chronic type B dissections will be complicated by an aneurysm,[w38] and ongoing research is directed at predicting patients at high risk of this complication, so that they can be targeted for earlier intervention.[22]

Chronic dissection is difficult to treat. Conventional open surgery has an appreciable death rate and poses considerable physiological challenges, including the need for posterolateral thoracotomy, single lung ventilation, cardiopulmonary bypass, hypothermia, heparinisation, cerebrospinal fluid drainage, and circulatory arrest to prevent stroke and paraplegia.[w39] The endovascular approach is associated with less morbidity and mortality; a systematic review of 810 patients found that one year survival is higher after endovascular stenting than after open surgery (endovascular surgery 93%; open surgery 79%).[23] However, the long term efficacy of an endovascular approach to preventing long term aortic related death is still unclear.

How should patients be followed up?

Ten year survival rates of patients who are discharged from hospital range from 30% to 60%.[24w25-w28 w40] The underlying pathophysiology of aortic medial disease and defective wall structure confers an ongoing risk of further dissection, aneurysmal degeneration, and rupture.[13] A prospective cohort study of 721 patients found this risk to be higher in women and that annual mortality was 12% once the aortic diameter exceeded 6 cm.[w41] Consequently, the European Society of Cardiology recommends regular cross sectional imaging of the aorta, preferably with magnetic resonance angiography, at one, three, and 12 months after discharge and every six to 12 months thereafter, depending on aortic size.[1] Various experts also advocate the combined use of echocardiography with axial imaging for routine surveillance.[w42] All patients should receive lifelong antihypertensive treatment, including β blockers, with a target blood pressure of 120/80 mm Hg.[25 26 27]

The sequelae of endovascular and open repair also merit surveillance. A small prospective cohort study reported that reintervention was needed in 27.5% of patients after open repair because of extension or recurrence of dissection, formation of a localised aneurysm remote from the original repair, graft dehiscence, aortic regurgitation, or infection.[28] A systematic review of the mid-term outcomes of endovascular treatment found high rates of reintervention for late morbidities, such as endoleak (8.1%), formation of a distal aneurysm (7.8%), and rupture (3.0%), thereby justifying mandatory postoperative surveillance.[29]

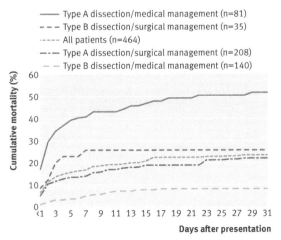

DeBakey classification

Type I	Originates in the ascending aorta; propagates at least to the aortic arch and often beyond it distally
Type II	Originates in and is confined to the ascending aorta
Type III	Originates in the descending aorta and extends distally down the aorta or, rarely, retrograde into the aortic arch and ascending aorta

Stanford classification

Type A	All dissections that affect the ascending aorta, regardless of the site of origin
Type B	All dissections that do not affect the ascending aorta

Fig 1 The Stanford and DeBakey classifications of aortic dissection. The dissection types are mainly differentiated by whether they affect the ascending aorta (the ascending aorta is affected in Stanford type A dissections, but not in Stanford type B dissections). Urgent surgical intervention is warranted when the ascending aorta is affected, and such cases are associated with higher mortality and morbidity than isolated descending aortic dissection[4]

Fig 2 Thirty day mortality according to dissection type and management strategy[w15]

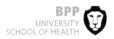

Contributors: SGT conceived the review, extracted evidence, and drafted the manuscript. AK, BOP and PJEH coauthored the article (including article direction, interpreting the literature, and editing the manuscript). MMT is guarantor.

Competing interests: All authors have completed the ICMJE uniform disclosure form at www.icmje.org/coi_disclosure.pdf (available on request from the corresponding author) and declare: no support from any organisation for the submitted work; no financial relationships with any organisations that might have an interest in the submitted work in the previous three years; no other relationships or activities that could appear to have influenced the submitted work.

Provenance and peer review: Not commissioned; externally peer reviewed.

Patient consent obtained.

A PATIENT'S PERSPECTIVE

I was relaxing at home one evening when I experienced sudden and extreme chest pain, which was followed by my left leg going numb. I called for an ambulance, which took me to the nearest hospital. After a computed tomography scan, I was diagnosed with a type A aortic dissection and transferred urgently to a regional vascular centre. The surgeons opened my chest and stitched a graft into the top of my aorta. Unfortunately, I had a mild stroke afterwards, which they had warned me about. I am still recovering from this but feel lucky to have survived, considering the high mortality rate.

I stayed well for a year but then developed chest pain and fever. This gradually worsened over four weeks and I was again admitted to my local hospital, where a computed tomography scan showed that I had pneumonia, pleural effusion, and now a type B dissection. They transferred me to the regional vascular centre, where the team decided that because this dissection was chronic and I was otherwise well, I did not need further intervention. I was investigated and treated for a bleeding stomach ulcer. I did well and was then discharged home but was readmitted a week later because I had recurrent chest pain and was coughing blood. A computed tomography scan found no clot in my lungs but showed that the aorta had increased in diameter from 5.9 cm to 7.9 cm. After three days in intensive care, where they controlled my blood pressure, I'm feeling better. I am still an inpatient at the regional vascular unit and am awaiting further surgery on my aorta. The surgeons have said that because of the complexity of my disease, I may be better suited to open rather than keyhole surgery.

UNANSWERED QUESTIONS AND ONGOING RESEARCH

- Which patients with uncomplicated type B dissection might benefit most from intervention? Research currently centres on defining a subgroup at greatest risk of future aneurysmal dilation despite best medical treatment (for example, aortic diameter >40 mm at presentation)[22]
- The INvestigation of STEnt Grafts in Aortic Dissection (INSTEAD) trial will report the long term outcomes of endovascular stent grafting for uncomplicated chronic type B dissection (conducted across seven European centres)[30]
- The Acute Dissection Stent-grafting or Best Medical Treatment (ADSORB) trial will report the success of endovascular stent grafting in patients randomised to best medical treatment with and without stent grafting for uncomplicated acute type B dissection
- The mid-term success of stent grafting for dissection will be clarified by publication of the results of postmarket registries (CAPTIVIA (NCT01181947) and VIRTUE (NCT01213589)

ADDITIONAL EDUCATIONAL RESOURCES

Resources for patients

- Patient UK information (www.patient.co.uk/doctor/Aortic-Dissection.htm)—A relatively in-depth summary for patients interested in the risk factors, diagnosis, and treatment of aortic dissection
- Mayo Clinic (www.mayoclinic.com/health/aortic-dissection/DS00605)—Detailed information about aortic dissection for patients explained in a stepwise fashion

Resources for healthcare professionals

- Hinchliffe RJ, Halawa M, Holt PJ, Morgan R, Loftus I, Thompson MM. Aortic dissection and its endovascular management. J Cardiovasc Surg (Torino) 2008;49:449-60
- Braverman AC. Acute aortic dissection: clinician update. Circulation 2010;122:184-8
- Kwolek CJ, Watkins MT. The INvestigation of STEnt Grafts in Aortic Dissection (INSTEAD) trial: the need for ongoing analysis. Circulation 2009;120:2513-4

TIPS FOR NON-SPECIALISTS

- Refer patients with confirmed aortic dissection (or symptomatic high risk patients) to a regional cardiovascular unit for urgent diagnostic investigation and treatment
- Young patients with a history of connective tissue disease (such as Marfan's disease) or congenital cardiovascular disease (such as bicuspid aortic valves) are at high risk
- Maintain systolic blood pressure at 100-120 mm Hg in patients with a history of dissection; prescribe antihypertensive drugs (including β blockers) and deal with other modifiable cardiovascular risk factors
- Ensure that patients with a history of dissection are enrolled in a surveillance programme at a regional cardiovascular unit

1 Erbel R, Alfonso F, Boileau C, Dirsch O, Eber B, Haverich A, et al. Diagnosis and management of aortic dissection. Eur Heart J 2001;22:1642-81.

2 Olsson C, Thelin S, Stahle E, Ekbom A, Granath F. Thoracic aortic aneurysm and dissection: increasing prevalence and improved outcomes reported in a nationwide population-based study of more than 14 000 cases from 1987 to 2002. Circulation 2006;114:2611-8.

3 Hinchliffe RJ, Halawa M, Holt PJ, Morgan R, Loftus I, Thompson MM. Aortic dissection and its endovascular management. J Cardiovasc Surg (Torino) 2008;49:449-60.

4 Nienaber CA, Eagle KA. Aortic dissection: new frontiers in diagnosis and management: Part I: from etiology to diagnostic strategies. Circulation 2003;108:628-35.

5 Januzzi JL, Isselbacher EM, Fattori R, Cooper JV, Smith DE, Fang J, et al. Characterizing the young patient with aortic dissection: results from the International Registry of Aortic Dissection (IRAD). J Am Coll Cardiol 2004;43:665-9.

6 Albornoz G, Coady MA, Roberts M, Davies RR, Tranquilli M, Rizzo JA, et al. Familial thoracic aortic aneurysms and dissections—incidence, modes of inheritance, and phenotypic patterns. Ann Thorac Surg 2006;82:1400-5.

7 Suzuki T, Mehta RH, Ince H, Nagai R, Sakomura Y, Weber F, et al. Clinical profiles and outcomes of acute type B aortic dissection in the current era: lessons from the International Registry of Aortic Dissection (IRAD). Circulation 2003;108(suppl 1):II312-7.

8 Von Kodolitsch Y, Schwartz AG, Nienaber CA. Clinical prediction of acute aortic dissection. Arch Intern Med 2000;160:2977-82.

9 Karthikesalingam A, Holt PJ, Hinchliffe RJ, Thompson MM, Loftus IM. The diagnosis and management of aortic dissection. Vasc Endovascular Surg 2010;44:165-9.

10 Ranasinghe AM, Strong D, Boland B, Bonser RS. Acute aortic dissection. BMJ 2011;343:d4487.

11 Collins JS, Evangelista A, Nienaber CA, Bossone E, Fang J, Cooper JV, et al. Differences in clinical presentation, management, and outcomes of acute type a aortic dissection in patients with and without previous cardiac surgery. Circulation 2004;110(11 suppl 1):II237-42.

12 Hiratzka LF, Bakris GL, Beckman JA, Bersin RM, Carr VF, Casey DE Jr, et al. 2010 ACCF/AHA/AATS/ACR/ASA/SCA/SCAI/SIR/STS/SVM guidelines for the diagnosis and management of patients with Thoracic Aortic Disease: a report of the American College of Cardiology Foundation/ American Heart Association Task Force on Practice Guidelines, American Association for Thoracic Surgery, American College of Radiology, American Stroke Association, Society of Cardiovascular Anesthesiologists, Society for Cardiovascular Angiography and Interventions, Society of Interventional Radiology, Society of Thoracic Surgeons, and Society for Vascular Medicine. Circulation 2010;121:e266-369.

13 Rogers AM, Hermann LK, Booher AM, Nienaber CA, Williams DM, Kazerooni EA, et al. Sensitivity of the aortic dissection detection risk score, a novel guideline-based tool for identification of acute aortic dissection at initial presentation: results from the international registry of acute aortic dissection. Circulation 2010;123:2213-8.

14 Ince H, Nienaber CA. Diagnosis and management of patients with aortic dissection. Heart 2007;93:266-70.

15 Nienaber CA, von Kodolitsch Y, Nicolas V, Siglow V, Piepho A, Brockhoff C, et al. The diagnosis of thoracic aortic dissection by noninvasive imaging procedures. N Engl J Med 1993;328:1-9.

16 Svensson LG, Kouchoukos NT, Miller DC, Bavaria JE, Coselli JS, Curi MA, et al. Expert consensus document on the treatment of descending thoracic aortic disease using endovascular stent-grafts. Ann Thorac Surg 2008;85(1 suppl):S1-41.

17 Tsai TT, Trimarchi S, Nienaber CA. Acute aortic dissection: perspectives from the International Registry of Acute Aortic Dissection (IRAD). Eur J Vasc Endovasc Surg 2009;37:149-59.

18 Tsai TT, Fattori R, Trimarchi S, Isselbacher E, Myrmel T, Evangelista A, et al. Long-term survival in patients presenting with type B acute aortic dissection: insights from the International Registry of Acute Aortic Dissection. Circulation 2006;114:2226-31.

19 Dake MD, Kato N, Mitchell RS, Semba CP, Razavi MK, Shimono T, et al. Endovascular stent-graft placement for the treatment of acute aortic dissection. N Engl J Med 1999;340:1546-52.

20 Trimarchi S, Nienaber CA, Rampoldi V, Myrmel T, Suzuki T, Bossone E, et al. Role and results of surgery in acute type B aortic dissection: insights from the International Registry of Acute Aortic Dissection (IRAD). Circulation 2006;114(1 suppl):I357-64.

21 Eggebrecht H, Nienaber CA, Neuhauser M, Baumgart D, Kische S, Schmermund A, et al. Endovascular stent-graft placement in aortic dissection: a meta-analysis. Eur Heart J 2006;27:489-98.

22 Chan YC, Clough RE, Taylor PR. Predicting aneurysmal dilatation after type B aortic dissection. Eur J Vasc Endovasc Surg 2011;42:464-6.

23 Subramanian S, Roselli EE. Thoracic aortic dissection: long-term results of endovascular and open repair. Semin Vasc Surg 2009;22:61-8.

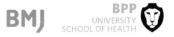

24 Umana JP, Lai DT, Mitchell RS, Moore KA, Rodriguez F, Robbins RC, et al. Is medical therapy still the optimal treatment strategy for patients with acute type B aortic dissections? *J Thorac Cardiovasc Surg* 2002;124:896-910.

25 Nienaber CA, Von Kodolitsch Y. Therapeutic management of patients with Marfan syndrome: focus on cardiovascular involvement. *Cardiol Rev* 1999;7:332-41.

26 Finkbohner R, Johnston D, Crawford ES, Coselli J, Milewicz DM. Marfan syndrome. Long-term survival and complications after aortic aneurysm repair. *Circulation* 1995;91:728-33.

27 Silverman DI, Burton KJ, Gray J, Bosner MS, Kouchoukos NT, Roman MJ, et al. Life expectancy in the Marfan syndrome. *Am J Cardiol* 1995;75:157-60.

28 Fattori R, Bacchi-Reggiani L, Bertaccini P, Napoli G, Fusco F, Longo M, et al. Evolution of aortic dissection after surgical repair. *Am J Cardiol* 2000;86:868-72.

29 Thrumurthy SG, Karthikesalingam A, Patterson BO, Holt PJ, Hinchliffe RJ, Loftus IM, et al. A systematic review of mid-term outcomes of Thoracic Endovascular Repair (TEVAR) of chronic type B aortic dissection. *Eur J Vasc Endovasc Surg* 2011;42:632-47.

30 Nienaber CA, Rousseau H, Eggebrecht H, Kische S, Fattori R, Rehders TC, et al. Randomized comparison of strategies for type B aortic dissection: the INvestigation of STEnt Grafts in Aortic Dissection (INSTEAD) trial. *Circulation* 2009;120:2519-28.

Related links

bmj.com/archive

Previous clinical reviews

- Laparoscopic colorectal surgery (2011;343:d8029)
- Managing infants who cry excessively in the first few months of life (2011;343:d7772)
- Managing motion sickness (2011;343:d7430)
- Osteoarthritis at the base of the thumb (2011;343:d7122)
- Inherited cardiomyopathies (2011;343:d6966)

bmj.com

- Get CME credits for this article

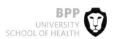

Extracorporeal life support

Alan M Gaffney, specialist registrar in anaesthesia[1,3],

Stephen M Wildhirt, professor of cardiothoracic surgery[2],

Michael J Griffin, consultant anaesthetist[3],

Gail M Annich, associate professor paediatric critical care medicine[4],

Marek W Radomski, professor of pharmacology[1]

[1]School of Pharmacy and Pharmaceutical Sciences, Trinity College, Dublin, Ireland

[2]Department of Thoracic, Cardiac, and Vascular Surgery, University of Tübingen, Tübingen, Germany

[3]Mater Misericordiae University Hospital, Dublin, Ireland

[4]C S Mott Children's Hospital, University of Michigan Health System, Ann Arbor, Michigan 48109, USA

Correspondence to: Marek W Radomski marek.radomski@tcd.ie

Cite this as: BMJ 2010;341:c5317

DOI: 10.1136/bmj.c5317

http://www.bmj.com/content/341/bmj.c5317

Extracorporeal life support (ECLS) is a variation of cardiopulmonary bypass. Whereas cardiopulmonary bypass facilitates open heart surgery for a number of hours, extracorporeal life support maintains tissue oxygenation for days to weeks in patients with life threatening respiratory or cardiac failure (or both).

As technology advances, indications increase, and the numbers of specialist centres rise, more doctors are likely to find themselves assessing patients for early referral, discussing this support option with relatives, directly or indirectly managing patients on extracorporeal life support, and providing follow-up outpatient and community based care. During the recent H1N1 influenza A pandemic, one third of patients admitted to the intensive care unit with severe respiratory failure required extracorporeal life support.[1]

Evidence from case series, cohort studies, registry database analyses, and randomised controlled trials form the basis of this overview.

What happens during extracorporeal life support?

The circuit consists of tubing taking deoxygenated blood from the patient, a pump, an artificial lung, a heat exchanger, and tubing returning oxygenated blood to the patient (fig 1). Venous-venous cannulation is used for isolated respiratory failure (tissue hypoxia secondary to hypoxaemia), whereas venous-arterial cannulation is used for cardiac failure (tissue hypoxia secondary to hypoperfusion) with or without respiratory failure (table 1).

Venous-venous

A double lumen cannula is commonly placed in a major vein. Deoxygenated blood flows from the venae cavae and oxygenated blood is returned to the right atrium (fig 1). Alternatively, separate inflow and outflow cannulas may be used (fig 2A).

Blood is removed distal to the right atrium and returned directly into the right atrium in an attempt to reduce mixing of deoxygenated with oxygenated blood, and to reduce recirculation of oxygenated blood within the circuit. It is impossible to prevent all mixing and recirculation, and

SOURCES AND SELECTION CRITERIA

We searched PubMed, Embase, and the Cochrane Library for systematic reviews, randomised trials, large population based studies, case controlled studies, case series, scientific and clinical reviews, evidence based guidelines, and published consensus statements between 1996 and 2010. We used the search terms "extracorporeal membrane oxygenation", "extracorporeal circulation", and "extracorporeal life support". We also consulted the registry database of the Extracorporeal Life Support Organization, personal databases, reference collections, and contemporary textbooks.

so, in the absence of pulmonary gas exchange, arterial oxyhaemoglobin saturation as low as 80% is common. Adequate oxygen delivery to the tissue, therefore, requires a sufficiently high cardiac output and a haematocrit above 40%.[2]

Venous-arterial

Cannulas are placed in a major artery and one or more major veins. Venous blood is oxygenated and pumped back directly into the arterial circulation, bypassing both the heart and lungs.

Femoral arterial cannulation is common in adults (fig 2B), whereas the carotid artery is commonly cannulated in infants (fig 2C). In femoral artery cannulation a distal down flow cannula may be needed to prevent leg ischaemia, whereas in carotid cannulation, collateral circulation must be relied on for adequate brain perfusion.

Existing transthoracic cardiopulmonary bypass cannulas may be used where extracorporeal life support is needed immediately after open heart surgery (fig 2D).

In the presence of native heart function, oxygenated blood may not reach the proximal aorta, and this results in cardiac and upper body hypoxaemia (fig 2B). An increase in blood flow rate, a change to venous-venous extracorporeal life support, or placement of an extravenous return cannula may be needed.

Anticoagulation

Because of blood-surface interaction, an infusion of unfractionated heparin is necessary to prevent thrombosis within the circuit and embolism to the patient.

Ventilation

Positive end expiratory pressure is applied to the lungs and the ventilator is set to deliver low tidal volumes, low inspiratory pressures, and a low inspired oxygen fraction. These so called rest settings help to prevent ventilator induced lung injury, oxygen toxicity, and ventilator associated haemodynamic compromise.[3] Prevention of further lung injury may be the major advantage of extracorporeal life support.

SUMMARY POINTS

- Extracorporeal life support is a type of cardiopulmonary bypass that supports the lungs, heart, or both for days to weeks in patients in intensive care with reversible life threatening respiratory or cardiac disease

- Venous-venous cannulation is used for respiratory failure and venous-arterial cannulation for cardiac failure (with or without respiratory failure)

- Bleeding and thrombosis are the most common serious complications

- Extracorporeal life support is used in children and adults; neonates with respiratory failure have the highest survival rates

- Timing of extracorporeal life support is important—the specialist centre should be consulted early in the course of illness

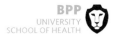

Which patients benefit?

Extracorporeal life support is a support modality rather than a treatment in itself. Its use is restricted to highly specialised centres. It is invasive, complex, resource intensive, and can be associated with serious complications. Extracorporeal life support is, therefore, mostly reserved for patients with a high risk of death who have failed conventional management and where the underlying respiratory or cardiac disease is reversible. It has also been used as a bridge to transplant and placement of a ventricular assist device, to aid weaning from cardiopulmonary bypass, and as an adjunct to cardiopulmonary resuscitation.

The greatest number of cases and highest survival rates have been reported in neonates with respiratory failure (table 2). Most of the evidence supporting extracorporeal life support for other age groups and indications consists of case reports, case series, and analyses of the Extracorporeal Life Support Organization database, although some randomised controlled trials have been reported. Randomised controlled trials are difficult to conduct given the relatively low numbers of patients requiring extracorporeal life support across many centres, the heterogeneity of underlying pathologies, and the speed of technological advances.

Children

The first cases of successful extracorporeal life support management of "moribund infants" were reported in 1974.[4] Thereafter, case series and cohort studies reported improved outcomes, when compared with standard care, in neonates supported with extracorporeal life support for respiratory and cardiac failure. Analysis of cases registered with the Extracorporeal Life Support Organization showed similar improved outcomes.[5 6 7 8]

Four randomised trials met inclusion criteria for a recent Cochrane Collaboration review of extracorporeal life support for severe respiratory failure in newborn infants.[9 10 11 12 13] Risk of mortality was typically reduced by 44% in infants given extracorporeal life support. The authors concluded that a policy of using extracorporeal life support resulted in "significantly improved survival without increased risk of severe disability."

Extracorporeal life support undertaken for cardiac failure constitutes less than a quarter of reported cases in children. No prospective randomised controlled trials have assessed effectiveness in this population. However, case series and registry analyses suggest that extracorporeal life support, where available, benefits children with severe life threatening cardiac failure.

Adults

Extracorporeal life support was first used successfully in an adult patient in 1972.[14] In 1979, a randomised prospective multicentre trial of conventional ventilation versus the addition of venous-arterial extracorporeal life support in 90 adults with severe acute respiratory failure reported high mortality (about 90%) in both groups. This is probably a reflection of the deleterious ventilatory strategies used at the time, venous-arterial rather than venous-venous cannulation, and older technologies.[15] Since then, many case series have shown improved success in adults.[16 17 18 19] Recently, a multicentre randomised controlled trial of conventional ventilator support versus extracorporeal life support for severe adult respiratory failure in 180 patients was published (the conventional ventilation or extracorporeal membrane oxygenation (ECMO) for severe adult respiratory failure (CESAR) trial).[2] Of patients allocated to consideration for extracorporeal life support, 63% survived to six months without disability compared with 47% of those allocated to conventional care. Those randomised to the intervention arm were managed in a single centre where 75% went on to receive extracorporeal life support. Patients in the control arm received conventional ventilation in the referring centres.

Table 1 Commonly used terms

Abbreviation	Definition	Details
ECLS	Extracorporeal life support	Encompasses all extracorporeal technologies and life support components including oxygenation, carbon dioxide removal, and haemodynamic support; renal and liver support may also be incorporated
ECMO	Extracorporeal membrane oxygenation	Older traditional term for extracorporeal life support that omits reference to inherent additional life supports such as haemodynamic support and carbon dioxide removal
VV ECLS	Venous-venous extracorporeal life support	Deoxygenated blood is drained from one or more major vein and oxygenated blood returned to the right atrium; supports respiratory function only and requires native heart function to deliver oxygenated blood to the tissues
VA ECLS	Venous-arterial extracorporeal life support	Deoxygenated blood is drained from one or more major vein and oxygenated blood pumped back into a major artery, thus providing tissue perfusion in the absence of adequate native heart function
ECPR	Extracorporeal cardiopulmonary resuscitation	Extracorporeal life support instituted during, and as an adjunct to, conventional cardiopulmonary resuscitation
ECCO2R	Extracorporeal membrane carbon dioxide removal	Selective carbon dioxide removal

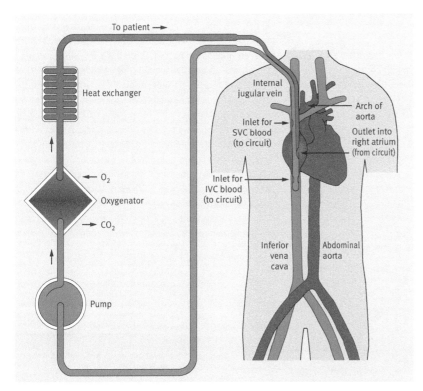

Fig 1 Double lumen cannula version of venous-venous extracorporeal life support for respiratory failure: deoxygenated blood from both the superior and inferior venae cavae passes into one lumen of the double lumen cannula. Blood flows in tubing to a pump and on to an oxygenator and heat exchange unit, before being returned to the right atrium through the second lumen with an oxyhaemoglobin concentration approaching 100%. Here, oxygenated blood mixes with deoxygenated blood that has bypassed the double lumen cannula. This mixture of oxygenated and deoxygenated blood (oxyhaemoglobin saturation of around 80%) is pumped by the heart through the non-functioning lungs into the aorta and on to the organs and tissues of the body. Blue: intravascular deoxygenated blood; red: intravascular oxygenated blood; dark red: intravascular and intracardiac mixed oxygenated and deoxygenated blood; IVC: inferior vena cava; SVC: superior vena cava

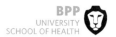

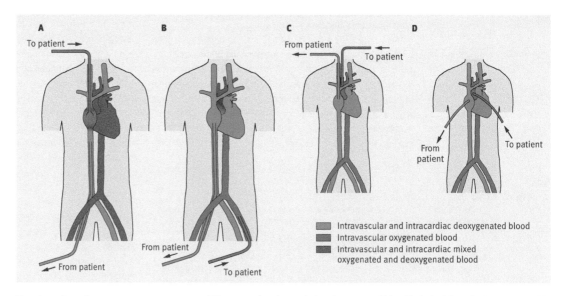

Fig 2 A: an alternative venous-venous extracorporeal life support (ECLS) cannulation; deoxygenated blood is drained from the femoral vein with oxygenated blood being returned to the right atrium. B-D: various venous-arterial configurations. B: blood is drained from the femoral vein and returned to the femoral artery where oxygenated blood flows in a retrograde direction up along the aorta; when some residual cardiac function remains, oxygenated ECLS blood mixes with deoxygenated blood ejected from the left ventricle. C: a cannulated carotid artery, a site often used in infants. D: transthoracic right atrial and aortic cardiopulmonary bypass cannulas. Blue: intravascular and intracardiac deoxygenated blood; red: intravascular oxygenated blood; dark red: intravascular and intracardiac mixed oxygenated and deoxygenated blood

No randomised controlled trials have compared extracorporeal life support with conventional care in adults with cardiac failure. Most evidence supporting adult cardiac extracorporeal life support comes from non-randomised trials, case series, and the Extracorporeal Life Support Organization registry database, as is the case for children.

Cardiopulmonary resuscitation
Extracorporeal life support has been instituted emergently during in-hospital cardiopulmonary resuscitation in children and adults. Case series have reported variable survival rates, and overall survival to hospital discharge rates of 29% in adults, 38% in neonates, and 39% in paediatric patients are reported in the Extracorporeal Life Support Organization registry database (table 2).[19 20 21]

Cost effectiveness
Where randomised controlled trials have incorporated economic evaluations into the study design, extracorporeal life support has been demonstrated to be as cost effective as other life extending technologies in common use in intensive care units in developed countries.[2 9 22 23 24]

What are the main complications?
Bleeding (7-34%) and thrombosis (8-17%) are the most common serious complications.[25] Because of blood-surface interaction, clots can form in the circuit and embolise with potentially devastating consequences. Systemic infusion of unfractionated heparin and the use of heparin bonded circuits help to reduce thrombus formation but bleeding risk is then increased. The delicate balance between haemostasis and thrombosis requires frequent clinical and laboratory monitoring with replacement of coagulation factors, fibrinogen, platelets, and antithrombin III, as necessary. Monitoring and appropriate treatment for disseminated intravascular coagulation (2-5%), haemolysis (7-12%), and fibrinolysis is also needed. Cannulation (7-20%) and surgical site bleeding (6-34%) are common. Invasive procedures and operations should be avoided.[26] Intracranial bleeding (1-11%), especially in neonates; gastrointestinal haemorrhage (1-4%); and pulmonary haemorrhage (4-8%) may also occur.[27]

All organ systems can be affected by hypoxia and hypoperfusion before and during extracorporeal life support.

Table 2 Survival after extracorporeal life support (ECLS)[25]

Neonatal*		
Group	Number of ECLS episodes	Survival to discharge or transfer (%)
Respiratory	24 017	75
Cardiac	4 103	39
ECPR	586	38
Paediatric*		
Group	Number of ECLS episodes	Survival to discharge or transfer (%)
Respiratory	4 635	56
Cardiac	5 026	47
ECPR	1 128	39
Adult*		
Group	Number of ECLS episodes	Survival to discharge or transfer (%)
Respiratory	2 121	53
Cardiac	1 238	34
ECPR	476	29

Neonatal: <1 month; paediatric: 1 month to 18 years; adult: >18 years.
ECPR: ECLS as adjunct to cardiopulmonary resuscitation.

Table 3 Most common underlying diagnoses needing extracorporeal life support[25]

Age group	Diagnosis
Respiratory system	
Neonates	Meconium aspiration syndrome
	Congenital diaphragmatic hernia
	Sepsis
	Persistent pulmonary hypertension of the newborn
	Respiratory distress syndrome
Children and adults	Viral pneumonia
	Bacterial pneumonia
	Aspiration
	Adult respiratory distress syndrome (ARDS)
	Acute respiratory failure (non-ARDS)
Cardiac system	
Neonates, children, and adults	Congenital defect
	Cardiac arrest
	Cardiomyopathy
	Myocarditis

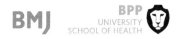

The brain is particularly vulnerable to damage by each of the above mechanisms and so, in addition to haemorrhage, seizures (2-10%) and infarction (1-8%) are common complications.

Despite these problems, extracorporeal life support is becoming ever safer, especially when appropriately selected patients are managed in specialised units with well trained and experienced staff supported by multidisciplinary teams.

When should patients be referred?

Extracorporeal life support should be considered in patients with severe, life threatening respiratory or cardiac failure that does not respond to conventional intensive care management. The disease process must be reversible or, failing this, the patient should be a candidate for transplantation or ventricular assist device placement.

Table 3 lists the most common underlying diseases in patients reported to the Extracorporeal Life Support Organization registry. Indications and contraindications vary among centres and continue to change as experience accrues and technology improves. Extracorporeal life support may be relatively contraindicated in patients who: are considered to be too far into the course of their disease; have been on conventional treatment for too long (usually >7-10 days); have pre-existing conditions that affect quality of life or that may be incompatible with normal life if the patient recovers (for example, brain injury, end stage malignancy, risk of systemic bleeding with anticoagulation); or are too young or too small (<32 weeks' gestational age, <2 kg).[28]

Although there are indices and scoring systems that help clinicians to determine the most appropriate time to consult with referral centres or to start extracorporeal life support

(table 4), these serve only as guides and are neither rigidly nor universally applied. Referring hospitals should become familiar with their local specialist centre's referral guidelines. In all cases, early discussion with the specialist centre is imperative to ensure appropriate patient selection

and timely transfer.

What are the long term effects?

Survivors of extracorporeal life support are more likely than the general population to have neurodevelopmental deficits, behavioural problems, and respiratory morbidities. However, when compared with the conventional care arms of randomised controlled trials, no between-group differences are seen for these outcomes.[2] [29] Patients require rehabilitation and multidisciplinary follow-up after discharge from hospital. A high index of suspicion for late manifestations of neurodevelopmental problems must be maintained.

Conclusion

Extracorporeal life support is a life saving intensive care resource when used in appropriately selected patients by well trained personnel in well organised centres. Advances in technology and development of antithrombogenic surfaces will continue to lower the complication rates associated with extracorporeal life support, allowing more patients to benefit from its use.

A PATIENT'S PERSPECTIVE

I heard about swine flu but just regarded it as something other people got and serious for people with an underlying medical condition. I was healthy.

I woke up one night with a temperature, aches, pains, a cough, and I felt weak. Things got worse as the week went on. I coughed up blood and had diarrhoea. On the tenth day my lips and hands turned blue. I was admitted to hospital, then sedated and ventilated. My lungs continued to deteriorate and the only option left on day 20 was extracorporeal membrane oxygenation (ECMO). My family told me that signing the consent form was the most difficult decision they had ever made.

The colour of the blood in the tubes frightened them at first. I remained on extracorporeal membrane oxygenation for 60 days. My only memory is of my mum and sister on one occasion. When the sedation was stopped I was frightened and confused. I was shocked to find out that swine flu had caused this.

I find it very difficult to comprehend the severity of my illness. I get tired quite easily and breathless from simple everyday tasks but I will make a full recovery and lead a normal life, which I find amazing.

ONGOING AND FUTURE RESEARCH

- Research into the modification of extracorporeal life support surfaces is ongoing with the goal of preventing thrombosis in the absence of heparin anticoagulation
- Although the conventional ventilation or ECMO (extracorporeal membrane oxygenation) for severe adult respiratory failure (CESAR) trial showed that management of adults with severe respiratory failure in an extracorporeal life support referral centre is superior to conventional management in referring centres, further trials are needed to confirm increased survival attributable to extracorporeal life support alone
- Trials are needed to define the use of extracorporeal life support in acute myocardial infarction (MI)
- Trials of whole body cooling during extracorporeal life support to prevent neurological disability are ongoing
- Trials are warranted to compare outcomes between extracorporeal life support and high frequency oscillatory ventilation

---

Table 4 Respiratory failure severity scores

Indicators	Extracorporeal life support considered	Extracorporeal life support initiated
Oxygenation index (neonates) = ((FiO2 x MAP)/PaO2) x 100	20	40
PF ratio: PaO2/FiO2	<150 on 90% oxygen	<80 on 90% oxygen (and Murray score of 3-4)
Murray score[30]		
Average score over all four parameters:		
1) PF ratio (mm Hg) on 100% oxygen: 300=0; 225-299=1; 175-224=2; 100-174=3; <100=4	2-3	3-4
2) Chest radiograph: normal=0; 1 point per quadrant infiltrated		
3) Positive end expiratory pressure (cm H2O): 5=0; 6-8=1; 9-11=2; 12-14=3; 15=4		
4) Lung compliance (ml/cm H2O): 80=0; 60-79=1; 40-59=2; 20-39=3; 19=4		

FiO2: fraction of inspired oxygen

MAP: mean airway pressure (cm H2O)

PaO2: partial pressure of oxygen in arterial blood (mm Hg)

mm Hg: millimetres of mercury

cm H2O: centimetres of water

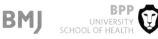

We are grateful to María José Santos-Martínez, Edmund Carton, and Peter Rycus for their valued contributions, and to Rafal Krol of the Medical Photography Department of the Mater Misericordiae University Hospital for preparing the figures.

Contributors: MWR originated the idea. AG searched the literature, wrote the first draft of the manuscript and finalised all revisions. GMA, MJG, MWR, and SMW made revisions and suggestions to the drafts. MWR is guarantor.

Funding: The work was supported by grants from Science Foundation Ireland (MWR) and the Health Research Board and Health Service Executive, Ireland (AMG).

Competing interests: All authors have completed the Unified Competing Interest form at www.icmje.org/coi_disclosure.pdf (available on request from the corresponding author) and declare that all authors had: no financial support for the submitted work from anyone other than their employer; no financial relationships with commercial entities that might have an interest in the submitted work; no spouses, partners, or children with relationships with commercial entities that might have an interest in the submitted work; and no non-financial interests that may be relevant to the submitted work.

Provenance and peer review: Not commissioned; externally peer reviewed.

1   Davies A, Jones D, Bailey M, Beca J, Bellomo R, Blackwell N, et al. Extracorporeal membrane oxygenation for 2009 influenza A(H1N1) acute respiratory distress syndrome. *JAMA* 2009;302:1888-95.
2   Peek GJ, Mugford M, Tiruvoipati R, Wilson A, Allen E, Thalanany MM, et al. Efficacy and economic assessment of conventional ventilatory support versus extracorporeal membrane oxygenation for severe adult respiratory failure (CESAR): a multicentre randomised controlled trial. *Lancet* 2009;374:1351-63.
3   Ventilation with lower tidal volumes as compared with traditional tidal volumes for acute lung injury and the acute respiratory distress syndrome. The Acute Respiratory Distress Syndrome Network. *N Engl J Med* 2000;342:1301-8.
4   Bartlett RH, Gazzaniga AB, Jefferies MR, Huxtable RF, Haiduc NJ, Fong SW. Extracorporeal membrane oxygenation (ECMO) cardiopulmonary support in infancy. *Trans Am Soc Artif Intern Organs* 1976;22:80-93.
5   Stolar CJ, Snedecor SM, Bartlett RH. Extracorporeal membrane oxygenation and neonatal respiratory failure: experience from the extracorporeal life support organization. *J Pediatr Surg* 1991;26:563-71.
6   Morton A, Dalton H, Kochanek P, Janosky J, Thompson A. Extracorporeal membrane oxygenation for pediatric respiratory failure: five-year experience at the University of Pittsburgh. *Crit Care Med* 1994;22:1659-67.
7   Green TP, Timmons OD, Fackler JC, Moler FW, Thompson AE, Sweeney MF. The impact of extracorporeal membrane oxygenation on survival in pediatric patients with acute respiratory failure. Pediatric Critical Care Study Group. *Crit Care Med* 1996;24:323-9.
8   Combes A, Leprince P, Luyt CE, Bonnet N, Trouillet J, Léger P, et al. Outcomes and long-term quality-of-life of patients supported by extracorporeal membrane oxygenation for refractory cardiogenic shock. *Crit Care Med* 2008;36:1404-11.
9   Mugford M, Elbourne D, Field D. Extracorporeal membrane oxygenation for severe respiratory failure in newborn infants. *Cochrane Database Syst Rev* 2008;3:CD001340.
10 UK collaborative randomised trial of neonatal extracorporeal membrane oxygenation. UK Collaborative ECMO Trial Group. *Lancet* 1996;348:75-82.
11 O'Rourke PP, Crone RK, Vacanti JP, Ware JH, Lillehei CW, Parad RB, et al. Extracorporeal membrane oxygenation and conventional medical therapy in neonates with persistent pulmonary hypertension of the newborn: a prospective randomized study. *Pediatrics* 1989;84:957-63.
12 Bartlett RH, Roloff DW, Cornell RG, Andrews AF, Dillon PW, Zwischenberger JB. Extracorporeal circulation in neonatal respiratory failure: a prospective randomized study. *Pediatrics* 1985;76:479-87.
13 Bifano E, Hakanson D, Hingre R, Gross S. Prospective randomized controlled trial of conventional treatment or transport for ECMO in infants with persistent pulmonary hypertension (PPHN). *Pediatr Res* 1992;31:196A.
14 Hill JD, O'Brien TG, Murray JJ, Dontigny L, Bramson ML, Osborn JJ, et al. Prolonged extracorporeal oxygenation for acute post-traumatic respiratory failure (shock-lung syndrome). Use of the Bramson membrane lung. *N Engl J Med* 1972;286:629-34.
15 Zapol WM, Snider MT, Hill JD, Fallat RJ, Bartlett RH, Edmunds LH, et al. Extracorporeal membrane oxygenation in severe acute respiratory failure. A randomized prospective study. *JAMA* 1979;242:2193-6.
16 Rich PB, Awad SS, Kolla S, Annich G, Schreiner RJ, Hirschl RB, et al. An approach to the treatment of severe adult respiratory failure. *J Crit Care* 1998;13:26-36.
17 Lindén V, Palmér K, Reinhard J, Westman R, Ehrén H, Granholm T, et al. High survival in adult patients with acute respiratory distress syndrome treated by extracorporeal membrane oxygenation, minimal sedation, and pressure supported ventilation. *Intensive Care Med* 2000;26:1630-7.
18 Hemmila MR, Rowe SA, Boules TN, Miskulin J, McGillicuddy JW, Schuerer DJ, et al. Extracorporeal life support for severe acute respiratory distress syndrome in adults. *Ann Surg* 2004;240:595-607.
19 Thiagarajan RR, Brogan TV, Scheurer MA, Laussen PC, Rycus PT, Bratton SL. Extracorporeal membrane oxygenation to support cardiopulmonary resuscitation in adults. *Ann Thorac Surg* 2009;87:778-85.
20 Tajik M, Cardarelli MG. Extracorporeal membrane oxygenation after cardiac arrest in children: what do we know? *Eur J Cardiothorac Surg* 2008;33:409-17.
21 del Nido PJ, Dalton HJ, Thompson AE, Siewers RD. Extracorporeal membrane oxygenator rescue in children during cardiac arrest after cardiac surgery. *Circulation* 1992;86(5 suppl):II300-4.
22 Roberts TE. Economic evaluation and randomised controlled trial of extracorporeal membrane oxygenation: UK collaborative trial. The Extracorporeal Membrane Oxygenation Economics Working Group. *BMJ* 1998;317:911-6.
23 Petrou S, Bischof M, Bennett C, Elbourne D, Field D, McNally H. Cost-effectiveness of neonatal extracorporeal membrane oxygenation based on 7-year results from the United Kingdom Collaborative ECMO Trial. *Pediatrics* 2006;117:1640-9.
24 Mahle WT, Forbess JM, Kirshbom PM, Cuadrado AR, Simsic JM, Kanter KR. Cost-utility analysis of salvage cardiac extracorporeal membrane oxygenation in children. *J Thorac Cardiovasc Surg* 2005;129:1084-90.
25 Extracorporeal Life Support Organization (ELSO) Extracorporeal Life Support (ECLS) registry report international summary. 2010.
26 Oliver WC. Anticoagulation and coagulation management for ECMO. *Semin Cardiothorac Vasc Anesth* 2009;13:154-75.
27 Marasco SF, Preovolos A, Lim K, Salamonsen RF. Thoracotomy in adults while on ECMO is associated with uncontrollable bleeding. *Perfusion* 2007;22:23-6.
28 Extracorporeal Life Support Organization. ELSO guidelines for cardiopulmonary extracorporeal life support. Version 1:1. 2009. www.elso.med.umich.edu.
29 Bennett CC, Johnson A, Field DJ, Elbourne D. UK collaborative randomised trial of neonatal extracorporeal membrane oxygenation: follow-up to age 4 years. *Lancet* 2001;357:1094-6.
30 Murray JF, Matthay MA, Luce JM, Flick MR. An expanded definition of the adult respiratory distress syndrome. *Am Rev Respir Dis* 1988;138:720-3.

Related links

bmj.com/archive

Previous articles in this series
- Managing diabetic retinopathy (*BMJ* 2010;341:c5400)
- Investigating and managing pyrexia of unknown origin in adults (*BMJ* 2010;341:c5470)
- Investigation and management of uveitis (*BMJ* 2010;341:c4976)
- Chronic pelvic pain in women (*BMJ* 2010;341:c4834)
- Head and neck cancer—Part 2: Treatment and prognostic factors (*BMJ* 2010;341:c4690)

ADDITIONAL EDUCATION RESOURCES

Resources for healthcare professionals
- Extracorporeal Life Support Organization (ELSO) (www.elso.med.umich.edu)—International consortium of extracorporeal life support specialists and centres. Maintains a registry database of patients managed with this technique; develops and publishes patient management, training, and organisational management guidelines; produces reports to participating centres
- Van Meurs K, Lally KP, Peek G, Zwischenberger JB, eds. ECMO: extracorporeal cardiopulmonary support in critical care. "The red book". 3rd ed. Extracorporeal Life Support Organization, 2005

Resources for patients
- University of Michigan. Family guide to neonatal extracorporeal membrane oxygenation (ECMO) (www.med.umich.edu/ecmo/patient/NeoECMO.pdf); Family guide to pediatric ECMO (www.med.umich.edu/ecmo/patient/PedECMO.pdf); Family guide to adult ECMO (www.med.umich.edu/ecmo/patient/AdultECMO.pdf)—Provide family and friends of patients with easy to understand information regarding extracorporeal life support

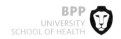

Refeeding syndrome: what it is, and how to prevent and treat it

Hisham M Mehanna, consultant and honorary associate professor, and director[1][2], Jamil Moledina, senior house officer [3], Jane Travis, Macmillan specialist dietitian[4]

[1]Institute of Head and Neck Studies and Education, Department of Otorhinolaryngology—Head and Neck Surgery, University Hospital, Coventry CV2 2DX

[2]Heart of England Foundation Trust, Birmingham

[3]Department of Otorhinolaryngology—Head and Neck Surgery, University Hospital, Coventry

[4]Department of Dietetics, University Hospital, Coventry

Correspondence to: H M Mehanna
Hisham.Mehanna@uhcw.nhs.uk

Cite this as: BMJ 2008;336:1495

DOI: 10.1136/bmj.a301

http://www.bmj.com/content/336/7659/1495

Refeeding syndrome is a well described but often forgotten condition. No randomised controlled trials of treatment have been published, although there are guidelines that use best available evidence for managing the condition. In 2006 a guideline was published by the National Institute for Health and Clinical Excellence (NICE) in England and Wales. Yet because clinicians are often not aware of the problem, refeeding syndrome still occurs.[1]

This review aims to raise awareness of refeeding syndrome and discuss prevention and treatment. The available literature mostly comprises weaker (level 3 and 4) evidence, including cohort studies, case series, and consensus expert opinion.[2] Our article also draws attention to the NICE guidelines on nutritional support in adults, with particular reference to the new recommendations for best practice in refeeding syndrome.[3] These recommendations differ in parts from—and we believe improve on—previous guidelines, such as those of the Parenteral and Enteral Nutrition Group of the British Dietetic Association (box 1).[4]

What is refeeding syndrome?

Refeeding syndrome can be defined as the potentially fatal shifts in fluids and electrolytes that may occur in malnourished patients receiving artificial refeeding (whether enterally or parenterally[5]). These shifts result from hormonal and metabolic changes and may cause serious clinical complications. The hallmark biochemical feature of refeeding syndrome is hypophosphataemia. However, the syndrome is complex and may also feature abnormal sodium and fluid balance; changes in glucose, protein, and fat metabolism; thiamine deficiency; hypokalaemia; and hypomagnesaemia.[1][6]

How common is refeeding syndrome?

The true incidence of refeeding syndrome is unknown—partly owing to the lack of a universally accepted definition. In a study of 10 197 hospitalised patients the incidence of severe hypophosphataemia was 0.43%, with malnutrition being one of the strongest risk factors.[7] Studies report a 100% incidence of hypophosphataemia in patients receiving

SUMMARY POINTS

- Refeeding syndrome is a potentially fatal condition, caused by rapid initiation of refeeding after a period of undernutrition
- It is characterised by hypophosphataemia, associated with fluid and electrolyte shifts and metabolic and clinical complications
- Awareness of refeeding syndrome and identification of patients at risk is crucial as the condition is preventable and the metabolic complications are avoidable
- Patients at high risk include chronically undernourished patients and those who have had little or no energy intake for more than 10 days
- Refeeding should be started at a low level of energy replacement. Vitamin supplementation should also be started with refeeding and continued for at least 10 days
- Correction of electrolyte and fluid imbalances before feeding is not necessary; it should be done alongside feeding

SOURCES AND SELECTION CRITERIA

We used the terms "refeeding", "syndrome", and "hypophosphataemia" to search the databases Medline, Embase, PubMed, Cochrane, CINAHL, and AMED (Allied and Complementary Medicine Database), as well as cross checking with reference lists, textbooks, and personal reference lists. We assessed the 151 identified papers for relevance. We assessed the quality of evidence in original articles according to guidelines published on the Evidence-Based On-Call website.[2]

total parenteral nutrition solutions that do not contain phosphorus. When solutions containing phosphate are used, the incidence can decrease to 18%.[8]

Several prospective and retrospective cohort studies of hyperalimentation in intensive care units have documented the occurrence of refeeding syndrome.[6][9] In a well designed prospective cohort study of a heterogeneous group of patients in intensive care units, 34% of patients experienced hypophosphataemia soon after feeding was started (mean (standard deviation) 1.9 (1.1) days).[10] Many case reports have highlighted the potentially fatal nature of the condition.[11][12] However, it is often not recognised or maybe inappropriately treated, especially on general wards.[1][6]

How does refeeding syndrome develop?

Prolonged fasting

The underlying causative factor of refeeding syndrome is the metabolic and hormonal changes caused by rapid refeeding, whether enteral or parenteral. The net result of metabolic and hormonal changes in early starvation is that the body switches from using carbohydrate to using fat and protein as the main source of energy, and the basal metabolic rate decreases by as much as 20-25%.[13]

During prolonged fasting, hormonal and metabolic changes are aimed at preventing protein and muscle breakdown. Muscle and other tissues decrease their use of ketone bodies and use fatty acids as the main energy source. This results in an increase in blood levels of ketone bodies, stimulating the brain to switch from glucose to ketone bodies as its main energy source. The liver decreases its rate of gluconeogenesis, thus preserving muscle protein. During the period of prolonged starvation, several intracellular minerals become severely depleted. However, serum concentrations of these minerals (including phosphate) may remain normal. This is because these minerals are mainly in the intracellular compartment, which contracts during starvation. In addition, there is a reduction in renal excretion.

Refeeding

During refeeding, glycaemia leads to increased insulin and decreased secretion of glucagon. Insulin stimulates glycogen, fat, and protein synthesis. This process requires minerals such as phosphate and magnesium and cofactors such as thiamine. Insulin stimulates the absorption of potassium into the cells through the sodium-potassium

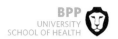

ATPase symporter, which also transports glucose into the cells. Magnesium and phosphate are also taken up into the cells. Water follows by osmosis. These processes result in a decrease in the serum levels of phosphate, potassium, and magnesium, all of which are already depleted. The clinical features of the refeeding syndrome occur as a result of the functional deficits of these electrolytes and the rapid change in basal metabolic rate.

What electrolytes and minerals are involved in the pathogenesis?

Phosphorus

Phosphorus is predominantly an intracellular mineral. It is essential for all intracellular processes and for the structural integrity of cell membranes. In addition, many enzymes and second messengers are activated by phosphate binding. Importantly it is also required for energy storage in the form of adenosine triphosphate (ATP). It regulates the affinity of haemoglobin for oxygen and thus regulates oxygen delivery to tissues. It is also important in the renal acid-base buffer system.

In refeeding syndrome, chronic whole body depletion of phosphorus occurs. Also, the insulin surge causes a greatly increased uptake and use of phosphate in the cells. These changes lead to a deficit in intracellular as well as extracellular phosphorus. In this environment, even small decreases in serum phosphorus may lead to widespread dysfunction of cellular processes affecting almost every physiological system (see box A on bmj.com).[14]

Potassium

Potassium, the major intracellular cation, is also depleted in undernutrition. Again, serum concentration may remain normal. With the change to anabolism on refeeding, potassium is taken up into cells as they increase in volume and number and as a direct result of insulin secretion. This results in severe hypokalaemia. This causes derangements in the electrochemical membrane potential, resulting in, for example, arrhythmias and cardiac arrest.

Magnesium

Magnesium, another predominantly intracellular cation, is an important cofactor in most enzyme systems, including oxidative phosphorylation and ATP production. It is also necessary for the structural integrity of DNA, RNA, and ribosomes. In addition, it affects membrane potential, and deficiency can lead to cardiac dysfunction and neuromuscular complications.[18]

Glucose

Glucose intake after a period of starvation suppresses gluconeogenesis through the release of insulin. Excessive administration may therefore lead to hyperglycaemia and its sequelae of osmotic diuresis, dehydration, metabolic acidosis, and ketoacidosis. Excess glucose also leads to lipogenesis (again as a result of insulin stimulation), which may cause fatty liver, increased carbon dioxide production, hypercapnoea, and respiratory failure.[15]

Vitamin deficiency

Although all vitamin deficiencies may occur at variable rates with inadequate intake, thiamine is of most importance in complications of refeeding. Thiamine is an essential coenzyme in carbohydrate metabolism. Its deficiency result in Wernicke's encephalopathy (ocular abnormalities, ataxia, confusional state, hypothermia, coma) or Korsakoff's syndrome (retrograde and anterograde amnesia, confabulation).[19]

Sodium, nitrogen, and fluid

Changes in carbohydrate metabolism have a profound effect on sodium and water balance. The introduction of carbohydrate to a diet leads to a rapid decrease in renal excretion of sodium and water.[20] If fluid repletion is then instituted to maintain a normal urine output, patients may rapidly develop fluid overload. This can lead to congestive cardiac failure, pulmonary oedema, and cardiac arrhythmia.

How can refeeding syndrome be prevented?

Identification of high risk patients is crucial (boxes 2 and 3).[3][4] Any patient with negligible food intake for more than five days is at risk of developing refeeding problems. Patients may be malnourished as a result of reduced intake (for example, owing to dysphagia, anorexia nervosa, depression, alcoholism); reduced absorption of nutrition (as in, for example, inflammatory bowel disease, coeliac disease); or increased metabolic demands (for example, in cancer, surgery). High risk patients include those who have been chronically undernourished, especially those who also have diminished physiological reserve. Patients with dysphagia (for example, as a result of stroke) in particular may be at high risk.

BOX 2 PATIENTS AT HIGH RISK OF REFEEDING SYNDROME [1][3][4]

- Patients with anorexia nervosa
- Patients with chronic alcoholism
- Oncology patients
- Postoperative patients
- Elderly patients (comorbidities, decreased physiological reserve)
- Patients with uncontrolled diabetes mellitus (electrolyte depletion, diuresis)
- Patients with chronic malnutrition:
  - -Marasmus
  - -Prolonged fasting or low energy diet
  - -Morbid obesity with profound weight loss
  - - High stress patient unfed for >7 days
  - -Malabsorptive syndrome (such as inflammatory bowel disease, chronic pancreatitis, cystic fibrosis, short bowel syndrome)
- Long term users of antacids (magnesium and aluminium salts bind phosphate)
- Long term users of diuretics (loss of electrolytes)

BOX 1 WHY USE THE NICE GUIDELINES ON REFEEDING SYNDROME?

- The guidelines are the most recent comprehensive review of the literature on refeeding syndrome
- The guideline development group was strongly multidisciplinary with wide ranging consultation with both professional and patient stakeholders
- The guidelines clearly identified points of good practice and areas for further research
- The new guidelines give explicit clinical criteria for patients "at risk" and "highly at risk" of developing refeeding syndrome, enabling better identification and prevention
- For patients with electrolyte deficits the new guidelines recommend immediate start of nutritional support at a lower rate, rather than waiting till the electrolyte imbalance has been corrected (as was recommended by previous guidelines), thus potentially avoiding further nutritional deterioration in patients

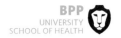

The figure summarises how to prevent and treat refeeding syndrome. To ensure adequate prevention, the NICE guidelines recommend a thorough nutritional assessment before refeeding is started.[3] Recent weight change over time, nutrition, alcohol intake, and social and psychological problems should all be ascertained. Plasma electrolytes (especially phosphate, sodium, potassium, and magnesium) and glucose should be measured at baseline before feeding and any deficiencies corrected during feeding with close monitoring.[3]

The NICE guidelines recommend that refeeding is started at no more than 50% of energy requirements in "patients who have eaten little or nothing for more than 5 days." The rate can then be increased if no refeeding problems are detected on clinical and biochemical monitoring (level D recommendation—see box 3).

For patients at high risk of developing refeeding syndrome, nutritional repletion of energy should be started slowly (maximum 0.042 MJ/kg/24 hours) and should be tailored to each patient. It can then be increased to meet or exceed full needs over four to seven days. In patients who are very malnourished (body mass index ≤14 or a negligible intake for two weeks or more), the NICE guidelines recommend that refeeding should start at a maximum of 0.021 MJ/kg/24 hours, with cardiac monitoring owing to the risk of cardiac arrhythmias (level D recommendation).[3] This explicit specification of the rate of refeeding in severely malnourished patients should help avoid complications arising from rapid refeeding and is an improvement on previous guidelines.[4] The NICE guidelines also state that correcting electrolyte and fluid imbalances before feeding is not necessary and that this should be done along with feeding. This is a change from previous guidelines[4] and potentially avoids prolongation of malnourishment and its effects on patients.

All guidelines recommend that vitamin supplementation should be started immediately, before and for the first 10 days of refeeding. Circulatory volume should also be restored. Oral, enteral, or intravenous supplements of the potassium, phosphate, calcium, and magnesium should be given unless blood levels are high before refeeding. Good quality studies on the exact levels of supplementation are lacking, however, and so the required levels of these supplements cited by NICE (figure) are only level D recommendations.[3]

Electrolyte levels should be measured once daily for one week, and at least three times in the following week. Urinary electrolytes could also be checked to help assess body losses and to guide replacement.

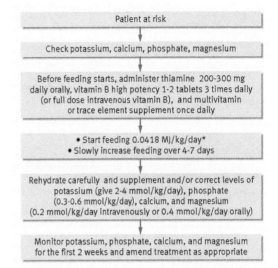

*If patient is severely malnourished (for example, body mass index (kg/m²) ≤14) or if intake is negligible for ≥2 weeks, start feeding at maximum of 0.0209 MJ/kg/day

Guidelines for management. Adapted from the guidelines of NICE[3] and the British Association of Parenteral and Enteral Nutrition[4]

How can refeeding syndrome be detected and treated?

Refeeding syndrome is detected by considering the possibility of its existence and by using the simple biochemical investigations described above. If the syndrome is detected, the rate of feeding should be slowed down and essential electrolytes should be replenished. The hospital specialist dietetics team should be involved.

The best method for electrolyte repletion has not yet been determined. Hypophosphataemia, hypomagnesaemia, and hypokalaemia in hospitalised patients are ideally treated with intravenous supplementation (table), but this is not without risks. A prospective comparative cohort study of 27 patients with severe hypophosphataemia showed the safety of administering 15-30 mmol phosphate over three hours via a central venous catheter in an intensive care unit.[16] However, the researchers reported the need for repeated doses in most patients. Terlevich et al reported efficacy of 50 mmol phosphate infused into a peripheral vein over 24 hours in 30 patients with no pre-existing renal dysfunction on general wards.[17] Further infusions may be required and so careful monitoring of blood levels is required. Caution is needed in patients with existing renal impairment, hypocalcaemia (which may worsen), or hypercalcaemia (which may result in metastatic calcification).

Fluid repletion should be carefully controlled to avoid fluid overload as described earlier. Sodium administration should be limited to the replacement of losses. In patients at high risk of cardiac decompensation, central venous pressure and cardiac rhythm monitoring should be considered.

Conclusion

Adherence to the NICE guidelines for preventing and treating refeeding syndrome (boxes 2 and 3) should reduce the incidence and associated complications of the syndrome. Further research is needed to determine the true incidence of refeeding syndrome and to ascertain the best management protocols.

Recommendation for phosphate and magnesium supplementation[3 4 6 13]

Mineral	Dose
Phosphate	
Maintenance requirement	0.3-0.6 mmol/kg/day orally
Mild hypophosphataemia (0.6-0.85 mmol/l)	0.3-0.6 mmol/kg/day orally
Moderate hypophosphataemia (0.3-0.6 mmol/l)	9 mmol infused into peripheral vein over 12 hours
Severe hypophosphataemia (<0.3 mmol/l)	18 mmol infused into peripheral vein over 12 hours
Magnesium	
Maintenance requirement	0.2 mmol/kg/day intravenously (or 0.4 mmol/kg/day orally)
Mild to moderate hypomagnesaemia (0.5-0.7 mmol/l)	Initially 0.5 mmol/kg/day over 24 hours intravenously, then 0.25 mmol/kg/day for 5 days intravenously
Severe hypomagnesaemia (<0.5 mmol/l)	24 mmol over 6 hours intravenously, then as for mild to moderate hypomagnesaemia (above)

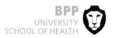

BOX 3 CRITERIA FROM THE GUIDELINES OF THE NATIONAL INSTITUTE FOR HEALTH AND CLINICAL EXCELLENCE FOR IDENTIFYING PATIENTS AT HIGH RISK OF REFEEDING PROBLEMS (LEVEL D RECOMMENDATIONS*)[3]

Either the patient has one or more of the following:

- Body mass index (kg/m^2) <16
- Unintentional weight loss >15% in the past three to six months
- Little or no nutritional intake for >10 days
- Low levels of potassium, phosphate, or magnesium before feeding

Or the patient has two or more of the following:

- Body mass index <18.5
- Unintentional weight loss >10% in the past three to six months
- Little or no nutritional intake for >5 days
- History of alcohol misuse or drugs, including insulin, chemotherapy, antacids, or diuretics

Recommendations derived from low grade evidence—mainly cohort and case series studies—and from consensus expert opinion

AREAS FOR FUTURE RESEARCH

- Formulation of consensus definitions and outcomes for reporting studies on nutrition
- Large multicentre studies concentrating on homogeneous, well defined study samples
- High quality trials to identify the best replacement and treatment regimens for phosphate and other minerals for refeeding syndrome

We thank Chuka Nwokolo (Department of Gastroenterology, University Hospital, Coventry) for his efforts and comments in reviewing this article.

Contributors: HMM planned the article, did the searches, evaluated the evidence, and wrote and reviewed the manuscript; he is also the guarantor. JM did the searches, evaluated the evidence, and helped with writing the article. JT did the searches, evaluated the evidence, and reviewed the manuscript.

Competing interests: None declared.

Provenance and peer review: Commissioned; externally peer reviewed.

1 Hearing SD. Refeeding syndrome. *BMJ* 2004;328:908-9.
2 Evidence-Based On-Call Database. *Levels of evidence* . 2007. www.eboncall.org/content/levels.html
3 National Institute for Health and Clinical Excellence. *Nutrition support in adults* . Clinical guideline CG32. 2006. www.nice.org.uk/page.aspx?o=cg032
4 Dewar H, Horvath R. Refeeding syndrome. In: Todorovic VE, Micklewright A, eds. *A pocket guide to clinical nutrition* . 2nd ed. British Dietetic Association, 2001.
5 Solomon SM, Kirby DF. The refeeding syndrome: a review. *JPEN J Parenter Enteral Nutr* 1990;14:90-7.
6 Crook MA, Hally V, Pantelli JV. The importance of the refeeding syndrome. *Nutrition* 2001;17:632-7.
7 Camp MA, Allon M. Severe hypophosphatemia in hospitalised patients. *Mineral & Electrolyte Metabolism* 1990;16:365-8.
8 Martinez MJ, Matrinez MA, Montero M, Campelo E, Castro I, Inaraja MT. Hypophosphatemia in postoperative patients on total parenteral nutrition:influence of nutritional support teams. *Nutr Hosp* 2006;21:657-60.
9 Hayek ME, Eisenberg PG. Severe hypophosphatemia following the institution of enteral feedings. *Arch Surg* 1989;124:1325-8.
10 Marik PE, Bedigan MK. Refeeding hypophosphataemia in an intensive care unit: a prospective study. *Arch Surg* 1996;131:1043-7.
11 Silvis SE, Paragas PD. Parasthesias, weakness, seizures, and hypophosphatemia in patients receiving hyperalimentation. *Gastroenterology* 1972;62:513-20.
12 Weinsier RL, Krumdieck CL. Death resulting from overzealous total parenteral nutrition: the refeeding syndrome revisited. *Am J Clin Nutr* 1980;34:393-9.
13 McCray S, Walker S, Parrish CR. Much ado about refeeding. *Practical Gastroenterology* 2004;XXVIII(12):26-44.
14 Knochel JP. The pathophysiology and clinical charactertistics of severe hypophosphatemia. *Arch Intern Med* 1977;137:203-20.
15 Klein CJ, Stanek GS, Wiles CE. Overfeeding macronutrients to critically ill adults: metabolic complications. *J Am Diet Assoc* 1998;98:795-806.
16 Perrault MM, Ostrop NJ, Tierney MG. Efficacy and safety of intravenous phosphate replacement in critically ill patients. *Ann Pharmacother* 1997;31:683-8.
17 Terlevich A, Hearing SD, Woltersdorf WW, Smyth C, Reid D, Mccullagh E, et al. Refeeding syndrome: effective and safe treatment with Phosphates Polyfusor. *Aliment Pharmacol Ther* 2003;17:1325-9.
18 Wacker WEC, Parisi AF. Magnesium metabolism. *N Engl J Med* 1968;278:658-63.
19 Reuler JB, Girard DE, Cooney TG. Wernicke's encephalopathy. *N Engl J Med* 1985;312:1035-9.
20 Veverbrants E, Arky RA. Effects of fasting and refeeding: I. Studies on sodium, potassium and water excretion on a constant electrolyte and fluid intake. *J Clin Endocrinol Metab* 1969;29:55-62.

BMJ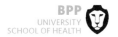

The role of interventional radiology in trauma

Ian A Zealley, consultant radiologist, Sam Chakraverty, consultant radiologist

¹Department of Radiology, Ninewells Hospital and Medical School, Dundee DD1 9SY

Correspondence to: I A Zealley ian. zealley@nhs.net

Cite this as: BMJ 2010;340:c497

DOI: 10.1136/bmj.c497

http://www.bmj.com/content/340/bmj.c497

Most preventable deaths from trauma are caused by unrecognised and therefore untreated haemorrhage, particularly in the abdomen. Haemorrhage causes early deaths, and the associated hypovolaemic shock leads to secondary brain injury and contributes to late death from multiorgan failure.[1] Early management is focused on resuscitation and the diagnosis and treatment of life threatening bleeding to prevent the lethal metabolic disturbance triad of acidosis, hypothermia, and coagulopathy.[2]

Many aspects of immediate trauma care suffer from a lack of high quality prospective research. This review is based predominantly on evidence from retrospective cohort series and is subject to the limitations inherent in this type of level 2 research.[3] There are no prospective randomised controlled trials of interventional radiology in major trauma. Although the volume of level 2 evidence is substantial and contains few contradictory findings, no robust level 1 evidence yet exists. This review aims to summarise the evidence supporting the use of interventional radiological techniques in the management of haemorrhage caused by blunt abdominal trauma.

What is the role of interventional radiology in abdominal trauma?

Interventional radiology uses minimally invasive endovascular techniques to stem haemorrhage. Endovascular haemostasic techniques are established in non-trauma clinical scenarios. In trauma, the main application is to control endovascular haemorrhage by blocking bleeding vessels (transcatheter arterial embolisation (fig 1) or relining them (stent grafting) (fig 2). The objective is to stop the bleeding without the physiological stress of surgery.

SUMMARY POINTS

- Interventional radiological techniques to stop bleeding are a minimally invasive alternative to surgery in blunt abdominal trauma
- In haemodynamically stable patients with trauma, interventional radiology has an established role in the management of solid organ injuries
- In haemodynamically unstable patients with trauma, interventional radiology is effective in stemming haemorrhage from pelvic fractures
- Recent series suggest that in a wider range of haemodynamically unstable patients interventional radiological techniques may further reduce the number of patients needing surgery
- The overall quality of the evidence for interventional radiological and surgical interventions in trauma is poor

Transcatheter arterial embolisation is now an accepted adjunct to non-operative and surgical management protocols in trauma. This parallels its increasing use in other settings of life threatening haemorrhage, such as gastrointestinal and postpartum haemorrhage.[4][5] Insertion of a stent graft is a well established technique in the management of traumatic rupture of the thoracic aorta.[6]

What injuries are sustained in blunt abdominal trauma?

The frequency of injury to different structures varies among studies. A recent prospective series in which 224 patients with sustained blunt abdominal trauma had computed tomography regardless of their haemodynamic status provides an illustration of patterns of injury (table).[7]

How does interventional radiology compare with surgery for control of haemorrhage after abdominal trauma?

The key question is: what evidence indicates the clinical scenarios in which interventional radiology for stopping haemorrhage is as good as or better than surgery in terms of morbidity and mortality? The evidence base is relatively poor. For transparency, we usually state the type of study and sample size—for example: (a) the evidence that saving a damaged spleen by using embolisation to avoid splenectomy is weak as it is based only on a study of 17 subjects, and (b) single centres reporting their own outcomes may choose to present them in a positive light.

Spleen

Splenectomy used to be the standard treatment for a damaged spleen. However, asplenic patients have impaired short and long term immunity. Unplanned splenectomy for iatrogenic surgical injury carries a twofold to 10-fold increase in the incidence of postoperative infection and double the risk of mortality.[8] A retrospective review of 196 patients with trauma injury found that splenectomy carried a 50% increased risk of postoperative infections.[9]

Several studies suggest that in haemodynamically stable patients embolisation achieves the same survival and reduces the need for splenectomy. A series of 154 patients found that the survival rate of 85% with embolisation was closely similar to the 82% survival in historical controls who had had splenectomy.[10] A Norwegian centre reported outcomes for 133 patients with splenic injuries before and after the introduction of embolisation to the trauma service.[11] The change in practice reduced the laparotomy rate from 55% to 30% and increased the rate of spleen salvage from 57% to 70%. The overall survival rate was stable at 85-89%; the survival rate in the United Kingdom for comparable patients is 78%.[1]

Importantly, embolisation does not obliterate the spleen. A prospective study of 17 patients found that half the splenic bulk was preserved[12] and that serological measures of immune function were normal. Embolisation may preserve splenic function, avoiding the short and long term risks of splenectomy.

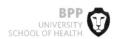

Complications in a retrospective series of 140 patients included recurrent haemorrhage in 11%, symptomatic infarct leading to splenectomy in 2%, and abscess in 4%.[13] Two smaller series with a total of 36 patients describe similar outcomes and also report fever in 56% and left pleural effusion in 31%[14 15]—a form of mild post-embolisation syndrome similar to that seen after tumour embolisation and attributed to tissue infarction.

Liver

For haemodynamically unstable patients with liver injuries the standard approach is rapid "damage control" surgery with extensive packing of liver injuries.[16] Bleeding from central hepatic or portal veins also requires surgical repair, even in haemodynamically stable patients.[17] In this setting embolisation is a potentially attractive adjunctive therapy for patients with ongoing haemorrhage. In one retrospective series seven patients with liver injuries had angiography after damage control surgery; six of these had ongoing bleeding, and embolisation was successful in all seven patients, with no late rebleeds.[18]

The potential impact of interventional radiology is shown in a review of outcomes for 114 patients with liver injuries before and after the introduction of embolisation to a trauma service in Norway.[19] In haemodynamically unstable patients, angiography and embolisation were performed immediately after damage control surgery. In haemodynamically stable patients with high grade injuries, angiography was performed immediately if there was clinical or computed tomography evidence of ongoing bleeding. The change in practice reduced the laparotomy rate from 58% to 34% and lowered the complication rate by 40% (including abscess, biloma, and bile leak). The survival rate was stable at 89-90%; the survival rate in the UK for comparable patients is 78%.[1]

High grade liver injuries cause extensive vascular and biliary disruption that may be exacerbated by treatment. Focal necrosis of devitalised liver tissue is seen after embolisation, especially with extensive injuries; subsequent abscess formation may require percutaneous drainage or surgical intervention.[20 21] A retrospective study of 71 patients receiving embolisation for hepatic trauma found that complications occurred in 61% (major hepatic necrosis in 42%, abscess in 17%, gallbladder necrosis in 7%, and bile leak in 20%).[20] Surprisingly, mortality in patients with major hepatic necrosis was lower than in those without (7% v 20%, P for difference=0.1).

Kidney

Injuries involving the renal arteries usually occur in conjunction with other solid organ injuries, and require intervention.[22] Embolisation is performed as selectively as possible to maximise preservation of viable, perfused renal tissue. Surgical treatment of similar injuries will often involve nephrectomy.

Recent reports indicate that embolisation is an effective haemostatic technique for these injuries. Initial haemostasis was achieved in all 43 patients reported in three retrospective series.[22 23 24] Rebleeding occurred in three patients (two of whom were treated with further embolisation), and abscess occurred in one patient. Ultimately, delayed nephrectomy was performed in five of the 43 patients but there were no deaths.[22 23 24]

Pelvic fracture

Bleeding from pelvic fractures may originate from bone, muscle, and large vessels. This adversely influences the prognosis for the severely injured patient (mortality can exceed 25%),[25] so

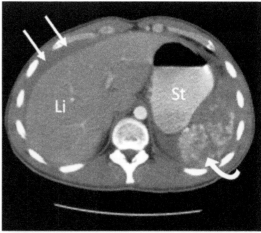

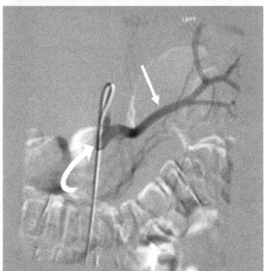

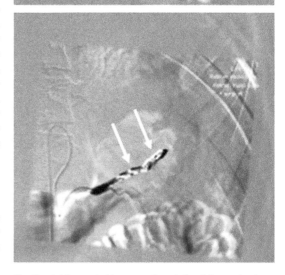

Fig 1 Top: Axial computed tomogram through the abdomen showing free intraperitoneal blood (straight arrows) and shattered spleen fragments (curved arrow); Li=liver, St= stomach. Centre: Angiogram showing catheter tip in origin of the splenic artery (curved arrow) and main splenic artery opacified with contrast material (straight arrow). Bottom: Angiogram showing complete occlusion of the main splenic artery after insertion of multiple metal coils (arrows) and gelatin slurry via the catheter. Temporary embolisation agents such as biodegradable gelatin are profoundly thrombogenic. The commonest permanent agents are metal coils incorporating microscopic filaments that encourage thrombosis.

prompt effective management is essential. Pelvic fractures are often associated with other abdominal injuries, emphasising

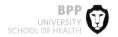
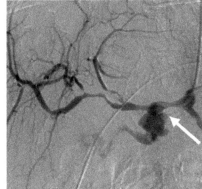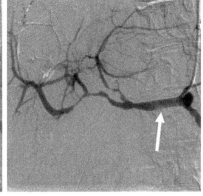

Fig 2 Left: Angiogram showing haemorrhage (arrow) from the hepatic artery. Right: Angiogram showing relining of the hepatic artery by insertion of a stent graft (arrow), which has stopped the haemorrhage while maintaining arterial blood flow to the liver.

Distribution of injuries by site among 224 patients with blunt abdominal injury in whom the injury was identified on computed tomography[7]

Site	Percentage of patients with identified injury	
	All patients	Haemodynamically unstable subgroup
Spleen	35	53
Liver	24	44
Kidney	13	15
Pancreas	12	0
Bowel perforation	9	6
Pelvic fracture	22	15

the importance of computed tomography in planning effective treatment.[26]

Surgical exploration and control of pelvic bleeding is technically challenging[25] and may disrupt the useful tamponade effect of existing haematoma (fig 3). Endovascular treatment for bleeding pelvic fracture has become an established and reliable technique.[27] In one retrospective study, angiography identified pelvic arterial bleeding in 19 of 26 haemodynamically unstable patients; it also identified that fitting surgical external fixator devices led to avoidable delays to angiography and haemostasis.[28] Pelvic fractures may instead be temporarily immobilised with sheet-wrap techniques to facilitate prompt assessment with computed tomography and subsequent angiography.

Complications of embolisation may be difficult to distinguish from the consequences of the injury itself. A retrospective series of 31 patients reported gluteal necrosis in three patients, all of whom had sustained degloving injuries of the buttock, although the embolisation may have contributed.[29] Another retrospective series—of 100 patients with pelvic fracture of whom 67 received embolisation—found a similar incidence of early complications (skin necrosis, perineal infection, nerve injury) in patients with and without embolisation.[30] Long term complications such as claudication, skin ulceration, and regional pain were also similar across treatment groups, although regional paraesthesia was more common after embolisation.[30]

Might interventional radiology be beneficial for the most severely injured patients?

Although interventional radiology for pelvic bleeding in haemodynamically unstable patients is gaining acceptance, the standard approach to other organ injuries in these patients remains surgery, without prior computed tomography.

The most widely adopted guidelines for management of haemodynamically unstable patients with blunt abdominal trauma advocate laparotomy without computed tomography

or attempted endovascular management.[31] Similarly, 97% of trauma surgeons in the United States consider haemodynamic instability to be an indication for immediate splenectomy in blunt splenic injury.[32] The concept that haemodynamically unstable patients should not have computed tomography but should instead proceed direct to laparotomy is widely accepted but not based on any evidence.[1]

However, this philosophy of care is challenged by the speed and clinical utility of modern multidetector computed tomography scanners. Laparotomy allows review and repair of injuries to solid organs and hollow viscera, but assessment of some commonly injured areas such as the retroperitoneum and pelvis is limited.[25] Some patients have bleeding in these regions identified on computed tomography only after surgery has failed, resulting in delayed diagnosis and delayed effective treatment.

Some centres now incorporate multidetector computed tomography into their trauma algorithms even for unstable patients. One prospective study examined outcomes in 252 haemodynamically stable and unstable patients with blunt abdominal trauma who all had immediate computed tomography, with management decisions taken jointly by a senior surgeon and interventional radiologist.[7] Twenty eight of the 34 haemodynamically unstable patients had active bleeding sites identified, and 13 had embolisation alone for liver, renal, splenic, and/or pelvic injuries. All survived without surgery. Six patients had no active bleeding identified on computed tomography and were successfully managed non-operatively. The survival rate was 31/34 (89%), with laparotomy performed in 15/34 and embolisation in 13/34. The three deaths occurred in patients initially treated surgically. Thus surgery was avoided in over half of these severely injured patients, all of whom would have had immediate laparotomy in most centres. If further prospective studies replicate these findings open surgery might be avoidable in some of the most severely injured patients. Early computed tomography was essential to the success of the management strategy described in this study.

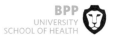

Another study evaluated 19 patients with multiple injuries who exhibited a transient haemodynamic response to initial fluid resuscitation.[26] These patients all had embolisation rather than surgery. Although the average systolic blood pressure at the time of embolisation was 80 (range 65-90) mm Hg, only one patient died from haemorrhage related to their abdominal injuries. A notable feature of this study was that the average time from admission to the start of angiography was only 92 minutes, during which the clinical evaluation, assessment of response to fluid, and computed tomography were performed. By contrast, a 2007 National Confidential Enquiry into Patient Outcome and Death (NCEPOD) that reviewed trauma services in England and Wales found that the average time from admission to computed tomography was 2.3-3.0 hours.[1]

These two small studies suggest that indications for interventional radiology might be expanded to include some haemodynamically unstable patients who would have surgery according to current management algorithms.

What are the barriers to progress in interventional radiology in the United Kingdom?

Despite numerous technological advances in traumatology, surgery, anaesthesia, and radiology the mortality from major trauma has not changed over the past 30 years and is particularly poor in the United Kingdom.[33] Incorporation of interventional radiological techniques into the management of severe injury is intuitively desirable as the additional trauma of surgery is avoided. The use of interventional radiology may increase the number of patients who are successfully managed non-operatively or act as a bridge to definitive surgery in initially unstable patients.[34]

The main barrier to progress is the absence of good evidence. Use of interventional radiology to treat ruptured berry aneurysms is well proved because prospective study designs have several hours' leeway in which to make treatment decisions after the initial subarachnoid haemorrhage. In major trauma, treatment decisions have to be made immediately

so study designs must allow this. Further, in contrast to subarachnoid or myocardial infarction, major trauma is not a discrete diagnosis with straightforward diagnostic criteria. Past research studies into thrombolysis for acute management of myocardial infarction were reasonably easy to organise because the treatment was simple to deliver and could be done by relatively junior medical staff at all times of the day and night. But the numerous possible injury combinations in major trauma require the collaboration of experienced staff from several disciplines (traumatology, anaesthesia, surgery, orthopaedics, radiology) to deliver high quality care.[1] Securing agreement among all members of these teams at several institutions for good recruitment into prospective randomised trials poses a substantial challenge that has not yet been overcome. In addition, serious problems exist regarding consent for research in hyperacute clinical scenarios where patients are usually attending without next of kin. Only after all these challenges have been overcome will it be possible to develop reliable triage tools to decide on early surgery, early endovascular treatment, or conservative management for individual patients.

In the United Kingdom administrative and cultural obstacles are also present. A review of trauma services in the 2007 NCEPOD report described very poor availability of senior clinicians and poor access to immediate computed tomography and interventional radiology.[1] Review of the records of 795 trauma patients found that surgery had been performed in 110 cases but embolisation in only one; perhaps limited awareness accompanies limited availability. The report recommended substantial changes to the organisation of trauma care in the UK and consideration of centralisation of relevant skills and resources to optimise patient care in the future.[1] If these recommendations are met this reorganisation would facilitate future high quality UK research into many of the management areas of major trauma, including clarifying the role of interventional radiology alongside fluid resuscitation and surgery.

Figure 4 illustrates the management pathway used at our institution for treating haemodynamically unstable patients who have blunt abdominal trauma. At any time the senior surgeon involved can divert the patient direct to the operating theatre. The target time from admission to computed tomography is one hour. Resuscitation continues during transfers and scanning; radiology rooms have piped gases and anaesthetic trolleys.

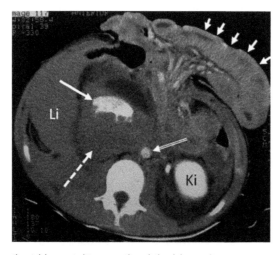

Fig 3 Axial computed tomogram through the abdomen of a haemodynamically unstable patient after surgical exploration had failed to identify a source of bleeding. Laparotomy released the abdominal tamponade on a retroperitoneal haematoma (dashed arrow), prompting further haemorrhage from the injured right kidney. Extravasation of intravenous contrast (white material, solid arrow) indicates rapid active bleeding. Expansion of the haematoma during surgery prevented reinsertion of the bowel (short arrows) into the abdomen. The liver (Li), normal left kidney (Ki), and constricted "shock" aorta (hollow arrow) are also labelled. The bleeding vessels were successfully treated with embolisation, but the patient died of multiorgan failure caused by the preceding prolonged hypovolaemic shock.

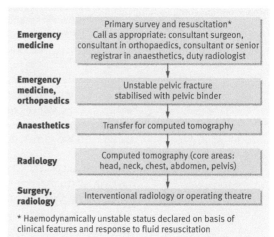

Emergency medicine	Primary survey and resuscitation* Call as appropriate: consultant surgeon, consultant in orthopaedics, consultant or senior registrar in anaesthetics, duty radiologist
Emergency medicine, orthopaedics	Unstable pelvic fracture stabilised with pelvic binder
Anaesthetics	Transfer for computed tomography
Radiology	Computed tomography (core areas: head, neck, chest, abdomen, pelvis)
Surgery, radiology	Interventional radiology or operating theatre

* Haemodynamically unstable status declared on basis of clinical features and response to fluid resuscitation

Fig 4 Management pathway used at authors' institution for treating haemodynamically unstable patients who have blunt abdominal trauma. Pathway shows decision making on key events, with each responsible specialty (senior level) indicated on the left

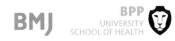

The authors acknowledge the substantial contribution made by the peer reviewers, Professor Jon Moss (Glasgow) and David Kessel (Leeds), to the development of this manuscript.

Contributors: IAZ received the commission to write the article and did the literature search and reviewed the literature. The authors wrote the article jointly. IAZ is the guarantor.

Competing interests: All authors have completed the Unified Competing Interest form at www.icmje.org/coi_disclosure.pdf (available on request from the corresponding author) and declare (1) no financial support for the submitted work from anyone other than their employer; (2) no financial relationships with commercial entities that might have an interest in the submitted work; (3) their spouses, partners, or children have no relationships with commercial entities that might have an interest in the submitted work; (4) no non-financial interests that may be relevant to the submitted work.

Provenance and peer review: Commissioned; externally peer reviewed.

Patient consent not required (patient anonymised, dead, or hypothetical).

1 National Confidential Enquiry into Patient Outcome and Death. Trauma: who cares? 2007. www.ncepod.org.uk/2007report2/Downloads/SIP_report.pdf.
2 Zacharias SR, Offner P, Moore EE, Burch J. Damage control surgery. AACN Clin Issues 1999;10:95-103.
3 Scottish Intercollegiate Guidelines Network. SIGN 50: a guideline developer's handbook. 2008. www.sign.ac.uk/pdf/sign50.pdf.
4 Scottish Intercollegiate Guidelines Network. Management of acute upper and lower gastrointestinal haemorrhage. (National clinical guideline 105.) www.sign.ac.uk/guidelines/fulltext/105/index.html.
5 Healthcare Commission. Investigation into 10 maternal deaths at, or following delivery at, Northwick Park Hospital, North West London NHS Trust, between April 2002 and April 2005. 2006. www.cqc.org.uk/_db/_documents/Northwick_tagged.pdf.
6 Hershberger RC, Aulivola B, Murphy M, Luchette FA. Endovascular grafts for treatment of traumatic injury to the aortic arch and great vessels. J Trauma 2009;67:660-71.
7 Fang JF, Wong YC, Lin BC, Hsu YP, Chen MF. Usefulness of multidetector computed tomography for the initial assessment of blunt abdominal trauma patients. World J Surg 2006;30:176-82.
8 Cassar K, Munro A. Iatrogenic splenic injury. J R Coll Surg Edinb 2002;47:731-41.
9 Wiseman J, Brown CVR, Weng J, Salim A, Rhee P, Demetriades D. Splenectomy for trauma increases the rate of early postoperative infections. Am Surg 2006;72:947-50.
10 Duchesne JC, Simmons JD, Schmeig RE Jr, McSwain NE Jr, Bellows CF. Proximal splenic artery angioembolization does not improve outcomes in treating blunt splenic injuries compared with splenectomy: a cohort analysis. J Trauma 2008;65:1346-53.
11 Gaarder C, Dormagen JB, Eken T, Skaga NO, Klow NE, Pillgram-Larsen J, et al. Nonoperative management of splenic injuries: improved results with angioembolization. J Trauma 2006;61:192-8.
12 Tominaga GT, Simon FJ, Dandan IS, Schaffer KB, Kraus JF, Kan M, et al. Immunologic function after splenic embolization, is there a difference? J Trauma 2009;67:289-95.
13 Haan J, Biffl W, Knudson MM, Davis KA, Oka T, Majercik S, et al. Splenic embolization revisited: a multicenter review. J Trauma 2004;56:542-7.
14 Ekeh AP, McCarthy MC, Woods RJ, Haley E. Complications arising from splenic embolization after blunt splenic trauma. Am J Surg 2005;189:335-9.
15 Wu SC, Chen RJ, Yang AD, Tung CC, Lee KH. Complications associated with embolization in the treatment of blunt splenic injury. World J Surg 2008;32:476-82.
16 Velmahos GC, Toutouzas K, Radin R, Chan L, Rhee P, Tillou A, et al. High success with nonoperative management of blunt hepatic trauma: the liver is a sturdy organ. Arch Surg 2003;138:475-81.
17 Holden A. Abdomen—interventions for solid organ injury. Injury 2008;39:1275-89.
18 Johnson JW, Gracias VH, Gupta R, Guillamondegui O, Reilly PM, Shapiro MB, et al. Hepatic angiography in patients undergoing damage control laparotomy. J Trauma 2002;52:1102-6.
19 Gaarder C, Naess PA, Eken P, Skaga NO, Pillgram-Larsen J, Klow NE, et al. Liver injuries—improved results with a formal protocol including angiography. Injury 2007;38:1075-83.
20 Dabbs D, Stein DM, Scalea TM. Major hepatic necrosis: a common complication after angioembolization for treatment of high-grade liver injuries. J Trauma 2009;66:621-9.
21 Kozar RA, Moore JB, Niles SE, Holcomb JB, Moore EE, Cothren CC, et al. Complications of non-operative management of high grade blunt hepatic injuries. J Trauma 2005;59:1066-71.
22 Chow SJD, Thompson KJ, Hartman JF, Wright ML. A 10-year review of blunt renal artery injuries at an urban level 1 trauma centre. Injury 2008;40:844-50.
23 Sofocleous CT, Hinrichs C, Brountzos E, Kaul S, Kannarkat G, Bahramipour P, et al. Angiographic findings and embolotherapy in renal arterial trauma. Cardiovasc Intervent Radiol 2005;28:39-47.
24 Dinkel H-P, Danuser H, Triller J. Blunt renal trauma: minimally invasive management with microcatheter embolization experience in nine patients. Radiology 2002;223:723-30.
25 Frevert S, Dahl B, Lonn L. Update on the roles of angiography and embolisation in pelvic fracture. Injury 2008;39:1290-4.
26 Hagiwara A, Murata A, Matsuda T, Matsuda H, Shimazaki S. The usefulness of transcatheter arterial embolization for patients with blunt polytrauma showing transient response to fluid resuscitation. J Trauma 2004;57:271-7.
27 Agolini SF, Shah K, Jaffe J, Newcomb J, Rhodes M, Reed JF 3rd. Arterial embolization is a rapid and effective technique for controlling pelvic fracture hemorrhage. J Trauma 1997;43:395-7.
28 Miller PR, Moore PS, Mansell E, Meredith WJ, Chang MC. External fixation or arteriogram in bleeding pelvic fracture: initial therapy guided by markers of arterial hemorrhage. J Trauma 2003;54:437-43.
29 Tottereman A, Dormagen JB, Madsen JE, Klow N-E, Skaga NO, Roise O. A protocol for angiographic embolization in exsanguinating pelvic trauma. Acta Orthopaedica 2006;77:462-8.
30 Travis T, Monsky WL, London J, Danielson M, Brock J, Wegelin J, et al. Evaluation of short-term and long-term complications after emergent internal iliac artery embolization in patients with pelvic trauma. J Vasc Interv Radiol 2008;19:840-7.
31 American College of Surgeons. ATLS, advanced trauma life support program for doctors. American College of Surgeons . ACS, 2008.
32 Fata P, Robinson L, Fakhry SM. A survey of EAST member practices in blunt splenic injury: a description of current trends and opportunities for improvement. J Trauma 2005;59:836-42.
33 Kessel DO, Nicholson AA. Trauma services must improve. BMJ 2008;336:1205, doi:10.1136/bmj.a168.
34 Gibson DE, Canfield CM, Levy PD. Selective nonoperative management of blunt abdominal trauma. J Emerg Med 2006;31:215-21.

PATHWAYS AND PROTOCOLS FOR MANAGING MAJOR TRAUMA

- All centres should develop robust communication pathways that ensure that management decisions in major trauma cases are as far as possible taken by experienced specialists in trauma surgery, anaesthetics, and diagnostic and interventional radiology
- Clinicians practising in non-specialist centres should identify the most appropriate specialist centre in their vicinity to discuss management protocols for major trauma, including blunt abdominal trauma. Subjects for discussion should include developing pathways of admission that bypass non-specialist centres where possible, and criteria and mechanisms for transferring patients whose outcome is likely to be improved by transfer
- Clinical management protocols and pathways should be developed in the knowledge that most major trauma in the United Kingdom presents outside normal working hours

---

ADDITIONAL EDUCATIONAL RESOURCES

- National Confidential Enquiry into Patient Outcome and Death. Trauma: who cares? 2007. www.ncepod.org.uk/2007report2/Downloads/SIP_report.pdf. The report is free with no registration required.
- Royal College of Radiologists. Standards for providing a 24-hour interventional radiology service. 2008. www.rcr.ac.uk/docs/radiology/pdf/Stand_24hr_IR_provision.pdf

---

AREAS FOR FUTURE RESEARCH

- Development and execution of study designs that prospectively randomise trauma patients to treatment arms (rather than retrospective series)
- Evaluation of the impact of immediate computed tomography for all patients with blunt abdominal trauma followed by non-operative management, interventional radiology, or damage control surgery, compared with traditional management algorithms
- For patients with blunt abdominal trauma who are in hypovolaemic shock, determination of the potential for interventional radiology to replace surgery by randomising patients either to (a) traditional immediate surgery or to (b) immediate computed tomography followed by embolisation with or without subsequent surgery, or surgery with or without subsequent embolisation

More titles in The BMJ Clinical Review Series

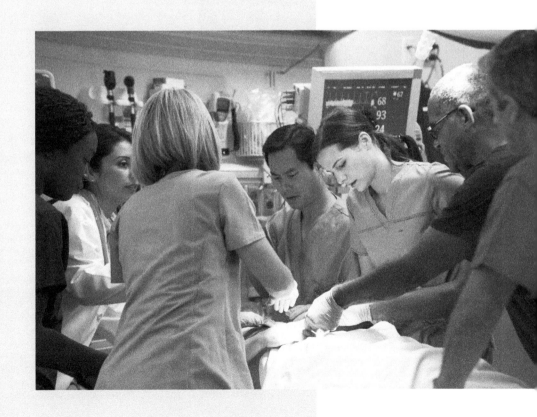

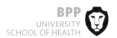

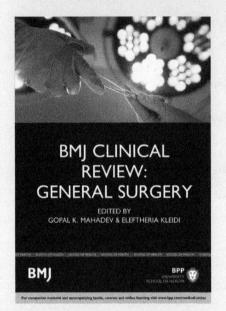
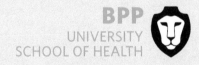

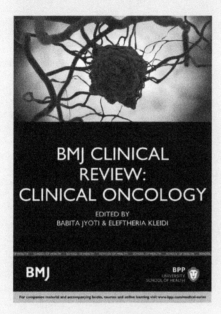

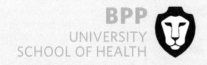

More titles in
The BMJ Clinical Review Career Series

This volume covers a range topics in the management and treatment of cancer.

Subjects dealt with include:
- The changing epidemiology of lung cancer with a focus on screening using low dose computed tomography
- Identifying brain tumours in children and young adults
- Prostate cancer
- Screening and the management of clinically localized disease
- The management of women at high risk of breast cancer
- Head and neck cancer with reference to epidemiology, presentation, prevention, treatment and prognostic factors
- Malignant and premalignant lesions of the penis
- Melanoma and advances in radiotherapy.
- Melanoma and advances in radiotherapy.

£29.99
August 2015
Paperback
978-1-472739-32-2

BPP
UNIVERSITY
SCHOOL OF HEALTH

www.bpp.com/medical-series

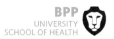
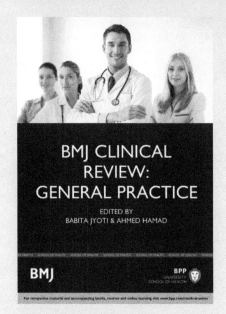
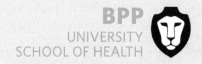

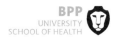

More titles in
The BMJ Clinical Review Series

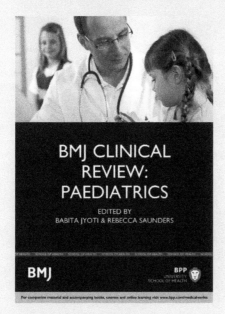

BMJ CLINICAL REVIEW: PAEDIATRICS

EDITED BY
BABITA JYOTI & REBECCA SAUNDERS

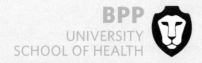

For companion material and accompanying books, courses and online learning visit www.bpp.com/medical-series

£29.99
July 2015
Paperback
978-1-472739-34-6

This book draws together a collection of current review articles published in the BMJ on clinically important Paediatric topics. Among the many subjects covered in this volume dealing with issues relating to the clinical care of children are contributions on:

- Managing common breastfeeding problems in the community
- The diagnosis of autism in childhood
- Issues relating to obesity in children including epidemiology, measurement, risk factors, screening, its prevention and management
- Identifying brain tumours in children and young adults
- Management of infantile colic
- The use and misuse of drugs and alcohol in adolescence
- Managing common symptoms of cerebral palsy in children
- The developmental assessment of children
- Allergic rhinitis in children
- Diagnosis and management of juvenile idiopathic arthritis

BPP
UNIVERSITY
SCHOOL OF HEALTH

www.bpp.com/medical-series

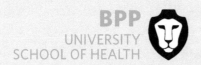
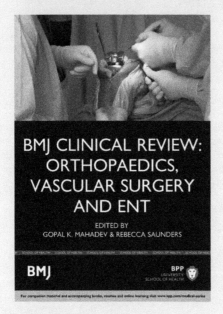

More titles in
The BMJ Clinical Review Series

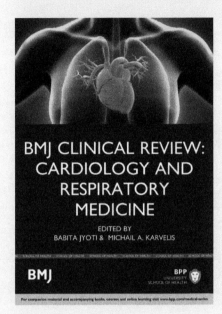

BMJ CLINICAL REVIEW: CARDIOLOGY AND RESPIRATORY MEDICINE

EDITED BY
BABITA JYOTI & MICHAIL A. KARVELIS

This volume presents a range of articles discussing significant issues in contemporary cardiology and respiratory medicine.

Among the topics covered are:
- Pre-participation screening for cardiovascular abnormalities in young competitive athletes
- The investigation and management of congestive heart failure
- Inherited cardiomyopathies
- Resistant hypertension
- The diagnosis and management of pulmonary hypertension
- Difficult to treat asthmatic conditions in adults
- Sarcoidosis
- How asbestos exposure affects the lungs.

£29.99
August 2015
Paperback
978-1-472738-89-9

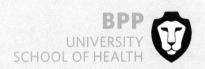

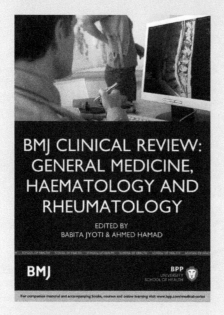
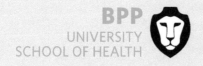

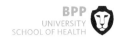

More titles in The Progressing your Medical Career Series

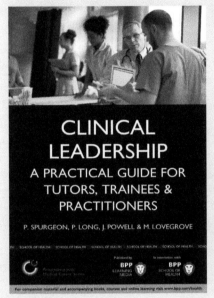

£24.99

June 2015

Paperback

978-1-472727-83-1

Are you a healthcare professional or student who wishes to acquire and develop your leadership and management skills? Do you recognise the role and influence of strong leadership and management in modern healthcare?

Clinical leadership is something in which all healthcare professionals can participate in, in terms of driving forward high quality care for their patients. In this up-to-date guide, the authors take you through the latest leadership and management thinking, and how this links in with the Clinical Leadership Competency Framework. As well as influencing undergraduate curricula this framework forms the basis of the leadership component of the curricula for all healthcare specialties, so a practical knowledge of it is essential for all healthcare professionals in training.

Using case studies and practical exercises to provide a strong work-based emphasis, this practical guide will enable you to build on your existing experiences to develop your leadership and management skills, and to develop strategies and approaches to improving care for your patients.

This book addresses:

- Why strong leadership and management are crucial to delivering high quality care;
- The theory and evidence behind the Clinical Leadership Competency Framework;
- The practical aspects of leadership learning in a wide range of clinical environments
- How clinical professionals and trainers can best facilitate leadership learning for their trainees and students within the clinical work-place.

Whether you are a student just starting out on your career, or an established healthcare professional wishing to develop yourself as a clinical leader, this practical, easy-to-use guide will give you the techniques and knowledge you require to excel.

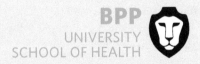

www.bpp.com/medical-series

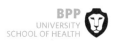

More titles in The Progressing your Medical Career Series

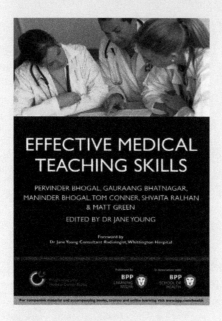

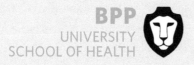

£19.99

September 2011

Paperback

978-1-445379-56-2

We can all remember a teacher that inspired us, encouraged us and helped us to excel. But what is it that makes a good teacher and are these skills that can be learned and improved?

As doctors and healthcare professionals we are all expected to teach, to a greater or lesser degree, and this carries a great deal of responsibility. We are helping to develop the next generation and it is essential to pass on the knowledge that we have gained during our experience to date.

This book aims to cover the fundamentals of medical education. It has been designed to be a guide for the budding teacher with practical advice, hints, tips and essential points of reflection designed to encourage the reader to think about what they are doing at each step.

By taking the time to read through this book and completing the exercises contained within it you should:

- Understand the needs of the learner
- Understand the skills required to be an effective teacher
- Understanding the various different teaching scenarios, from lectures to problem based teaching, and how to use them effectively
- Understand the importance and sources of feedback
- Be aware of assessment techniques, appraisal and revalidation

This book aims to provide you with a foundation in medical education upon which you can build the skills and attributes to become a competent and skilled teacher.

BPP
UNIVERSITY
SCHOOL OF HEALTH

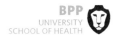
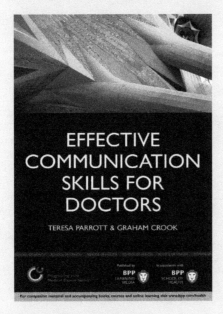
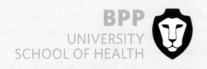

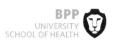
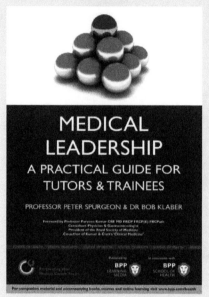
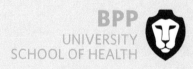

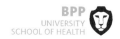
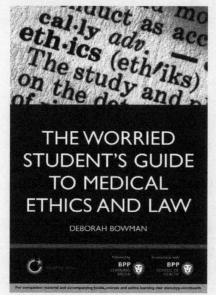
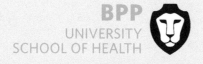

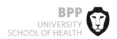
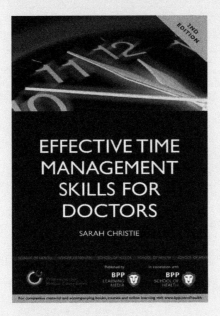
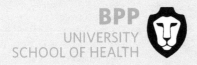

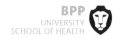
More titles in the Essential Clinical Handbook Series

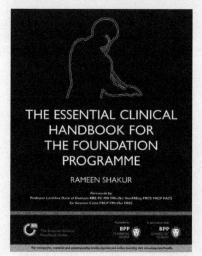

THE ESSENTIAL CLINICAL HANDBOOK FOR THE FOUNDATION PROGRAMME

RAMEEN SHAKUR

£24.99

October 2011

Paperback

978-1-445381-63-3

Unsure of what clinical competencies you must gain to successfully complete the Foundation Programme? Unclear on how to ensure your ePortfolio is complete to enable your progression to ST training?

This up-to-date clinical handbook is aimed at current foundation doctors and clinical medical students and provides a comprehensive companion to help you in the day-to-day management of patients on the ward. Together with this it is the first handbook to also outline clearly how to gain the core clinical competencies required for successful completion of the Foundation Programme. Written by doctors for doctors this comprehensive handbook explains how to successfully manage all of the common cases you will face during the Foundation Programme and:

- Introduces the Foundation Programme and what is expected of a new doctor especially with the introduction of Modernising Medical Careers

- Illustrates clearly the best way to manage, step-by-step, over 150 commonly encountered clinical diseases, including NICE guidelines to ensure a gold standard of clinical care is achieved.

- Describes how to successfully gain the core clinical competencies within Medicine and Surgery including an extensive list of differentials and conditions explained

- Explores the various radiology images you will encounter and how to interpret them

- Tells you how to succeed in the assessment methods used including DOP's, Mini-CEX's and CBD's

- Has step by step diagrammatic guide to doing common clinical procedures competently and safely.

- Outlines how to ensure your ePortfolio is maintained properly to ensure successful completion of the Foundation Programme.

- Provides tips and advice on how to start preparing now to ensure you are fully prepared and have the competitive edge for your CMT/ST application.

The introduction of the e-Portfolio as part of the Foundation Programme has paved the way for foundation doctors to take charge of their own learning and portfolio. Through following the expert guidance laid down in this handbook you will give yourself the best possible chance of progressing successfully through to CMT/ST training.

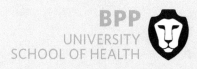

BPP
UNIVERSITY
SCHOOL OF HEALTH

www.bpp.com/medical-series

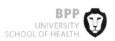

More titles in The Essential Clinical Handbook Series

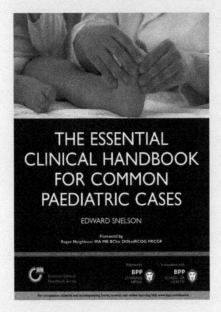

Not sure what to do when faced with a crying baby and demanding parent on the ward? Would you like a definitive guide on how to manage commonly encountered paediatric cases?

This clear and concise clinical handbook has been written to help healthcare professionals approach the initial assessment and management of paediatric cases commonly encountered by Junior Doctors, GPs, GP Specialty Trainee's and allied healthcare professionals. The children who make paediatrics so fun, can also make it more than a little daunting for even the most confident person. This insightful guide has been written based on the author's extensive experience within both a General Practice and hospital setting.

Intended as a practical guide to common paediatric problems it will increase confidence and satisfaction in managing these conditions. Each chapter provides a clear structure for investigating potential paediatric illnesses including clinical and non-clinical advice covering: background, how to assess, pitfalls to avoid, FAQs and what to tell parents. This helpful guide provides :

- A problem/symptom based approach to common paediatric conditions

- As essential guide for any doctor assessing children on the front line

- Provides easy-to-follow and step-by-step guidance on how to approach different paediatric conditions

- Useful both as a textbook and a quick reference guide when needed on the ward

This engaging and easy to use guide will provide you with the knowledge, skills and confidence required to effectively diagnose and manage commonly encountered paediatric cases both within a primary and secondary care setting.

September 2011
Paperback
978-1-445379-60-9

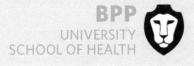